Current Research in HIV/AIDS

Current Research in HIV/AIDS

Edited by Spencer Brooks

STATES
ACADEMIC PRESS
www.statesacademicpress.com

States Academic Press,
109 South 5th Street,
Brooklyn, NY 11249, USA

Visit us on the World Wide Web at:
www.statesacademicpress.com

ISBN: 978-1-63989-137-5

Cataloging-in-Publication Data

Current research in HIV/AIDS / edited by Spencer Brooks.
p. cm.
Includes bibliographical references and index.
ISBN 978-1-63989-137-5
1. HIV infections--Research. 2. HIV (Viruses)--Research. 3. AIDS (Disease)--Research. I. Brooks, Spencer.
RC606.6 .C87 2022
616.979 2--dc23

Table of Contents

Preface

The main aim of this book is to educate learners and enhance their research focus by presenting diverse topics covering this vast field. This is an advanced book which compiles significant studies by distinguished experts in the area of analysis. This book addresses successive solutions to the challenges arising in the area of application, along with it; the book provides scope for future developments.

HIV stands for human immunodeficiency virus and AIDS stands for acquired immunodeficiency syndrome. HIV comprises two species of retrovirus that infect humans. They cause AIDS, a condition that leads to the failure of the immune system, which results in life-threatening opportunistic infections and cancers. After initial infection with HIV, a person may experience a brief period of influenza-like illness or there may be a prolonged period without symptoms. HIV is a sexually transmitted infection that spreads by contact with infected blood, vaginal fluids and semen. Non-sexual transmission may also occur from infected mother to her child during pregnancy or childbirth by exposure to her blood and through breast milk. This book includes some of the vital pieces of work being conducted across the world, on various topics related to HIV and AIDS. It is compiled in such a manner, that it will provide in-depth knowledge about the current researches in this field. Scientists and students actively engaged in this field will find this book full of crucial and unexplored concepts.

It was a great honour to edit this book, though there were challenges, as it involved a lot of communication and networking between me and the editorial team. However, the end result was this all-inclusive book covering diverse themes in the field.

Finally, it is important to acknowledge the efforts of the contributors for their excellent chapters, through which a wide variety of issues have been addressed. I would also like to thank my colleagues for their valuable feedback during the making of this book.

Editor

1

Three Decades of HIV/AIDS Pandemic: Challenges Faced by Orphans in Tembisa, South Africa

Pius Tangwe Tanga, Princess Khumalo and Priscilla Gutura

Abstract

This paper was extracted from a broader study conducted on the effectiveness of social support mechanisms provided to human immunodeficiency virus/acquired immunodeficiency syndrome (HIV/AIDS) orphans in Tembisa, Gauteng Province. Using a qualitative research design, an interview guide was designed for in-depth interviews, which were conducted with 12 HIV- and AIDS-affected and -infected orphans. In addition, a focus group discussion was run with 13 children's caregivers and two social workers were interviewed as key informants. Nevertheless, this paper discusses the challenges faced by orphans of HIV and AIDS. Maslow's hierarchy of needs was used as the theoretical framework of the study. The findings indicate that the death of a parent signifies the disruption of the basic pattern of a child's life living in the urban area where the role of extended families does not exist as compared to rural areas where a child belongs to the whole village. There are challenges that are impacting on the daily lives of the HIV/AIDS-affected and -infected orphans. Notably, the participants' narratives suggested that there were challenges in terms of health, shelter, education and food. It is concluded therefore that the war against the impacts of HIV and AIDS is still far from being achieved.

Keywords: HIV and AIDS, social support, challenges, orphans, caregivers, social workers

1. Introduction

Human immunodeficiency virus (HIV) and acquired immunodeficiency syndrome (AIDS) is one of the major public health challenges and it is a pandemic worldwide [1]. Statistics released by Statistics South Africa showed that the population of the country was estimated at 54.96 million by mid-2015 with approximately 48% being male and 52% female [2]. Furthermore,

Statistics SA showed that the estimated overall HIV prevalence rate is approximately 11.2% of the total South African population. The total number of people living with HIV is estimated at approximately 6.19 million in 2015. For adults aged 15–49 years, an estimated 16.6% of the population is HIV positive [2].

Further, HIV/AIDS has increased the number of orphans enormously to the extent that the United Nations in 2000 defines an orphan as a child who has lost one parent. This is because, when the first parent is killed by the disease, the next one follows within a short period of time. The death of both parents leads the child to be called a double orphan [3]. However, in most African nations, the fact of the matter is that the burden of parental death from AIDS is the greatest with 12.3 million children under the age of 15 having lost one or both parents to AIDS [4]. There is an estimation that 12 million children aged 17 and younger in the sub-Saharan Africa have lost one or both parents mainly due to HIV/AIDS [5]. This sordid truth is not far-fetched even in the Southern African region. Then, it was concluded that these children are often left in the care of caregivers who have limited resources and abilities to care and provide for their psychosocial needs [6].

The General Household Survey in 2007 identified approximately 3.7 million orphans (children without both parents) living in South Africa. This survey also indicated that the number of children who had lost both parents had increased over the previous 5 years (2002–2006) and of further interest was that during 2006, 77% of all orphans were of school-going age—7 years and above.

Substantially, there are international articles that place primary responsibility of the welfare of children on parents or guardians and extended families. These are the Convention of the Rights of the Child (CRC) (Article 5) and the African Charter on the Rights and Welfare of the Child (AC) (Articles 9 (3) and 18). However, the African norms and values just like the aforementioned articles also articulate such child-welfare values. Even Kawewe [6] argues that in many African traditions the extended family is part and parcel of child rearing with the villagers and community members playing a role as the child is viewed as belonging to everyone. He further concludes that the AIDS pandemic defies the concept of the analogy 'it takes a village to raise a child' as many communities can no longer cope with those in need of care. As a result, children are left without caregivers. Some are left in alternative care such as adoption, non-relative care or institutionalization.

South Africa is a signatory to the Declaration of Commitment of the United Nations General Assembly Special Session on Children held in 2002 (UNGASS). One of the articles of the Declaration states that

> By 2003 develop, and by 2005 implement national policies and strategies to:
>
> Build and strengthen governmental family and community capacities to provide supportive environments for orphans and boys and girls infected and affected by HIV and tAIDS including by providing appropriate counselling and psycho-social support, ensuring their enrolment in school and access to shelter, good nutrition, health and social services on an equal basis with other children, to protect orphans and vulnerable children from all forms of abuse, violence, exploitation, discrimination, trafficking and loss of inheritance. (Article 65)

In the past few years of the post-apartheid regime, profound political and social changes have been seen in South Africa, with the government taking the lead in introducing significant social welfare policy changes [7]. Major objectives of social welfare policies in South Africa are alleviating poverty and enabling the previously disadvantaged communities to have access to basic social services [8]. The social security system (mainly social grants) is the government's chief initiative in tackling poverty and inequality through which, according to [9], it has over 16 million beneficiaries accessing the social grants provided for by the government. Among these grants is a grant for children known as the Foster Care Grant.

The Foster Care Grant is also used to provide support for children orphaned by HIV and AIDS; it is orphans who have lost both parents who are the most likely to be receiving the grant, providing that children remain in the care of foster parents [10]. Partially reflecting the effects of a deepening HIV and AIDS pandemic, since 10 years ago, when HIV-related orphaning rates started rising rapidly, the use of the Foster Care Grant changed. The number of Foster Care Grant beneficiaries rose from 43,000 in 1997 to 300,000 in 2006 [11]. As of 30 April 2016, approximately 545,000 children were receiving the Foster Care Grant [9].

The Sowetan reported that the Social Development Minister Bathabile Dlamini, in Gugulethu, had highlighted that caregivers were reported to be misusing social grants [12]. According to the government, these social assistance grants are to assist caregivers to give orphans (in this case, HIV and AIDS orphans) a better life, a chance to be respectable members of the community and reduce poverty. However, a number of studies carried out so far have indicated that child poverty is still exceedingly high [13, 14]. According to UNICEF's report on the level of child poverty, it was clearly indicated that poverty was deepening in various parts of South Africa [4]. It was further argued that poverty and unemployment are key concerns that impact on a family's capacity to care for their children [7]. They also noted that previous inequalities in education, health care and basic infrastructure have also contributed to the backlog in present services [7]. The vulnerability of children, especially those living in poor areas, is compounded by HIV and AIDS.

A number of researchers [15, 16] have indicated that the HIV and AIDS pandemic is one of the greatest threats to the realization of child rights in South Africa and sub-Saharan Africa. Research by the Children's Institute demonstrates some of the multiple vulnerabilities faced by children before the death of caregivers [17]. Children often take on the responsibility of caring for sick adults and are unable to attend school or study because of the difficulties at home. In short, children's experiences of orphanhood and its compounded vulnerabilities begin long before the death of a significant adult. It is not surprising that many of the subsequent experiences of children who have been orphaned are poverty-related—such as an inability to afford school fees and school uniforms, prolonged experiences of hunger, inadequate housing and poor access to water [17]. On the other hand, Meintjes and Hall [18] reported that although the government and civil society have expressed concern about the growing number of children living in child-headed households, there is little evidence to support this fear.

The Department of Social Development provides care and support to orphans and vulnerable children and their caregivers and these include child-care forums, community-based drop-ins, home-based care centres, early childhood development programmes, among others. For the purpose of this study, support mechanisms refer to all social support given to HIV and AIDS orphans in Tembisa Child and Family Welfare Society Organization. This assistance might be from social workers, care workers or givers and other members of society, offering support to orphans affected and infected with HIV and AIDS. The need for continuing social welfare policy reform processes and providing support mechanisms for responding to orphans and vulnerable children in South Africa is critical for policymakers. This research therefore evaluated the social support provided to HIV and AIDS orphans in Tembisa, Gauteng. A huge emphasis is placed on the challenges faced. The study focused more on the challenges faced by female caregivers as they form the bulk of Tembisa Child and Family Welfare Society's caseloads and the HIV and AIDS orphans in their care.

2. The research problem

The AIDS epidemic has affected many children in South Africa leaving them either affected or infected [19]. These children are left behind with the greatest challenge of all which is figuring out how to survive, they are left with responsibilities way beyond their capacities, and they lack financial, emotional, physical, mental and material support to care for themselves. In addition, they are left under the care of people who are financially, emotionally, physically or mentally incapable to care for them [20]. The government has put forward means to assist these children to cope with the difficulties of life, but regardless of these there is still a need to determine how effective the measures put forward are assisting.

The majority of orphans and vulnerable children in South Africa are left in the care of old and weak women or sickly caregivers. The government has made recommendable success in combating abject poverty and hunger through social assistance programme [21]. Even after such measures, issues such as fraud still hover around and most caregivers and orphans are still battling with meeting challenges of day-to-day living. However, [21] continues to argue that the high prevalence of HIV and AIDS among caregivers has worsened the challenges of child poverty. The government in 2005 enacted the Children's Act 38 of 2005 which provided under Section 155 and 156 for the orphans of whatever nature to be associated with Foster Care Grants. The grant was to assist foster parents put the orphaned children through school, clothe them and shelter them. Due to the backlogs in many organizations assisting with the application of these grants and the misuse of such grants by some foster parents, the survival of HIV and AIDS orphans is still a struggle far from being won. The previous inequalities in education, health care and basic infrastructure have highly contributed in caregivers being unable to care for orphans and orphaned children [21].

3. Theoretical framework

This study is anchored on Maslow's theory of human needs [22]. Maslow's theory of human needs depicts the hierarchy in a manner where needs in the lower level should be met before an individual can progress and satisfy the needs in the next level. This theory has five levels of needs, the lowest being the most basic need that a body cannot survive without and the top of the pyramid the least basic human need [23]. The lowest level of the pyramid is physiological needs, safety and security needs, love and belonging needs; at the top of the pyramid are esteem needs and self-actualization. Once a need is satisfied an individual will be able to go to the next need [24].

This theory is relevant in this study as HIV/AIDS orphans have needs that should be met in order to fulfil their responsibilities. Orphans are driven by several factors to strive to satisfy the bottom need, and then move on up the hierarchy. Therefore, through understanding their challenges as AIDS orphans, ways of motivating them to fulfil their lives can be developed and implemented.

4. Research area and methodology

Data presented in this paper were collected from Tembisa and the participants included HIV/AIDS orphans and their caregivers and social workers. The purpose was to get views from both the orphans themselves and the people who cared for these orphans. It is believed that once the researcher has developed an understanding of the rationale behind the choice of engaging in any form of research (either qualitative or quantitative), he designs the study [25]. Therefore, a qualitative research design was selected for this study. The goal of this method was to learn about the phenomenon and get in-depth information and feelings of the participants.

The study was conducted in Tembisa Township in the East Rand of the Gauteng province in South Africa. The township is just a few kilometres outside the Kempton Park and the second largest township in Gauteng after Soweto. Its population is estimated to be a little over 500,000. The township came about during the apartheid era as a beacon of hope to the black families who were evicted from their homes. Many people live in poverty and in shacks or the recently built houses from the government (Reconstruction and Development Programme). Tembisa Child and Family Welfare Society provides social services to the township, especially for HIV/AIDS orphans and their caregivers.

This study was only limited to HIV and AIDS orphans being serviced by Tembisa Child and Family Welfare Society and also residing there. The study also targeted the caregivers of the orphans and the social workers who were servicing them. Therefore, this research made use of 13 caregivers, two social workers and 12 orphans. For the purpose of this study, the non-probability procedure in the form of purposive sampling was utilized to select the sample. The orphans were selected purposefully from the database of HIV and AIDS orphans receiving services from Tembisa Child and Family Welfare Society. The samples were drawn from the caseloads of social workers.

The study used semi-structured interviews with the aid of interview guides. The interview guide consisted of non-directive unstructured questions which were written in English, but the interviews were conducted in both English and Zulu. The questions on the research guide were meant to guide the researcher to keep to the objectives of the study. The interviews conducted were recorded with an audio recorder to make it easy to capture all the data and also to avoid misquoting the participants.

Focus groups were also used as a method of collecting data and they targeted care givers. Focus groups are a means of understanding how people feel or think about an issue [26] and can help understand how people feel about the issue being studied. Participants in the focus groups were allowed to share their perceptions, points of views, experiences and wishes without any pressure. An environment that is tolerant and non-threatening to all participants was created. Once the research reached a point of saturation [27], the data collection process was concluded.

Qualitative data analysis was used. Data analysis was explained as the process of bringing order, structure and meaning to a mass of data collected [26]. Qualitative data analysis according to Ref. [26] is a search for general statements about relationships in different categories of data. The researchers went through the transcripts of the collected data with the use of a translator. Data analysis was done through the process of thematic analysis. Through reading the transcripts, the researcher came up with the underlying meanings of the information gathered. This process was repeated until a list of topics was acquired. Topics were then clustered together into baskets and were labelled as 'major topics', 'unique topics' and 'leftovers'. Data were then categorized into themes after finding the most descriptive wording for the topics [26].

In line with the ethical requirements of research, the researchers consulted with relevant authorities to gain access to research components. In order to gain access to the participants, the researchers firstly gained permission from the university in the form of an ethical clearance certificate. Other ethical procedures, including informed consent, anonymity and confidentiality, as well as participant debriefing were put into place during and after data collection. Potential respondents were verbally informed at the start of the study that their participation was completely voluntary and verbal consent of their participation was obtained. Caregivers provided verbal consent for themselves and their children. The children themselves gave consent for their participation and child-friendly language was used.

5. Results

This section provides the findings of the study, according to the themes that emerged. Firstly, the biographical information of the participants is laid out. Thereafter, the challenges faced by orphans, caregivers and social workers are presented.

5.1. Biographical characteristics of participants

Interviews were held with 12 orphans within the age range of 10–18 (both affected and/infected with HIV and AIDS). In terms of gender, these children were proportionately selected, that is, they consisted of six males and six females. A total number of eight children interviewed were both affected and infected with HIV and AIDS and four indicated that they were affected only. Seven of the orphans were maternal orphans with unknown fathers, two were paternal orphans with unknown mothers and three of them were double orphans.

The population of orphaned children in Tembisa is very high with Tembisa Child and Family Welfare Society recording a number of more than 3000 families every year. The average dependency ratio in most of these families is 1:3. In all cases reported to the organization, of every 10 children, eight are orphans affected or infected by HIV and AIDS. Furthermore, amongst 13 participants who were in the focus group discussions, there were three child-care workers and 10 caregivers. All of the participants were female black Africans. The participants' ages ranged from the age of 21–65 years. Two social workers were also interviewed as key informants.

5.2. Challenges faced by HIV and AIDS orphans

The study aimed at investigating the challenges that were being faced in the provision of psychosocial support to HIV and AIDS orphans and the results of these are highlighted in this section.

5.2.1. Theme one: poor health

HIV and AIDS has in the past presented a continuum of complex health issues that ranged from protecting personal health to ensuring that societies have adequate supplies of health care. In Tembisa, the main hospital (Tembisa Hospital) has a facility specifically for children infected with HIV and AIDS. All the children participating in the study who were on anti-retro viral medication or immune boosters claimed to attend *check-ups* at the hospital (Masakhane clinic). Child F stated:

> I started taking Anti Retro Viral treatment at the age of 5 (now 15 years old). It has been a routine for me and they are now like a part of me. My aunt usually takes me to the clinic for my check-up, but when she is not available to do so I go on my own…

Caregivers reported to understand the need to keep the children under constant monitoring to ensure that they did not default on their medication. It was, however, an agreement with most of the participants in the focus group that keeping track of what the children ate and did during school hours was difficult. They reported that because these are children and they like to experiment, they eat most of the things that they are told not to eat at the hospital. They eat these things behind the caregivers' backs. Such defaults only come to light when the children's viral loads spiral after hospital check-up.

Furthermore, the caregivers mentioned that they could not afford nutritious food to give the children. The two social workers who were interviewed also highlighted that the health of orphans deteriorated at times because of lack of nutritious food to eat which is required by those who were living with the virus. One of the social workers said:

> When we send the children for assessments to our doctor or the nurses here, we usually find out that the child's health would have deteriorated in terms of their CD4 count. This is usually caused by the children not eating the right food they are supposed to eat for example vegetables and fruits. (Social Worker 1)

5.2.2. Theme two: inadequate shelter

Of all the children in the study, five reported to be residing in either '*shacks*' or as tenants in outside rooms. Four children reported to be staying in their parental homes and three reported that they lived in the homes of extended family members and that their parents never owned houses of their own. One child stated that:

> I live with my three siblings in my grandmother's house. My mother used to live with us before she fell sick and passed away. Lucky for us, we are the only family my grandmother has now. (Child D)

For most of these children, though the case is quite different and another child highlighted that:

> My aunt has four children of her own and they are girls. She and my mother stayed together in our shack from the time I was born. The shack is two roomed and had one bedroom which my aunt and cousins sleep in. Two of my cousins now have children… there is hardly any space… (Child H).

5.2.3. Theme three: poor school performance

The loss of a parent due to any disease is not easy for a child. Losing a parent to HIV and AIDS is not easy for most children as they suffer from psychosocial effects and often lose concentration at school. Seven of the children interviewed were aware that their parents died of HIV and AIDS and two of these witnessed the illness and death of their parents. Child B reported:

> I was twelve and the eldest. I would help to wash and dress my mother. She was very sick but did not want to go to the hospital until it was too late… She passed away at home in my presence (sobs)…

The child reported that during the time her mother was sick, she went to school occasionally so as to help look after her. Her performance at school dropped a lot that she had to repeat some grades. Four years later, she still remembered the death of her mother like it was yesterday.

In all the interviews, the children indicated that when their parents had the HIV- and AIDS-related sicknesses, their performances in school were affected. Four of the participants suffered through absenteeism from school and hence missed out on some lessons and important tests. Others (six) had to drop out of school after the death of their parents and re-start at a later stage in a new school with present caregivers. Some (two) because of family circumstances were forced to enter into the system and be institutionalized, hence resulting in stigmatization by other learners in those schools. These and other factors have resulted in lower performance by most HIV and AIDS orphans as well as the overburden placed on caregivers to address their needs.

The caregivers also highlighted that the children's performance at school were poor. One caregiver mentioned that:

> At one point I was called by the principal of the school because of the poor performance of my sister's child I am staying with. The principal mentioned that the child was so brilliant but after the death of her mother her grades were getting lower and lower (Caregiver AA)

5.2.4. Theme four: food insecurity

Health and nutrition statuses tend to decline as less money is often available to properly feed the household. One caregiver reported that the greatest challenge they had with caring for the orphans was that it was not easy having an extra mouth to feed with the present day economy. She stated that:

> I have five children of my own and when my brother died, his three children came to stay with me as his wife died too and I am the only family left. Two of his children are attending school and the youngest is at crèche... my salary was not enough to feed and clothe my children (Caregiver BB)

Through the organization's Family Preservation programme, many community children find a source of food security from the food parcels handed out every month. Normally, family preservation is meant to work with a family for at least 6 months and discharge afterwards. One social worker stated this:

> Some of our clients are placed on family preservation as a temporary measure whilst we work on processing their foster care applications which normally take longer than a year (Social Worker 2).

Tembisa is not an agrarian region; hence farming for food is not an option for many caregivers. None of the community members in the focus groups reported to have a backyard garden in their homes as they claimed that space was taken up by outside rooms which they used as a source of income.

Child B reported that she and her siblings stayed with their parents in the rural areas of Limpopo where life was simple and much cheaper. After the death of their mother, they had to move to Tembisa to stay with their maternal aunt as she was the only surviving family they knew. She described life in Gauteng (Tembisa to be precise) as very expensive as their aunt had to put food on the table every day, clothe them, pay bills and school fees. When asked how they survived, one care giver said that, 'We wait a long time to have foster care grants paid out and most of us are unemployed and survive on part time jobs that give us less than R500.00 a month...'

Another caregiver also highlighted that, '... if it were not for the outside rooms I built from a loan I got from the bank last year, life would be very hard for us... Rental money from tenants helps us...'. For most orphans, the loss of parents meant no more income in the house.

6. Discussion

The aim of the paper was to explore the challenges faced by HIV and AIDS orphans in Tembisa. The data obtained in the study is aligned with the literature which portrays orphan-related challenges which are impacting on the daily lives of the HIV/AIDS-affected and -infected orphans. Notably, the participants' narratives suggested that there were challenges in terms of health, shelter, education and food. According to [27], the death of a parent signifies the disruption of the basic pattern of a child's life. With death comes the challenge of meeting the child's basic needs.

The study highlights that the HIV/AIDS pandemic leaves a trajectory of orphans under the care of overloaded elderly women to assume an inexplicably major role in societal provisions, while undermining their engagement in civil society. This relates to what was outlined that many orphans are being cared for by the already structurally marginalized women, particularly elderly grandmothers often living in destitution [1].

The extended family network that has traditionally existed in Africa and South Africa is finding itself increasingly under strain because of HIV/AIDS [28]. The Department of Social Development in 2012 outlined that the HIV and AIDS pandemic has disrupted family, community and social structures, and has led to a marked increase in the number of orphans and other vulnerable children. The findings of the study strongly support the available literature that argues that children orphaned by HIV and AIDS depend mainly on their extended families to meet their basic needs.

In the case of infected children, their health is determined by the nutrition they get and getting access to their treatments at the right times. Lack of proper finances was found to be a big challenge as most caregivers were either unemployed or at the age of pension. The findings further suggest that although the government has placed certain supports such as social assistance grants, their inaccessibility makes it hard for caregivers to support HIV and AIDS orphans. Increasing poverty can cause a degradation of the immediate family environment and increases health risks whilst reducing its ability to obtain health services [29].

The results of the study also showed that the education of the orphans is disrupted. As [30] put it across, the loss of a productive family member is likely to be a financial burden and might push a family into poverty, increasing the likelihood that a child orphaned by AIDS will miss out on school. More literature confirms this, that, educationally, as poverty and HIV/AIDS reinforce each other, many orphans are denied the right to an education [31, 32]. UNICEF [33] showed that children orphaned by AIDS may miss out on school enrolment, have their schooling interrupted or perform poorly in school as a result of their situation. However, the figures released in 2013 by UNICEF revealed that in most countries in sub-Saharan Africa, the gap between school attendance of orphans and non-orphans has significantly narrowed, although progress varies across the region.

The study indicates that the physiological needs of the orphans are not being met. As Maslow's hierarchy of needs outline, if the physiological needs are not met, the human body cannot function properly and will ultimately fail. These needs are thought to be the most important; they should be met first. Therefore, the plight of orphans could be addressed in the same manner where their basic needs are met for them to get fulfilled.

Since the year 2002, there have been a diverse set of problems associated with the use of the foster care system to provide financial assistance to the country's increasing number of orphans [34]. There has been evidence that the social worker and court-based foster care system are not coping with the demand for foster care orders. In May 2011, the North Gauteng High Court ordered the Department of Social Development to design a comprehensive legal solution to the foster care crisis by 2014 [35]. This was due to the fact that a large number of Foster Care Grants had lapsed by 2009 leaving vulnerable children without assistance while social workers were unable to provide quality services to abused children due to higher foster care caseloads. At the same time, caregivers and children had to wait an unreasonably long time for their grants to be processed. Nevertheless, there has been criticism on the Department of Social Development for a slow and limited response to the crisis in the foster care system [36].

The current Foster Care Grant system demands that the applicant produces both parent's death certificates and affidavit stating who they are in relation to the child and why they are applying for the grant. It is with no reasonable doubt that some orphans are left in the care of extended relatives and grandmothers who have no clue who the fathers or sometimes mothers of the children are. Most of the orphaned children are left without birth registrations and caregivers face problems when trying to register the births of the children. While the access to the Child Support Grants has increased substantially over the years, the Foster Care Grant remains a favourable option for those who can access it because it is more than three times the amount of Child Support Grants [37].

Research by the Children's Institute demonstrates that the extension of the Child Support Grants to all children can play a critical role in supporting children through the AIDS pandemic in South Africa [38]. It argued that the current financial assistance offered by government to orphans (namely the Foster Care Grant) is inappropriate and inadequate in the face of HIV and AIDS because the number of foster care cases in many parts of South Africa already exceeds the capacity of social workers and courts. As a result, many orphans are unable to access Foster Care Grants. This is the case as Tembisa Child and Family Welfare Society where families have to wait a year or two before their applications are processed. At the time of processing, some children are already deceased or the prospective foster parents themselves. In other cases, the children end up moving to other areas as the prospective foster parents cannot afford to provide for them.

Even after the government has allowed for extension orders for foster care to be extended until the child turns 18 and not every 2 years, there is still many social workers and courts are facing in the bid to make foster care applications much faster for clients [39]. The continued use of the administratively complex foster care system for the provision of basic financial support for orphans brings the child protection system to its knees rendering it even less able to provide protection to children who really need it.

The Children's Institute further noted that the poverty of children is neither synonymous with nor exclusive to orphanhood [34]. According to them, a social security system, which provides grants to orphans under the age of 18 without providing adequate support to many other impoverished children whose parents are alive, is simply discriminatory. In other words, it fails to make provisions for the multitude of other children growing up in vulnerability due to HIV and AIDS. There are many South African children growing in the care of HIV- and AIDS-infected mothers or fathers and receive no social support from the state [40]. Their vulnerability is therefore not taken into consideration because one of the parents is still alive.

7. Conclusions and recommendations

Almost three decades into the HIV/AIDS pandemic, most people have an understanding of how AIDS-related deaths impact families [41]. From the discussion of the findings, it can be safely concluded that HIV and AIDS orphans in Tembisa face many challenges in terms of health, education, food and shelter. This means that the physiological needs of these orphans are not met. The fight for the impact of HIV and AIDS is far from being won even though the world has three decades of living in the era of this pandemic. There is therefore a need to provide for ongoing support systems for HIV and AIDS orphans.

While the broader literature confirms that extended families play an important role in care, other data highlight a high level of strain felt by carers. The findings show that caregivers themselves are struggling with dealing with the HIV and AIDS pandemic as they themselves are carriers who also have to deal with the loss of their children or parents, and are left with the burden of caring for orphans. The burden becomes unbearable because most of the caregivers are unemployed and those that are employed make a low income and have other dependents to care for. Accessing state assistance is sometimes a major problem as some orphans are left without birth registrations. Those that do get the assistance are either finding it not enough or as argued by researchers are misusing it. Therefore, the following recommendations are suggested:

- There is an urgent need for kinship caregivers to be given greater support, both financially and emotionally.
- Keeping the orphans and vulnerable children in education should remain a key role of the child care advocates.
- Health education to improve the orphans' knowledge of the dangers they put themselves in when they do not leave a healthy lifestyle. If HIV- and AIDS-infected children are taught how to live healthy lifestyles the re-occurrence of orphanhood due to HIV and AIDS could be stopped. Furthermore, a healthy lifestyle means a long, fruitful life, hence caregivers do not have to go through the pain of losing the children like they did the parents of the children.
- There should be interventions designed to address structural factors such as administration of the Foster Care Grant which may improve outcomes for both caregivers and children.
- Finally, interventions directed at families should take into account the abilities, needs and challenges faced by different types of caregiver, rather than generalizing such that food and shelter needs can be met.

8. Limitations of the study

Due to the purpose of the research, participants might have overemphasized their situation in a hope that the researcher might bring quality services in due course. On the other hand, the participants might have given socially acceptable answers in order to hide their situation and thereby distorting the data that were being collected. Also the fact that one of the researchers was part of the Tembisa Child and Family Welfare Society's social workers might have influenced some responses to be biased. However, the researchers had an informed consent with the participants whereby the aim and objectives of the study were clearly laid out. The participants were informed that the research was for academic purposes, hence the biasness was limited. This also developed trustworthiness among the participants as they were assured of privacy and confidentiality. The time frame of the research was also a limitation. Regarding the small sample that was used for the study, the findings are not conclusive and cannot be used to make generalizations about the population of interest. However, they develop an initial understanding and sound base for further decision-making.

Author details

Pius Tangwe Tanga*, Princess Khumalo and Priscilla Gutura

*Address all correspondence to: ptanga@ufh.ac.za

University of Fort Hare, Alice, South Africa

References

[1] Joint United Nations Programme on HIV/AIDS. The Gap Report. In. Geneva, Switzerland: UNAIDS; 2014.

[2] Statistics South Africa. Mid-year population estimates. [Internet]. 2015. Available from: http://beta2.statssa.gov.za/publications/P0302/P03022015.pdf [Accessed 2016-02-15].

[3] UNAIDS. Report on the global HIV/AIDS epidemic. [Internet] 2000. Available from http://data.unaids.org/pub/Report/2000/2000_gr_en.pdf [Accessed 2015-10-30].

[4] UNICEF. Measuring the Determinants of Childhood Vulnerability [internet]. 2014. Available from: http://data.unicef.org/hiv-aids/care-support [Accessed 2015-11-23].

[5] Nyangara F, Kalungwa Z, Obiero W, Thurman TR, Chapman J. Promoting a home-based program model for supporting children affected by HIV/AIDS: Evaluation of Tumaini project in Iringa region, Tanzania. MEASURE Evaluation. 2009.

[6] Kawewe SM. Reclaiming civil society and the plight of AIDS orphaned children and elderly women caregivers in sub-Saharan Africa: a global human rights dilemma for international social workers. Women in Welfare Education. 2006 Nov 1; 8:64–77.

[7] September R, Dinbabo M. Gearing up for implementation: A new Children's Act for South Africa. Practice. 2008; 1: 20(2):113–122.

[8] White Paper. Principles, guidelines, recommendations, proposed policies and programmes for developmental social welfare in South Africa. Republic of South Africa: Department of Welfare. 1997.

[9] South African Social Security Agency (SASSA). Statistical report on social grants. [Internet] 2016. Available from: www.sassa.gov.za [Accessed 2016-05-02].

[10] Leibbrandt M, Woolard I, Finn A, Argent J. Trends in South African income distribution and poverty since the fall of apartheid. 2010.

[11] Pauw K, Mncube L. Expanding the social security net in South Africa: Opportunities, challenge and constraints. Development Policy Research Unit (DPRU). Working Paper 07/127. University of Cape Town; 2007.

[12] Sowetan. Misuse of social grants is rife. [Internet] 2012. Available from: http://www.sowetanlive.co.za/news/2012/05/25/misuse-of-social-grants-is-rife [Accessed 2015-10-28].

[13] Barnes H, Noble M, Wright G, Dawes A. A geographical profile of child deprivation in South Africa. Child Indicators Research. 2009; 2:181–199. DOI: 10.1007/s12187-008-9026-2

[14] Wright G, Barnes H, Noble M, Dawes A. The South African index of multiple deprivation for children 2001 at database level. Pretoria: Department of Social Development. 2009.

[15] Kirby D, Laris BA, Rolleri L. Sex and HIV education programs for youth: their impact and important characteristics. 2006.

[16] Joint United Nations Programme on HIV/AIDS. Report on the Global Acquired Immunodeficiency Syndrome Epidemic. UNAIDS; 2008.

[17] Children's Institute. Analysis of the 2009/10 budgets of the nine provincial departments of Social Development: Are the budgets adequate to implement the Children's Act? [Internet]. 2009. Available from http://www.ci.org.za/depts/ci/pubs/pdf/rights/workpap/Childrens_Act_Budget_Analyss_2009_Prov_DSD_Votes_28May2009.pdf [Accessed 2015-08-25].

[18] Meintjies H, Hall K. Child Rights in Focus. University of Cape Town Children's Institute, CapeTown. 2009.

[19] Bradshaw D, Johnson L, Schneider H, Bourne D, Dorrington R. Orphans of the HIV/AIDS Epidemic. Burden of Disease Research Unit, Medical Research Council. 2002:1–4.

[20] Twine R, Collinson M A, Polzer-Ngwato T, Kahn K. Evaluating access to a child-oriented poverty alleviation intervention in Rural South Africa. Scandinavian Journal of Public Health. 2007; 35:118–127. DOI: 10.1080/14034950701430008

[21] Kaseke E. The role of social security in South Africa. Social Work. 2010; **53**: 159–168. DOI: 10.1177/0020872809355394

[22] Maslow A H. Motivation and Personality. (3rd ed.). New York, NY: Harper & Row. 1987.

[23] Huitt, W. Maslow's hierarchy of needs. Educational Psychology Interactive. Valdosta, GA: Valdosta State University. [Internet] 2007. Available from http://www.edpsycinteractive.org/topics/regsys/maslow.html [Accessed 2015-08-25].

[24] The Adler Group. Maslow's hierarchy of hiring pyramid: performance based hiring. [Internet] 2011. Available from: http://www.eremedia.com/ere/maslows-hierarchy-of-hiring-pyramid-according-to-adler/[Accessed 2015-10-31].

[25] Creswell JW. An Introduction to Qualitative Research. London: Sage; 2008.

[26] De Vos AS, Strydom H, Fouche CB, Delcourt SSL. Research at Grass Roots for the Social Science and Human Service Professions. 3rd edition. Pretoria: Van Schaick Publishers; 2005.

[27] Gambril E. Research on Social Work Practice. Englewood Cliffs, NJ: Prentice Hall; 2010.

[28] Ferreira M. HIV/AIDS and family well-being in Southern Africa: Towards an analysis of policies and responsiveness. United Nations Department of Economic and Social Affairs Division for Social Policy and Development Policy. Windhoek, Namibia. 2015.

[29] Nyawasha TS. Psychosocial Support to Orphans and Vulnerable Children. Word-mart. [Internet] 2006. Available from http://www.wordmart.com/html/psycho-social_support1.html [Accessed 2015-09-05].

[30] UNICEF, UNAIDS W. UNFPA and UNESCO. Children and AIDS: Fifth Stocktaking Report, 2010, Geneva, Switzerland. 2010.

[31] Lachman P, Poblete X, Ebigbo PO, Nyandiya-Bundy S, Bundy R P, Killian B, Doek J. Challenges facing child protection. Child Abuse and Neglect. 2002; 26:587–617. ISSN: 01452134.

[32] Subbarao K, Coury D. Reaching out to Africa's Orphans: A Framework for Public Action. World Bank Publications; Washington D.C, USA. 2004.

[33] UNICEF. Africa's Orphaned and Vulnerable Generations: Children Affected by AIDS. UNICEF; 2006.

[34] Children's Institute. *South African Child Gauge* [internet]. 2012. Available from: http://www.ci.org.za/depts/ci/pubs/pdf/general/gauge2012/sa_child_gauge2012.pdf (Accessed 2015-10-28).

[35] Proudlock P, Hall K, Meintjies H, Jamieson L. Children's Institute amicus curiae affidavit in Sithasolwazi Stemele & Minister for Social Development, Case No. 14/1/4-206/10, South Gauteng High Court, 2011. Retrieved from: www.ci.org.za.

[36] Business Day Live. NGOs criticise ministerial committee probing Foster Care Grants. [Internet]. 2014. Available from: http://www.bdlive.co.za/national/2014/10/24/ngos-criticise-ministerial-committee-probing-foster-care-grants [Accessed 2015-05-08].

[37] Jacobs M, Shung-King M, Smith C, editors. South African child gauge 2005. Children's Institute, University of Cape Town; 2005.

[38] Avert Organization. HIV and AIDS Information [internet]. 2004. Available from: www.avert.org. [Accessed 2015-11-20].

[39] Gray M. Back to basics: A critique of the strengths perspective in social work. Families in Society: The Journal of Contemporary Social Services. 2011 Jan 1; 92(1):5–11.

[40] Rosa S, Guthrie T. Extending the child support grant to all children under 18 years. ACCESS, Children's Institute, UCT. 2002.

[41] Kuo C, Operario D. Caring for AIDS orphaned children: An exploratory study of the challenges faced by carers in KZN, South Africa. Vulnerable Child Youth Studies. 2010; 5:344–352. DOI: 10.1080/17450128.2010.516372

2

HIV Infection and Infertility

Thana Khawcharoenporn and Beverly E. Sha

Abstract

Human immunodeficiency virus (HIV) infection has become a chronic and manageable disease since the availability of combination antiretroviral therapy (cART). Persons living with HIV are living longer with better quality of life. Given that worldwide many HIV-infected individuals are in the reproductive age, fertility and reproductive desire have emerged as clinically important issues among this population. Biological changes caused by HIV, including systemic illnesses, stress, and weight loss, may affect the function of reproductive organs and result in infertility. Newly diagnosed HIV infection may cause psychological trauma and decrease in sexual drive and sexual activity. Several HIV/acquired immune deficiency syndrome (AIDS)-related comorbidities have been reported to be associated with infertility. These include orchitis, acute epididymitis, and pelvic inflammatory disease caused by opportunistic pathogens and coinfections with sexually transmitted infections (STIs) acquired through a similar route of transmission as HIV. The common STIs caused by *Neisseria gonorrhoeae, Chlamydia trachomatis, Ureaplasma urealyticum, Treponema pallidum,* herpes simplex virus-2, and *Trichomonas vaginalis* can damage the reproductive system and cause infertility. Hypogonadism especially in men with AIDS is one of the important endocrine disorders that causes infertility. Although cART provides significant benefits in reducing morbidity and mortality among HIV-infected persons, some antiretroviral drugs, including nucleoside reverse transcriptase inhibitors, are toxic to cellular mitochondria and may affect the mitochondrial biogenesis of sperm and oocytes. HIV-infected individuals may have limited access to reproductive care given the severity of their disease, cost of care, stigmatization, and lack of specific HIV infection/infertility knowledge among their providers.

In the post–cART era, reproductive care has become an important issue to be co-managed with HIV care. Reproductive care includes not only comprehensively managing HIV infection but also minimizing the risk of horizontal HIV transmission in serodiscordant couples, providing suitable options for unprotected timed intercourse, intrauterine insemination with partner or donor sperm, in vitro fertilization with intracytoplasmic sperm injection (IVF/ICSI), embryo donation, and adoption. This chapter reviews potential effects of HIV infection, related opportunistic infections, and physical and psychological comorbidities on fertility; the impact of cART on fertility; and the management of reproductive issues among HIV-infected individuals.

Keywords: HIV, AIDS, Infection, Infertility

1. Introduction

There were approximately 37 million people living with human immunodeficiency virus (PLWHIV) globally at the end of 2014.[1] The course of HIV infection has changed from a deadly disease to a chronic and manageable disease since the introduction of combination antiretroviral therapy (cART) in the 1990s. The estimated life expectancy of a 20-year-old PLWHIV has increased from 30 years during 1996–1999 to 46 years during 2006–2008 according to the UK Collaborative HIV Cohort Study.[2] The increased life expectancy along with improved quality of life has led to increase in reproductive desire among this population.[3] Fertility of PLWHIV can be affected by HIV infection and associated infections. Infections can physically impact the anatomical structure and biological function of the reproductive system, whereas stress and psychiatric disorders related to HIV infection may lessen sexual drive and frequency of sexual intercourse. In addition, socioeconomic factors including limited financial means, difficulty accessing HIV care, and stigmatization can contribute to social withdrawal and reduced reproductive potential among PLWHIV. Management of reproductive health along with cART has become a necessary component of comprehensive HIV care in the post–cART era. The etiologies and epidemiology of HIV-related infertility, factors that may impact fertility, and management options and considerations for infertility among HIV-infected individuals are reviewed in this chapter.

2. Epidemiology of HIV-related infertility

The data on the magnitude and burden of HIV-related infertility derive mostly from studies conducted among HIV-infected women. A previous study using data from case–control studies and theoretical predictions from a model of the proximate determinants of fertility and HIV incidence in African countries demonstrated the 25–40% lower rate of fertility among HIV-infected women compared to HIV-negative women.[4] In a prospective cohort study from the United States during 1994–2002, women with HIV were less likely to conceive than uninfected women (pregnancy rates 7.4 vs.15.2 per 100 person-years, respectively).[5] Using demographic and health surveys between 2003 and 2007, the Joint United Nations Program on HIV/AIDS (UNAIDS) estimated that the global age-specific fertility ratio for HIV-infected women in the reproductive age group of 20–44 years is 0.53 to 0.76 compared to that of women without HIV.[6] A survey study conducted at HIV fertility clinics in the United Kingdom demonstrated a 40% prevalence of tubal factor infertility among HIV-infected women.[7] Despite the infertility in women living with HIV, pregnancy rates among this population have increased steadily over the past 10 years to between 4 and 6 pregnancies per 100 person-years, varying by region due to the advances in HIV treatment and mother-to-child transmission prevention.[8] This may reflect an increase in reproductive desire and/or unexpected pregnancies and indicate the need for reproductive health care, fertility management, and family planning along with HIV comprehensive care among PLWHIV.

3. HIV effects on fertility

There are several factors associated with HIV infection that can potentially affect fertility in PLWHIV. These factors can be categorized into biological factors, psychological factors, and social factors (Figure 1).

Factors associated with infertility

Biological factors

- Advanced age
- Degree of immunosuppression
- Poor adherence to cART
- Systemic illnesses
- Stress
- Weight loss
- Protracted anovulation and amenorrhea (women)
- Impairment of sperm parameters (men)
- Loss of germ cells within testes (men)
- Primary and secondary hypogonadism
- Sexually-transmitted infections
- Opportunistic infections
- Other genital tract infections
- NRTIs toxicity

Psychological factors

- Feeling of guilt and shame
- Being afraid of HIV transmission
- Awareness of challenges in pregnancy, birth and parenting in the context of HIV infection
- Concerns about personal health and cART efficacy

Social factors

- Financial problems
- Limited reproductive care access
- Social norms and values of reproductive care and HIV/AIDS
- HIV stigmatization
- Lack of knowledge among caring physicians
- Limited availability of assisted reproductive therapy

Note: AIDS, acquired immune deficiency syndrome; cART, combination antiretroviral therapy; HIV, human immunodeficiency virus; NRTIs, nucleoside reverse transcriptase inhibitors.

Figure 1. Factors associated with infertility among people living with human immunodeficiency virus

3.1. Biological factors

Demographic characteristics that have been reported to be associated with low rates of pregnancy among HIV-infected women include advanced age, white ethnicity (compared to black ethnicity), having CD4 cell count of less than 100 cells/mm^3, and poor adherence to cART. [8-10] Systemic illnesses from HIV and its related comorbidities, stress, and weight loss generally impact the reproductive potential of both sexes.[3] HIV-infected women are more likely than non-HIV-infected women to have protracted anovulation and amenorrhea.[11-14] The number of ovulatory cycles was found to correlate with the severity of immunosuppression and having an AIDS diagnosis. Although there have been no reports of ovarian aging or failure,[15] HIV-infected women may have reduced ovarian reserve.[16] In HIV-infected men, impairment of sperm parameters affecting fertility has been described. The impairment includes lower ejaculation volume, sperm count, and progressive motility (defined as the percent of sperm with forward motility) despite normal morphology compared to non-HIV-infected men.[17-19] Sperm concentration levels, total count, and motility were found to positively correlate with the height of the CD4 cell count, indicating the adverse effect of worsening immunodeficiency on these sperm parameters.[19] Other studies demonstrated that the semen of HIV-infected men was more viscous and contained fewer motile sperm but more round cells.[20] In addition, a study of testicular specimens from autopsy samples (1981–1998) revealed progressive loss of germ cells within the testes with prolonged survival with AIDS.[21] Although recent data indicate that cART significantly decreased total sperm count and progressive motility and increased the proportion of abnormal sperm forms,[22] these adverse effects are balanced by the overwhelming benefits of cART for immune reconstitution, morbidity and mortality reduction, and overall improvement of sperm characteristics associated with higher CD4 cell counts.

3.1.1. Hypogonadism and HIV/AIDS

Hypogonadism was recognized as a relatively common condition early in the HIV epidemic and characterized by a low level of testosterone among HIV-infected men. Hypogonadism can be categorized into primary hypogonadism, which is a disorder of the testes, and secondary hypogonadism, which is a disorder of the pituitary or hypothalamus. Hypogonadism can be associated with various signs and symptoms, including muscle wasting, weight loss, low bone mineral density, and decreased libido.[23] During the early course of HIV disease, men tend to have normal serum testosterone levels. As the disease progresses to AIDS, low serum testosterone levels become more frequent, particularly in those with more advanced immunosuppression (e.g., CD4 cell count less than 100 cells/mm^3). Early in the HIV epidemic, 30–50% of symptomatic HIV-infected men had low total serum testosterone levels, which significantly correlated with weight loss and CD4 cell depletion.[24-26] The prevalence of hypogonadism in HIV-infected men has decreased with cART initiation occurring at earlier stages of HIV infection. Effective HIV therapy can normalize testosterone levels over time.[27] Most cases of decreased testosterone levels in HIV-infected men are related to secondary hypogonadism.[24, 28] Other characteristics that have been reported to be associated with low testosterone levels include older age, a detectable HIV RNA level of greater than 10,000 copies/

mL, injection drug use, hepatitis C coinfection, high body mass index, and insulin resistance.[28-31] In addition, several medications commonly used among HIV-infected individuals can affect testosterone levels through varied mechanisms. Systemic glucocorticoids and megestrol acetate can cause hypogonadism by suppressing the hypothalamic–pituitary–gonadal axis, whereas a high dose of ketoconazole (at least 400 mg per day) directly inhibits steroidogenesis. Psychotropic medications can cause hyperprolactinemia and testosterone deficiency, whereas chronic use of alcohol, opiates, and marijuana can impair testosterone production.[32, 33]

Primary hypogonadism	Secondary hypogonadism
Congenital abnormalities	**Congenital abnormalities**
· Klinefelter's syndrome	· Congenital GnRH deficiency
· Other chromosomal abnormalities (e.g., 46, XY/XO; 47, XYY)	· Leptin or leptin receptor mutation
· Mutation in the FSH and LH receptor genes	· Gonadotropin subunit mutations
· Cryptorchidism	
· Disorders of androgen biosynthesis	
· Myotonic dystrophy	
· Congenital anorchia	
· Varicocele	
Acquired diseases	**Acquired diseases**
· Infectious orchitis	· Hyperprolactinemia
· Radiation	· Gonadal steroids
· Alkylating and antineoplastic agents	· Glucocorticoids
· Ketoconazole	· Continuous opiate administration
· Glucocorticoids	· Critical illness
· Dibromochloropropane	· Chronic systemic illness
· Trauma	· Anorexia nervosa
· Testicular torsion	· Diabetes mellitus
· Bilateral orchiectomy	· Obesity
· Autoimmune damage	· Pituitary adenoma
· Chronic systemic diseases	· Metastatic tumor damaging pituitary gland
· Cirrhosis	· Sarcoidosis
· Chronic kidney disease	· Hemochromatosis
· Idiopathic	· Tuberculous meningitis
	· Pituitary apoplexy
	· Trauma
	· Idiopathic

Note: FSH, follicle-stimulating hormone; GnRH, gonadotropin-releasing hormone; LH, luteinizing hormone.

Table 1. Causes of hypogonadism in males

HIV-infected men with symptomatic hypogonadism may present with loss of facial and body hair, decreased muscle mass and strength, diminished libido, impotence, testicular atrophy, gynecomastia, depression, low energy, and poor concentration.[34] Diagnosis of hypogonadism is made based on a clinical suspicion and low serum testosterone levels (generally less than 300 ng/dL). The screening test of choice is the serum total testosterone concentration (free plus protein-bound fractions). However, in some cases, the total testosterone levels may be normal, whereas the free levels may be low because of the higher sex hormone-binding globulin levels among HIV-infected persons. Thus, in a patient with suspected testosterone deficiency and serum total testosterone concentration in the lower half of the normal range (less than 500 ng/dL), the free testosterone levels should be assessed.[34] Testosterone levels should not be evaluated during an acute illness because of the transient decline of androgen levels related to the acute event. To distinguish between primary and secondary hypogonadism, follicle-stimulating hormone (FSH) and luteinizing hormone (LH) levels need to be measured. The elevated FSH and LH levels suggest primary hypogonadism, whereas normal or low levels of FSH and LH are consistent with secondary hypogonadism. Further evaluation should be geared toward diagnosing the possible causes of primary and secondary hypogonadism in HIV-infected men as detailed in Table 1.

3.1.2. Comorbid diseases and HIV/AIDS

3.1.2.1. Sexually Transmitted Infections (STIs)

The impact of STIs on fertility among PLWHIV depends on the local prevalence of the STIs. Given the common route of transmission of causative agents and immunosuppressive status caused by HIV, STIs tend to be more prevalent, to be more severe, to take longer to resolve, and to be more prone to treatment failure in HIV-infected persons compared to the general population. Common causative pathogens for STIs among PLWHIV include bacteria, such as *Neisseria gonorrhoeae, Chlamydia trachomatis, Ureaplasma urealyticum, Mycoplasma hominis, Mycoplasma genitalium, Treponema pallidum, Haemophilus ducreyi,* and *Klebsiella granulomatis*; viruses, such as hepatitis B and C viruses, herpes simplex virus (HSV), and human papillomavirus (HPV); and protozoa, such as *Trichomonas vaginalis*. The underlying pathogenesis for STI-related infertility is direct damage and subsequent anatomical and functional abnormalities of the genital organs, including the testes and epididymis in men and cervix, uterus, fallopian tubes, and ovaries in women. A previous study demonstrated that the DNA of STI pathogens was detected in semen of 45 of 241 asymptomatic men seeking an infertility investigation (19%) and was associated with a decrease in sperm concentration, motile sperm concentration, total sperm count, and neutral alpha-glucosidase concentration.[35]

Gonorrhea is a STI caused by *N. gonorrhea* and commonly manifests as urethritis in both sexes and pelvic inflammatory disease in women. The reported complications related to fertility of gonorrhea include urethral strictures and subsequent impairment of testicular functions in men.[36] Similarly, *C. trachomatis* can cause urethritis in both sexes and pelvic inflammatory disease in females. Epidemiologic data suggest that *C. trachomatis* may be associated with tubal obstruction and subsequent infertility in women.[37] The impact of Mycoplasma, that is, *U.*

urealyticum, *M. hominis*, and *M. genitalium*, on fertility is uncertain. *U. urealyticum* may cause infertility through its effects on sperm chromatin and DNA, whereas *M. genitalium* can attach to spermatozoa and can be transported to the female genital tract.[38, 39] Syphilis is caused by *T. pallidum* and is more prevalent among PLWHIV. Orchitis, epididymitis, and testicular mass have been reported as manifestations of syphilis in HIV-infected men.[40, 41] Although *H. ducreyi* and *K. granulomatis* do not directly affect the reproductive tract, they both cause ulcers and lymphadenopathy around the genital area, which may affect reproductive potential.

Chronic viral hepatitis B and C can cause impairment in sperm concentration, motility, morphology, and viability, whereas HPV primarily affects sperm motility.[42] The presence of HSV DNA in semen has been associated with decreased sperm concentration and reduced motility.[43] In HIV-infected women, chronic HPV infection increases the risk of cervical cancer development and possibly leads to infertility. An important protozoan *T. vaginalis* is the cause of vaginitis, endometritis, adnexitis, and pyosalpinx in women, which can lead to infertility and preterm birth and low birth weight of the newborn.[44] In men, it is associated with complications including urethritis, prostatitis, epididymitis, and infertility through inflammatory damage or interference with sperm function.[44]

3.1.2.2. Opportunistic Infections (OIs)

HIV-infected persons are at increased risk for opportunistic infections (OIs) depending on their degree of immunosuppression. Tuberculosis is a common OI in HIV-tuberculosis endemic locales and its prevalence is higher among PLWHIV compared to non-HIV-infected persons, regardless of the CD4 cell count. Genital tract infection caused by *Mycobacterium tuberculosis* contributes to infertility and poorer reproductive health outcomes in both sexes.[3] Salmonellosis, toxoplasmosis, and cryptococcosis can manifest as disseminated infections involving the genital organs. Although cytomegalovirus (CMV) can cause orchitis and epididymitis in HIV-infected men, there are no data on its effect on sperm characteristics.[42] Candidiasis is frequently reported among HIV-infected persons with CD4 cell counts less than 200 cells/mm^3. It is the cause of balanitis in men and vaginitis and cervicitis in women, which may affect fertility.

3.1.2.3. Other infections

Other infectious causes of orchitis in both HIV-infected and non-HIV-infected men include bacteria, such as *Escherichia coli*, *Klebsiella pneumoniae*, *Pseudomonas aeruginosa*, *Staphylococcus* spp., and *Streptococcus* spp., and viruses, such as mumps, varicella, coxsackievirus, and echovirus.[45] These infections may also contribute to infertility.

3.1.3. Antiretroviral agents

Nucleoside reverse transcriptase inhibitors (NRTIs) remain key components of recommended cART regimens. They inhibit HIV-1 reverse transcriptase, which reduces viral replication and improves disease control. However, these medications also inhibit mitochondrial DNA (mtDNA) synthesis and cause a decrease in polypeptides involved in electron transport, which can result in cell injury.[46] The degree of mitochondrial toxicity is specific to each NRTI. Theoretically, an HIV-infected person's fertility may be affected by NRTI use via the damage to mitochondrial biogenesis of gametes.[3] This is supported by the mtDNA depletion observed in sperm and oocytes of HIV-infected patients taking NRTIs and in low oocyte mtDNA in patients with ovarian insufficiency.[47-49] Data from epidemiologic studies are conflicting regarding the impact of cART on fertility. A prospective cohort from the United States reported the lower likelihood of conception associated with antiretroviral therapy among HIV-infected women,[5] whereas a more recent study from Africa demonstrated significantly higher pregnancy rates among HIV-infected women on cART compared to those not on cART.[50] However, these two studies were conducted in different settings and time, and specific behavioral and biological mechanisms were not explored. Zidovudine (azidothymidine, AZT) is the NRTI drug that has been studied the most. In animal studies, AZT has been shown to suppress cell division in the preimplantation mouse embryo, causing reduction in inner cell mass proliferation, greater number of resorptions, and fewer fetuses.[51, 52] A previous study demonstrated that exposure to NRTI transplacentally caused significant fetal mitochondrial damage in experimental monkeys.[53] Unfortunately, there have been no studies examining fertility effect of NRTIs in humans.

3.2. Psychological factors

Decrease in sexual activity after a new diagnosis of HIV infection is usually observed and may be accompanied by the feeling of guilt and shame and aggravated by the stigma related to HIV infection.[54] Individuals recently diagnosed with HIV infection reported to have decreased desire for or interest in sex relations. They also reported to use condom more consistently during sexual intercourse to avoid transmission of HIV to their partners.[55] Previous studies indicated that HIV-infected women often chose to avoid pregnancy.[56, 57] However, another study revealed that high-risk behaviors, unplanned pregnancies, and pregnancy termination remain prevalent among this population.[58] In the pre–cART era, there was a significant increase in the pregnancy termination rate from 3.5 to 6.3 per 100 women-years following a new HIV diagnosis in the United Kingdom and Ireland[56] and 47% of pregnancies were voluntarily terminated following a new HIV diagnosis in an Australian study.[57] The reasons for pregnancy termination may include challenges of pregnancy, birth and parenting in the context of HIV infection, concerns about increased risks of complications related to pregnancy and delivery, and risk of HIV transmission to the newborn. A previous study reported that unplanned pregnancy, lower CD4 cell count, and having an HIV-infected current partner were factors associated with the decision to terminate a pregnancy.[59] Following the introduction of cART with overall improvement in health and immune status of HIV-infected women, the rates of elective pregnancy termination after a HIV diagnosis were 22%-26% decreased from the pre–cART period.[60, 61] With the success of cART in preventing mother-to-child HIV transmission, HIV infection was reported to have no effect on desire for pregnancy among young urban African Americans aged 15–24 years.[62] Reproductive desire among PLWHIV may now be associated with personal health, cART, concern about HIV transmission, and social factors. Some HIV-infected persons have an increased desire for children as a way of concealing their HIV-infected status and improving their feelings of self worth. Others stated that their HIV diagnosis increased their desire for children at an earlier age and some chose to have children following advances in HIV care.[63-65]

3.3. Social factors

The HIV/AIDS epidemic has a significant impact on the economic and political stability of a nation. Awareness of HIV/AIDS at the population level may affect the age of sexual debut, frequency of sexual intercourse, safer sex and contraceptive practices, perceived value of marriage, social norms, and fertility intentions and choices of PLWHIV.[3] The dramatic improvement in the life expectancy of PLWHIV and reduction in HIV transmission rates following treatment of the infected partner have changed ethical considerations regarding childbearing in HIV-infected individuals. Early in the HIV/AIDS epidemic, pregnancy in HIV-infected women was considered morally problematic, whereas recently, the Ethics Committee of the American Society for Reproductive Medicine stated that it is ethical for health care providers to assist PLWHIV who seek pregnancy when optimal precautions to prevent HIV transmission are utilized.[66] Despite more opportunities for access to reproductive care, PLWHIV still face multiple obstacles. First, the severity of their disease, level of immunosuppression, presence of OIs, and other comorbid diseases may impair their fertility. Second, their HIV provider may have limited knowledge to counsel them on reproductive health issues, and infertility specialists may have limited expertise in providing care for HIV-infected persons. Third, HIV stigmatization could potentially preclude them from establishing reproductive care. Finally, assisted fertility therapy (AFT) is technically complicated in regard to HIV transmission prevention and costliness and may not be available in all settings.[3]

4. Fertility management

Fertility management for PLWHIV should be comprehensive and involve cART, specific management for factors associated with infertility, and AFT while minimizing the risk of horizontal and vertical transmission of HIV.

4.1. Combination antiretroviral therapy

With advances in the development of antiretroviral agents, cART has become more potent and effective, more tolerable and convenient to administer, and less toxic. Current guidelines recommend that PLWHIV should receive cART when they are willing and able to commit to treatment and understand the benefits and risks of therapy and the importance of adherence, regardless of the CD4 cell count level.[67] The benefits of early cART among persons with a CD4 cell count above 500 cells/mm^3 were demonstrated in a recent large-scale randomized trial that showed a reduction in mortality, AIDS-related events, and non–AIDS-related events in those started on cART immediately versus waiting until the CD4 cell count fell below 350 cells/mm^3.[68] The currently recommended initial cART regimens consist of a backbone of two NRTIs and any one drug from the following drug classes: non-NRTI, protease inhibitor with a booster, or integrase inhibitor with or without a booster.[67, 69, 70] The initial cART regimens recommended by different consensus guidelines are shown in Table 2. A patient-specific regimen from these lists will be chosen based on convenience of administration, adverse reactions, local availability, cost, and health plan coverage. The goals of cART are immunologic response, defined as an increase in CD4 cell count, and virologic response, defined as HIV RNA suppression below the lower limit of detection. By extending life expectancy and improving overall health, immunity, and quality of life from cART, cART is expected to improve fertility outcomes. Achieving a sustained virologic response is particularly important to reduce the risk of HIV horizontal and vertical transmission during conception attempts, pregnancy, and delivery.

DHHS 2015	EACS 2015	WHO 2013
ABC + 3TC + DTG	ABC + 3TC + DTG	TDF + FTC/3TC + EFV
TDF + FTC + DTG	TDF + FTC + DTG	
TDF + FTC + EVG/c or TAF + FTC + EVG/c	TDF + FTC + EVG/c	
TDF + FTC + RAL	TDF + FTC + RAL	
TDF + FTC + DRV/r	TDF + FTC + DRV/r	
	TDF + FTC + RPV	

Note: 3TC, lamivudine; ABC, abacavir; DHHS, the U.S. Department of Health and Human Services; DRV/r, ritonavir-boosted darunavir; DTG, dolutegravir; EACS, European AIDS Clinical Society; EFV, efavirenz; EVG/c, cobicistat-boosted elvitegravir; FTC, emtricitabine; RAL, raltegravir; RPV, rilpivirine; TAF, tenofovir alafenamide; TDF, tenofovir disoproxil fumarate; WHO, World Health Organization.

Table 2. Recommended first-line combination antiretroviral therapy regimens based on consensus guidelines

4.2. Specific management for factors associated with infertility

4.2.1. Management of biological factors

Immunosuppression and wasting syndrome can be improved by cART. In addition, PLWHIV who are taking cART with sustained immunologic and virologic responses will have reduced incidences of OIs, such as tuberculosis, salmonellosis, toxoplasmosis, cryptococcosis, CMV infection, and candidiasis. NRTIs selected for the backbone of a cART regimen should have the least toxicity on mitochondria to minimize the impact on oocytes and sperm. These "safer" NRTIs include tenofovir, abacavir, lamivudine, and emtricitabine.[67, 69, 70] Good general health and less physical stress are associated with normal ovulation and menstrual cycles in HIV-infected women, whereas cART improves overall sperm parameters among HIV-infected men. STIs, OIs, and other infections should be promptly diagnosed and treated to prevent damage to the genital organs. It is important that sex partners of patients with STIs should be counseled, tested, and treated accordingly.

Hypogonadism should be recognized early, correctly diagnosed, and treated in HIV-infected men. Testosterone treatment is indicated in men with low serum concentrations of testosterone and any of the following signs or symptoms including low libido and/or hypogonadal symptoms, low bone mineral density, low body mass, or weight loss despite virologic response to cART. Prior to initiation of testosterone replacement therapy, patients should be evaluated for coexisting depression and psychosocial stressors along with baseline laboratory studies including complete blood count, a metabolic panel, lipid panel, and a prostate-specific antigen (PSA). Long-term effects of suppression of the hypothalamic–pituitary–gonadal axis, promoting malignancy of the prostate gland and cardiovascular diseases, in those older than 60 years should be carefully monitored. Patients with a history of prostate cancer, a palpable prostate nodule, or an elevated PSA should not be prescribed testosterone replacement therapy.[34, 71] The routes of testosterone administration should be based on the patient's preference and include transdermal patch, gel, and intramuscular injection. For injections, the initial dose is 200 mg every 2 weeks or 100 mg every week. The dose can be titrated based on testosterone levels measured midway between injections aiming for the mid-normal reference range. Testosterone replacement therapy should continue as long as there are symptomatic benefits and no adverse effects.

4.2.2. Management of psychological and social factors

Knowledge about HIV and its epidemiology, routes of transmission, clinical course, long-term prognosis, and benefit of cART is critical to PLWHIV in reducing HIV transmission to their sexual partners and improvinge their adherence and outcomes. A previous study demonstrated that increased reproductive intention was associated with patient optimism regarding cART efficacy.[72] To overcome the challenges in pregnancy, birth, and parenting, PLWHIV should be informed about the recent advances in antenatal, perinatal, and postnatal care to prevent HIV transmission to their newborns. Family planning counseling should be provided to prepare them for child rearing and to cope with any problems they may face. Issues on reproductive care access for PLWHIV are very new for many developing countries, because the main goals for HIV care in these countries are currently improving access to HIV testing and treatment. Financial burdens, medical coverage, and availability of centers that can provide AFT need to be considered when developing and implementing local, regional, and national policies or guidelines for the reproductive care of PLWHIV. In the meantime, physicians who care for PLWHIV should update their knowledge to optimally assess and manage fertility issues among persons with HIV infection. HIV stigmatization may be reduced by campaigns and specific interventions that are appropriate and feasible for each locale.

4.3. Assisted fertility therapy

Relevant issues to be considered regarding fertility treatment in PLWHIV include risk of HIV horizontal transmission in serodiscordant heterosexual couples and methods to reduce HIV transmission. Generally, the rate of HIV heterosexual transmission is approximately 1 per

500 to 1 per 1,000 episodes of unprotected sexual intercourse.[3] However, the risk of transmission can increase significantly if there are genital tract infections from STIs or OIs, trauma with sex, lack of male circumcision, and high plasma HIV RNA levels in seropositive persons.[73, 74] Thus, a thorough evaluation is needed before AFT. History including a detailed history of their HIV infection and any associated complications, recent CD4 cell counts and HIV RNA levels, past and current cART regimens, history of antiretroviral drug resistance, ongoing HIV risk behaviors, and fertility problems should be obtained. Physical examination should focus on signs relevant to causes of infertility, genital organs, and Pap smear in women. An HIV-infected partner should be treated with cART until HIV RNA suppression has been achieved prior to AFT. Partners who have STIs need to be treated to reduce transmission risks of HIV and STI-associated pathogens. Trauma during sexual intercourse should be avoided or minimized, and safer sex practices should be encouraged outside the conception attempts. Proposed algorithm for fertility management among HIV-infected couples is shown in Figure 2.

Post-exposure prophylaxis (PEP) with cART in uninfected partners may be used after the unprotected sexual intercourse (conception attempt). Although there have not been well-designed studies in human that assess the efficacy of this intervention, the benefits of HIV transmission reduction have been shown in an animal study and a retrospective study of health care workers exposing to body fluids of HIV-infected persons.[75, 76] The recommended PEP regimens that are also safe if the pregnancy does occur are combined tenofovir, emtricitabine, and ritonavir-boosted atazanavir, ritonavir-boosted darunavir, or raltegravir.[77] PEP should be initiated as soon as possible after HIV exposure but within 48 hours and should be continued for 28 days. Because of its demonstrated efficacy, tenofovir–emtricitabine (TDF/FTC) once daily for pre-exposure prophylaxis (PrEP) administered to the seronegative partner is now the preferred approach to reduce the risk of HIV transmission among serodiscordant couples. Among heterosexual couples, pericoital tenofovir vaginal gel was the first PrEP intervention that showed a 39% efficacy at reducing HIV acquisition among high-risk South African women.[78] Several other randomized controlled trials have demonstrated the benefit of PrEP at reducing HIV acquisition among HIV-negative at-risk individuals including 1) the iPrEx study that demonstrated 44% reduction in the incidence of HIV among men who have sex with men taking daily oral TDF/FTC,[79] 2) the Partners-PrEP study that demonstrated 75% and 67% reduction in the incidence of HIV among serodiscordant couples taking daily oral TDF or TDF/FTC, respectively, in Africa,[80] and 3) the TDF2 study that demonstrated 62% reduction in the incidence of HIV among heterosexual men and women taking daily oral TDF/FTC in Botswana.[81] Pharmacokinetic data suggest that PrEP should begin at least 1 week before unprotected sex for optimal benefit. The uninfected partners who choose to take PEP and/or PrEP need to be regularly screened and monitored for HIV infection and adverse effects of the drugs in PEP and/or PrEP regimens.[67, 77]

In regards to limiting risk of HIV vertical transmission, cART given to HIV-infected women antenatally and avoiding breastfeeding can reduce the rate of transmission from 25–40% to less than 1%.[67] Invasive procedures, such as amniocentesis, chorionic villus sampling, and use of fetal scalp electrodes, should be avoided in HIV-infected women because these can

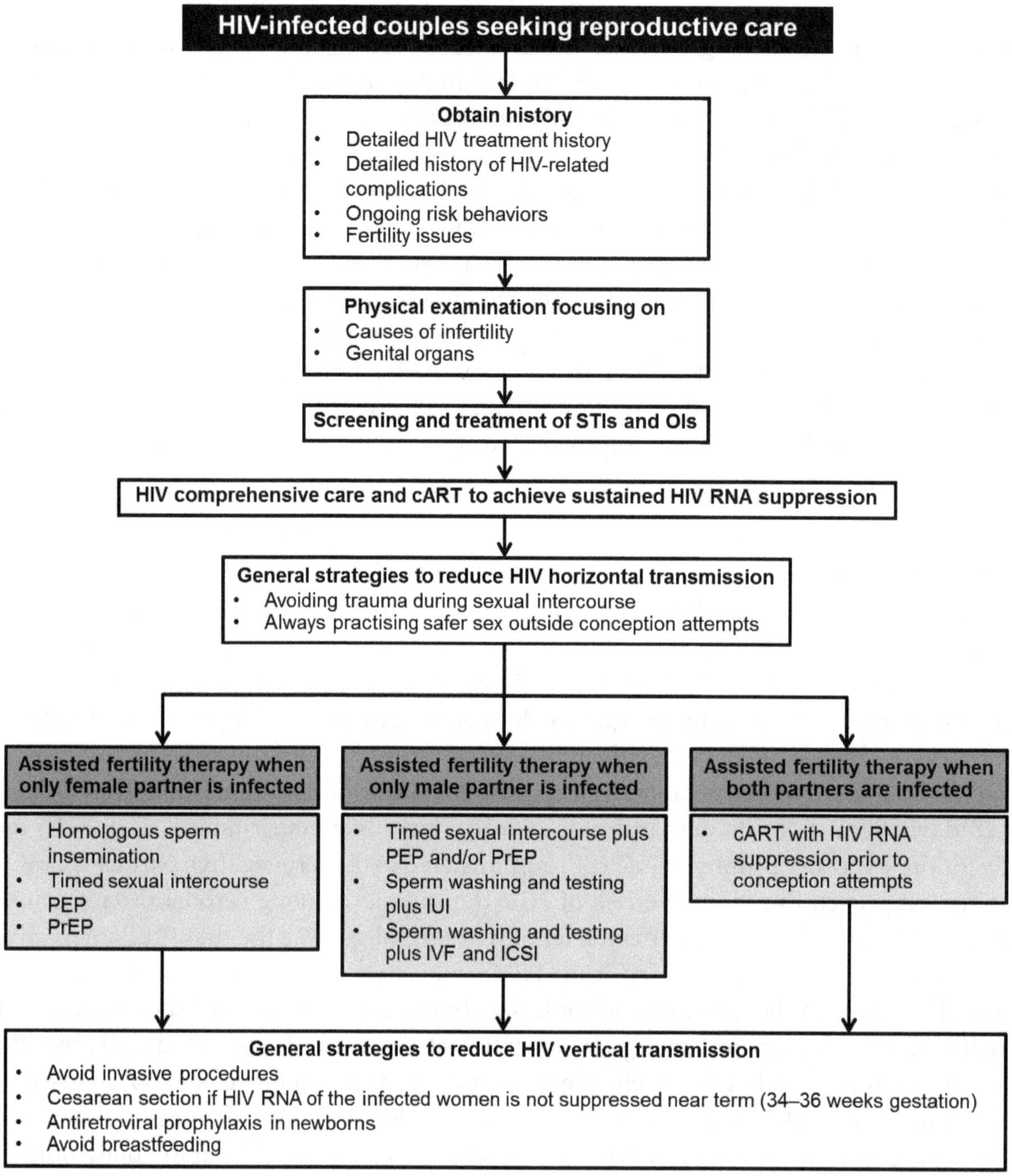

Note: cART, combination antiretroviral therapy; HIV, human immunodeficiency virus; ICSI, intracytoplasmic sperm injection; IUI, intrauterine insemination; IVF, in vitro fertilization; OIs, opportunistic infections; PEP, post-exposure prophylaxis; PrEP, pre-exposure prophylaxis; RNA, ribonucleic acid; STIs, sexually transmitted infections.

Figure 2. Proposed algorithm of fertility management in HIV-infected couples

increase the risk of fetal/infant exposure to maternal body fluids. Cesarean section instead of normal vaginal delivery can further reduce the risk of maternal-infant transmission in HIV-infected pregnant women whose HIV RNA has not been suppressed following cART. United States guidelines use a HIV RNA level of >1,000 copies/mL at 34–36 weeks gestation as a threshold for recommending Cesarean section, whereas European guidelines recommend a threshold of >50 copies/mL.[67, 69] Women who achieve virologic suppression near term can proceed with vaginal delivery without increased transmission risk. Antiretroviral prophylactic regimens for newborns of HIV-infected mothers should be prescribed based on the risk of transmission. In general, AZT is recommended for the first 4–6 weeks of life with additional medications added if the mother did not achieve viral suppression. HIV-infected mothers should not breastfeed their babies due to the risk of transmission via breast milk.

4.3.1. AFT when only the female partner is infected

If a woman is HIV infected and her male partner is uninfected, HIV transmission can be avoided by using homologous insemination with the male partner's sperm. However, if this option is not feasible, such as the desire to become pregnant naturally, couples should limit unprotected sexual intercourse to the time of ovulation (timed intercourse) using ovulation kits or basal body temperature monitoring to predict ovulation. These measures allow couples to limit the number of unprotected sexual encounters. In addition, the HIV-infected women should be on cART with a suppressed viral load. The male partner may choose to take PEP and/or PrEP to reduce the risk of HIV transmission; however, these options are not as safe as homologous insemination.[82]

4.3.2. AFT when only the male partner is infected

Conception between an HIV-infected man and his HIV-uninfected female partner is more complicated. The risk of HIV transmission can be reduced by using timed intercourse when the HIV-infected man's plasma HIV RNA is undetectable on cART. However, the HIV transmission of timed intercourse in this setting has been reported to be associated with inconsistent condom use outside the conception attempt.[83] Thus, the practice of timed intercourse alone to prevent HIV transmission to the female partner is not generally recommended in this setting.[82] Additional PEP and/or PrEP may be used to reduce HIV transmission. A study of serodiscordant couples, in which the woman was treated with oral tenofovir taken shortly before and after each unprotected sexual encounter, showed that none of the women became infected with HIV and pregnancy rates reached 75% after 12 attempts.[84] Based on available data, once-daily TDF/FTC for the women would generally be recommended throughout the conception period in countries where resources are available for PrEP.

Sperm preparation and testing prior to intrauterine insemination (IUI) have been described as methods to reduce the chance of HIV transmission to the uninfected female partner. The sperm preparation involves a three-step process.[3, 82] First, the liquefied semen is filtered through a Percoll gradient. Next, the isolated spermatozoa are washed to eliminate seminal plasma and hyperosmotic gradient media. Finally, a modified swim-up method recovers highly motile spermatozoa from leukocytes. After this process, the final sperm specimen is tested by polymerase chain reaction assays for the presence of HIV. If this final specimen tests negative, it is used for insemination. In men with severe dyspermia, the final swim-up step that removes infected leukocytes cannot be performed and thus the semen should be tested for HIV DNA. Utilizing this process, 1,600 inseminations were performed in 513 HIV-uninfected women and resulted in 228 pregnancies. At 1-year follow-up, none of the children older than 3 months of age and none of the mothers became HIV infected.[85] In addition, studies reviewing world-wide data in 2004 and data from several centers demonstrated no HIV transmission to the uninfected female partners who were inseminated using sperm washing and IUI.[86, 87]

There have been recent data supporting the use of IVF/ICSI to reduce HIV transmission to uninfected women. A 10-year retrospective study of 181 serodiscordant couples undergoing IVF/ICSI, in which sperm was prepared using a modified density-gradient centrifugation and the swim-up method, revealed no HIV infection among the uninfected women and their 170 children.[88] Another study from the Center for Reproductive Assisted Techniques for HIV in Europe reported no evidence of seroconversion in any uninfected partners or children on follow-up.[86] Unfortunately, these techniques are generally prohibitively expensive. Although the data on efficacy and safety of the AFT techniques are encouraging, the potential risk of HIV transmission is not completely eliminated and more studies are required. Until then, serodiscordant couples should also be counseled about other safer options, including using donor sperm, donor embryo, adoption, or not having children.[82] If couples want to have their own biological children, they should be informed about available risk reduction techniques and the availability of centers that can provide effective methods of sperm preparation and testing. Fertility centers should use approved study protocols with informed consent and provide appropriate follow-up of sexual partners and their children.

4.3.3. AFT when both partners are infected

While HIV seroconcordant couples do not have the same concerns about HIV transmission as do HIV serodiscordant couples, the risk of transmission of different strains of HIV between each other or superinfection exists. HIV superinfection in seroconcordant couples has been reported to increase the risk of HIV RNA rebound and decrease in CD4 cell count following immune reactivation.[89] The best way to minimize the risk of superinfection and optimize reproductive outcomes for couples and their offspring is to use cART to achieve HIV RNA suppression in both partners prior to conception attempts.

4.4. Healthcare workers and cross-contamination risks

Healthcare workers are at risk of exposure to blood-borne pathogens, including HIV through patient care. However, if standard universal precautions to prevent the transmission of infectious diseases are followed, the risk of acquiring these pathogens is very small and is not sufficient to deny reproductive services to PLWHIV. To date, there have been no reports of occupational HIV transmission to health care workers performing AFT, suggesting that the risk of transmission is extremely low. Theoretical concerns about contaminating other gametes and embryos stored in the same laboratory from cross-contamination have been raised. To date, no such event has been reported. To avoid this risk, it is recommended that samples from HIV-infected persons be processed in a separate laboratory or designated space within the main laboratory and to use a dedicated storage tank.[82]

5. Conclusions

Reproductive issues have become more relevant among PLWHIV who are living longer and are staying healthier on cART. Fertility outcomes of PLWHIV have been improving for the past decade, although they remain inferior to those of the general population. HIV can impact fertility in many ways that involve biological, psychological, and social factors. Assessing and managing fertility issues in HIV-infected individuals and couples involve the use of cART, diagnosing and correcting causes of infertility, and AFT, which has become more effective and safer. Further studies are needed to address the efficacy and safety of AFT techniques as well as the complex social and ethical challenges of fertility issues of HIV-infected persons. Healthcare workers caring for PLWHIV should be knowledgeable in both HIV infection and reproductive health because they may now be legally and ethically obligated to provide reproductive care and assistance to this population.

Author details

Thana Khawcharoenporn[1*] and Beverly E. Sha[2]

*Address all correspondence to: thanak30@yahoo.com

1 Division of Infectious Diseases, Faculty of Medicine, Thammasat University, Pathumthani, Thailand

2 Division of Infectious Diseases, Rush University Medical Center, Chicago, IL, USA

References

[1] UNAIDS. Fact Sheet 2015. Available at: www.unaids.org/en/resources/campaigns/HowAIDSchangedeverything/factsheet. Accessed 16 December 2015.

[2] May M, Gompels M, Delpech V, Porter K, Post F, Johnson M, et al. Impact of late diagnosis and treatment on life expectancy in people with HIV-1: UK Collaborative HIV Cohort (UK CHIC) Study. BMJ 2011; 343: d6016. doi: 10.1136/bmj.d6016.

[3] Kushnir VA, Lewis W. Human immunodeficiency virus/acquired immunodeficiency syndrome and infertility: emerging problems in the era of highly active antiretrovirals. Fertil Steril 2011; 96: 546–553.

[4] Zaba B, Gregson S. Measuring the impact of HIV on fertility in Africa. AIDS 1998; 12 Suppl 1: S41–S50.

[5] Massad LS, Springer G, Jacobson L, Watts H, Anastos K, Korn A, et al. Pregnancy rates and predictors of conception, miscarriage and abortion in US women with HIV. AIDS 2004; 18: 281–286.

[6] Chen WJ, Walker N. Fertility of HIV-infected women: insights from demographic and health surveys. Sex Transm Infect 2010; 86: ii22–ii27.

[7] Frodsham LC, Boag F, Barton S, Gilling-Smith C. Human immunodeficiency virus infection and fertility care in the United Kingdom: demand and supply. Fertil Steril 2006; 85: 285–289.

[8] Westreich D, Maskew M, Rubel D, MacDonald P, Jaffray I, Majuba P. Incidence of pregnancy after initiation of antiretroviral therapy in South Africa: a retrospective clinical cohort analysis. Infect Dis Obstet Gynecol 2012; 2012: 917059.

[9] Huntington SE, Thorne C, Bansi LK, Anderson J, Newell ML, Taylor GP, et al. Predictors of pregnancy and changes in pregnancy incidence among HIV-positive women accessing HIV clinical care. AIDS 2013; 27: 95–103.

[10] Lancaster KE, Kwok C, Rinaldi A, Byamugisha J, Magwali T, Nyamapfeni P, et al. Incident pregnancy and pregnancy outcomes among HIV-infected women in Uganda and Zimbabwe. Int J Gynaecol Obstet 2015; 131: 255–259.

[11] Chirgwin KD, Feldman J, Muneyyirci-Delale O, Landesman S, Minkoff H. Menstrual function in human immunodeficiency virus-infected women without acquired immunodeficiency syndrome. J Acquir Immune Defic Syndr Hum Retrovirol 1996; 12: 489–94.

[12] Cejtin HE, Kalinowski A, Bacchetti P, Taylor RN, Watts DH, Kim S, et al. Effects of human immunodeficiency virus on protracted amenorrhea and ovarian dysfunction. Obstet Gynecol 2006; 108: 1423–1431.

[13] Ellerbrock TV, Wright TC, Bush TJ, Dole P, Brudney K, Chiasson M. Characteristics of menstruation in women infected with HIV. Obstet Gynecol 1996; 87: 1030–1034.

[14] Harlow SC, Schuman P, Cohen M, Ohmit SE, Cu-Uvin S, Lin X, et al. Effect of HIV infection on menstrual cycle length. J Acquir Immune Defic Syndr 2000; 24: 68–75.

[15] Seifer DB, Golub ET, Lambert-Messerlian G, Springer G, Holman S, Moxley M, et al. Biologic markers of ovarian reserve and reproductive aging: application in a cohort study of HIV infection in women. Fertil Steril 2007; 88: 1645–1652.

[16] Coll O, Fiore S, Floridia M, Giaquinto C, Grosch-Wörner I, Guiliano M, et al. Pregnancy and HIV infection: a European consensus on management. AIDS 2002; 16 Suppl 2: S1–S18.

[17] White DJ, Mital D, Taylor S, St John JC. Sperm mitochondrial DNA deletions as a consequence of long term highly active antiretroviral therapy. AIDS 2001; 15: 1061–1062.

[18] Bujan L, Sergerie M, Moinard N, Martinet S, Porte L, Massip P, et al. Decreased semen volume and spermatozoa motility in HIV-1-infected patients under antiretroviral treatment. J Androl 2007; 28: 444–452.

[19] Nicopoullos JD, Almeida PA, Ramsay JW, Gilling-Smith C. The effect of human immunodeficiency virus on sperm parameters and the outcome of intrauterine insemination following sperm washing. Hum Reprod 2004; 19: 2289–2297.

[20] Crittenden JA, Handelsman DJ, Stewart GJ. Semen analysis in human immunodeficiency virus infection. Fertil Steril 1992; 57: 1294–1299.

[21] Shevchuk MM, Pigato JB, Khalife G, Armenakas NA, Fracchia JA. Changing testicular histology in AIDS: its implication for sexual transmission of HIV. Urology 1999; 53: 203–208.

[22] Nicopoullos JD, Almeida P, Vourliotis M, Gilling-Smith C. A decade of the sperm-washing programme: correlation between markers of HIV and seminal parameters. HIV Med 2011; 12: 195–201.

[23] Wanke CA, Silva M, Knox TA, Forrester J, Speigelman D, Gorbach SL. Weight loss and wasting remain common complications in individuals infected with human immunodeficiency virus in the era of highly active antiretroviral therapy. Clin Infect Dis 2000; 31: 803–805.

[24] Dobs AS, Dempsey MA, Ladenson PW, Polk BF. Endocrine disorders in men infected with human immunodeficiency virus. Am J Med 1988; 84: 611–616.

[25] Raffi F, Brisseau JM, Planchon B, Rémi JP, Barrier JH, Grolleau JY. Endocrine function in 98 HIV-infected patients: a prospective study. AIDS 1991; 5: 729–733.

[26] Christeff N, Gharakhanian S, Thobie N, Rozenbaum W, Nunez EA. Evidence for changes in adrenal and testicular steroids during HIV infection. J Acquir Immune Defic Syndr 1992; 5: 841–846.

[27] Dubé MP, Parker RA, Mulligan K, Tebas P, Robbins GK, Roubenoff R, et al. Effects of potent antiretroviral therapy on free testosterone levels and fat-free mass in men in a prospective, randomized trial: A5005s, a substudy of AIDS Clinical Trials Group Study 384. Clin Infect Dis 2007; 45: 120–126.

[28] Klein RS, Lo Y, Santoro N, Dobs AS. Androgen levels in older men who have or who are at risk of acquiring HIV infection. Clin Infect Dis 2005; 41: 1794–1803.

[29] Araujo AB, O'Donnell AB, Brambilla DJ, Simpson WB, Longcope C, Matsumoto AM, et al. Prevalence and incidence of androgen deficiency in middle-aged and older men: estimates from the Massachusetts Male Aging Study. J Clin Endocrinol Metab 2004; 89: 5920–5926.

[30] Grossmann M, Gianatti EJ, Zajac JD. Testosterone and type 2 diabetes. Curr Opin Endocrinol Diabetes Obes 2010; 17: 247–256.

[31] Zitzmann M. Testosterone deficiency, insulin resistance and the metabolic syndrome. Nat Rev Endocrinol 2009; 5: 673 681.

[32] Misra M, Papakostas GI, Klibanski A. Effects of psychiatric disorders and psychotropic medications on prolactin and bone metabolism. J Clin Psychiatry 2004; 65: 1607–1618.

[33] Cooper OB, Brown TT, Dobs AS. Opiate drug use: a potential contributor to the endocrine and metabolic complications in human immunodeficiency virus disease. Clin Infect Dis 2003; 37 Suppl 2: S132–S136.

[34] Bhasin S, Cunningham GR, Hayes FJ, Matsumoto AM, Snyder PJ, Swerdloff RS, et al. Testosterone therapy in men with androgen deficiency syndromes: an Endocrine Society clinical practice guideline. J Clin Endocrinol Metab 2010; 95: 2536–2559.

[35] Bezold G, Politch JA, Kiviat NB, Kuypers JM, Wolff H, Anderson DJ. Prevalence of sexually transmissible pathogens in semen from asymptomatic male infertility patients with and without leukocytospermia. Fertil Steril 2007; 87: 1087–1097.

[36] Ochsendrof FR. Sexually transmitted infections: impact on male fertility. Andrologia 2008; 40: 72–75.

[37] Eggert-Kruse W, Gerhard I, Näher H, Tilgen W, Runnebaum B. Chlamydial infection —a female and/or male infertility factor? Fertil Steril 1990; 53: 1037–1043.

[38] Reichart M, Kahane I, Bartoov B. In vivo and in vitro impairment of human and ram sperm nuclear chromatin integrity by sexually transmitted *Ureaplasma urealyticum* infection. Biol Reprod 2000; 63: 1041–1048.

[39] Svenstrup HF, Fedder J, Abraham-Peskir J, Birkelund S, Christiansen G. *Mycoplasma genitalium* attaches to human spermatozoa. Hum Reprod 2003; 18: 2103–2109.

[40] Michelson HE. Syphilis of the epididymis. JAMA 1919; 73: 1431–1433.

[41] Varma R, Baithun S, Alexander S, Goh BT. Acute syphilitic interstitial orchitis mimicking testicular malignancy in an HIV-1 infected man diagnosed by *Treponema pallidum* polymerase chain reaction. Int J STD AIDS 2009; 20: 65–66.

[42] Garolla A, Pizzol D, Bertoldo A, Menegazzo M, Barzon L, Foresta C. Sperm viral infection and male infertility: focus on HBV, HCV, HIV, HPV, HSV, HCMV, and AAV. J Reprod Immunol 2013; 100: 20–29.

[43] Neofytou E, Sourvinos G, Asmarianaki M, Spandidos DA, Makrigiannakis A. Prevalence of human herpes virus types 1-7 in the semen of men attending an infertility clinic and correlation with semen parameters. Fertil Steril 2009; 91: 2487–2494.

[44] Fichorova RN. Impact of *T. vaginalis* infection on innate immune responses and reproductive outcome. J Reprod Immunol 2009; 83: 185–189.

[45] Brookings C, Goldmeier D, Sadeghi-Nejad H. Sexually transmitted infections and sexual function in relation to male fertility. Korean J Urol 2013; 54: 149–156.

[46] Lewis W, Day BJ, Copeland WC. Mitochondrial toxicity of NRTI antiviral drugs: an integrated cellular perspective. Nat Rev Drug Discov 2003; 2: 812–22.

[47] Pavili L, Daudin M, Moinard N, Walschaerts M, Cuzin L, Massip P, et al. Decrease of mitochondrial DNA level in sperm from patients infected with human immunodeficiency virus-1 linked to nucleoside analogue reverse transcriptase inhibitors. Fertil Steril 2010; 94: 2151–2156.

[48] Lopez S, Coll O, Durban M, Hernandez S, Vidal R, Suy A, et al. Mitochondrial DNA depletion in oocytes of HIV-infected antiretroviral-treated infertile women. Antivir Ther 2008; 13: 833–838.

[49] May-Panloup P, Chretien MF, Jacques C, Vasseur C, Malthiery Y, Reynier P. Low oocyte mitochondrial DNA content in ovarian insufficiency. Hum Reprod 2005; 20: 593–597.

[50] Myer L, Carter RJ, Katyal M, Toro P, El-Sadr WM, Abrams EJ. Impact of antiretroviral therapy on incidence of pregnancy among HIV-infected women in Sub-Saharan Africa: a cohort study. PLoS Med 2010; 7: e1000229.

[51] Toltzis P, Mourton T, Magnuson T. Effect of zidovudine on preimplantation murine embryos. Antimicrob Agents Chemother 1993; 37: 1610–1613.

[52] Toltzis P, Marx CM, Kleinman N, Levine EM, Schmidt EV. Zidovudine-associated embryonic toxicity in mice. J Infect Dis 1991; 163: 1212–1218.

[53] Gerschenson M, Nguyen V, Ewings EL, Ceresa A, Shaw JA, St Claire MC, et al. Mitochondrial toxicity in fetal *Erythrocebus patas* monkeys exposed transplacentally to zidovudine plus lamivudine. AIDS Res Hum Retroviruses 2004; 20: 91–100.

[54] Delvaux T, Nöstlinger C. Reproductive choice for women and men living with HIV: contraception, abortion and fertility. Reprod Health Matters 2007; 15: 46–66.

[55] Agboghoroma CO, Giwa-Osagie OF. Management of infertility in HIV infected couples: a review. Afr J Reprod Health 2012; 16: 13–20.

[56] Stephenson JM, Griffioen A. The effect of HIV diagnosis on reproductive experience. Study Group for the Medical Research Council Collaborative Study of Women with HIV. AIDS 1996; 10: 1683–1687.

[57] Thackway SV, Furner V, Mijch A, Cooper DA, Holland D, Martinez P, et al. Fertility and reproductive choice in women with HIV-1 infection. AIDS 1997; 11: 663–667.

[58] Wilson TE, Massad LS, Riester KA, Barkan S, Richardson J, Young M, et al. Sexual, contraceptive, and drug use behaviors of women with HIV and those at high risk for infection: results from the Women's Interagency HIV Study. AIDS 1999; 13: 591–598.

[59] Floridia M, Tamburrini E, Tibaldi C, Anzidei G, Muggiasca ML, Meloni A, et al. Voluntary pregnancy termination among women with HIV in the HAART era (2002–2008): a case series from a national study. AIDS Care 2010; 22: 50–53.

[60] Townsend CL, Cortina-Borja M, Peckham CS, Tookey PA. Trends in management and outcome of pregnancies in HIV-infected women in the UK and Ireland, 1990–2006. BJOG 2008; 115: 1078–1086.

[61] Bongain A, Berrebi A, Mariné-Barjoan E, Dunais B, Thene M, Pradier C, et al. Changing trends in pregnancy outcome among HIV-infected women between 1985 and 1997 in two southern French university hospitals. Eur J Obstet Gynecol Reprod Biol 2002; 104: 124–128.

[62] Finocchario-Kessler S, Sweat MD, Dariotis JK, Anderson JR, Jennings JM, Keller JM, et al. Childbearing motivations, pregnancy desires, and perceived partner response to a pregnancy among urban female youth: does HIV-infection status make a difference? AIDS Care 2012; 24: 1–11.

[63] Craft SM, Delaney RO, Bautista DT, Serovich JM. Pregnancy decisions among women with HIV. AIDS Behav 2007; 11: 927–935.

[64] Nattabi B, Li J, Thompson SC, Orach CG, Earnest J. A systematic review of factors influencing fertility desires and intentions among people living with HIV/AIDS: implications for policy and service delivery. AIDS Behav 2009; 13: 949–968.

[65] Squires KE, Hodder SL, Feinberg J, Bridge DA, Abrams S, Storfer SP, et al. Health needs of HIV-infected women in the United States: insights from the women living positive survey. AIDS Patient Care STDS 2011; 25: 279–285.

[66] Ethics Committee of the American Society for Reproductive Medicine. Human immunodeficiency virus and infertility treatment. Fertil Steril 2010; 94: 11–15.

[67] Department of Health and Human Services. Guidelines for the use of antiretroviral agents in HIV-1-infected adults and adolescents. Available at: http://aidsinfo.nih.gov/guidelines. Accessed 3 January 2016.

[68] Lundgren JD, Babiker AG, Gordin F, Emery S, Grund B, Sharma S, et al. Initiation of antiretroviral therapy in early asymptomatic HIV infection. N Engl J Med 2015; 373: 795–807.

[69] European AIDS Clinical Society. The European Guidelines for treatment of HIV-infected adults in Europe. Available at: www.eacsociety.org/guidelines/eacs-guidelines/eacs-guidelines.html. Accessed 3 January 2016.

[70] World Health Organization. Consolidated guidelines on the use of antiretroviral drugs for treating and preventing HIV infection. Available at: www.who.int/hiv/pub/guidelines/arv2013/download/en/. Accessed 3 January 2016.

[71] Basaria S, Coviello AD, Travison TG, Storer TW, Farwell WR, Jette AM, et al. Adverse events associated with testosterone administration. N Engl J Med 2010; 363: 109–122.

[72] Kaida A, Lima VD, Andia I, Kabakyenga J, Mbabazi P, Emenyonu N, et al. The WHOMEN's Scale (Women's HAART Optimism Monitoring and EvaluatioN Scale v. 1) and the association with fertility intentions and sexual behaviours among HIV-positive women in Uganda. AIDS Behav 2009; 13: S72–S81.

[73] Galvin SR, Cohen MS. The role of sexually transmitted diseases in HIV transmission. Nat Rev Microbiol 2004; 2: 33–42.

[74] Laga M, Nzila N, Goeman J. The interrelationship of sexually transmitted diseases and HIV infection: implications for the control of both epidemics in Africa. AIDS 1991; 5: S55–S63.

[75] Otten RA, Smith DK, Adams DR, Pullium JK, Jackson E, Kim CN, et al. Efficacy of postexposure prophylaxis after intravaginal exposure of pig-tailed macaques to a human-derived retrovirus (human immunodeficiency virus type 2). J Virol 2000; 74: 9771–9775.

[76] Cardo DM, Culver DH, Ciesielski CA, Srivastava PU, Marcus R, Abiteboul D, et al. A case-control study of HIV seroconversion in healthcare workers after percutaneous exposure. Centers for Disease Control and Prevention Needlestick Surveillance Group. N Engl J Med 1997; 337: 1485–1490.

[77] Kuhar DT, Henderson DK, Struble KA, Heneine W, Thomas V, Cheever LW, et al. Updated US Public Health Service guidelines for the management of occupational exposures to human immunodeficiency virus and recommendations for postexposure prophylaxis. Infect Control Hosp Epidemiol 2013; 34: 875–892.

[78] Abdool Karim Q, Abdool Karim SS, Frohlich JA, Grobler AC, Baxter C, Mansoor LE, et al. Effectiveness and safety of tenofovir gel, an antiretroviral microbicide, for the prevention of HIV infection in women. Science 2010; 329: 1168–1174.

[79] Grant RM, Lama JR, Anderson PL, McMahan V, Liu AY, Vargas L et al. Preexposure chemoprophylaxis for HIV prevention in men who have sex with men. N Engl J Med 2010; 363: 2587–2599.

[80] Baeten JM, Donnell D, Ndase P, Mugo NR, Campbell JD, Wangisi J et al. Antiretroviral prophylaxis for HIV prevention in heterosexual men and women. N Engl J Med 2012; 367: 399–410.

[81] Thigpen MC, Kebaabetswe PM, Paxton LA, Smith DK, Rose CE, Segolodi TM, et al. Antiretroviral preexposure prophylaxis for heterosexual HIV transmission in Botswana. N Engl J Med 2012; 367: 423–434.

[82] Ethics Committee of American Society for Reproductive Medicine. Human immunodeficiency virus (HIV) and infertility treatment: a committee opinion. Fertil Steril 2015; 104: e1–e8.

[83] Mandelbrot L, Heard I, Henrion-Geeant E, Henrion R. Natural conception in HIV-negative women with HIV-infected partners. Lancet 1997; 349: 850–851.

[84] Vernazza PL, Graf I, Sonnenberg-Schwan U, Geit M, Meurer A. Preexposure prophylaxis and timed intercourse for HIV-discordant couples willing to conceive a child. AIDS 2011; 25: 2005–2008.

[85] Semprini AE, Levi-Setti P, Ravizza M, Pardi G. Assisted conception to reduce the risk of male-to-female sexual transfer of HIV in serodiscordant couples: an update [abstract]. Presented at the 1998 Symposium on AIDS in Women, Sao Paulo, Brazil, September 14–15, 1998.

[86] Bujan L, Hollander L, Coudert M, Gilling-Smith C, Vucetich A, Guibert J, et al. Safety and efficacy of sperm washing in HIV-1 serodiscordant couples where the male is infected: results from the European CREAThE network. AIDS 2007; 21: 1909–1914.

[87] Kambin S, Batzer F. Assisted reproductive technology in HIV serodiscordant couples. Sex Reprod Menopause 2004; 2: 92–100.

[88] Sauer MV, Wang JG, Douglas NC, Nakhuda GS, Vardhana P, Jovanovic V, et al. Providing fertility care to men seropositive for human immunodeficiency virus: reviewing 10 years of experience and 420 consecutive cycles of in vitro fertilization and intracytoplasmic sperm injection. Fertil Steril 2009; 91: 2455–2460.

[89] Smith DM, Richman DD, Little SJ. HIV superinfection. J Infect Dis 2005; 192: 438–444.

3

Anti-Retroviral–Based HIV Pre-Exposure Prophylaxis for Women: Recent Advances and Next Steps

Flavia Matovu Kiweewa, Kenneth K. Mugwanya and Francis Kiweewa

Abstract

There is a daunting challenge to prevent human immunodeficiency virus (HIV) acquisition in women at high risk of acquiring HIV. Of the 37 million people globally living with HIV, more than half are women. Women account for nearly 60% of adults with HIV in sub-Saharan Africa, where unprotected heterosexual sex is the primary driver of the epidemic. While male condoms are effective, they are not always used, and this is not something women can control. Women urgently need prevention tools they can decide to use, independent of a husband or partner. Pre-exposure prophylaxis (PrEP), in which HIV-uninfected persons with ongoing HIV risk use antiretroviral (ARV) medications as chemoprophylaxis against sexual HIV acquisition, is a promising new HIV prevention strategy. We review recent advances in the development of new biomedical HIV prevention interventions with a highlight of findings from pivotal clinical trials, as well as a discussion on future generation strategies for women.

Keywords: HIV, women, tenofovir, dapivirine, pre-exposure prophylaxis

1. Introduction

In 2015, 2.1 million people became newly infected with Human Immuno Deficiency Virus (HIV) and 1.1 million died from Acquired Immuno Deficiency Syndrome (AIDS) related illnesses [1]. According to the Joint United Nations Programme on HIV/AIDS (UNAIDS) Global Report, 70 percent of the 37 million people estimated to be living with HIV reside in sub-Saharan Africa [1]. In this setting, where unprotected heterosexual sex is the primary driver of the epidemic, women account for nearly 60 percent of adults with HIV.

While existing HIV-1 prevention interventions including behavior change, use of male and female condoms, treatment of sexually transmitted infections (STIs), male circumcision, and uptake of antiretroviral (ARV) treatment to reduce the infectiousness of persons with HIV-1 have gone a long way in controlling the spread of HIV-1 infection [2–6], HIV-1 rates in young women in resource limited settings remain unacceptably high [1]. This is in part, because many HIV-1 prevention methods require the participation or consent of a male partner. Women urgently need prevention tools they can decide to use, independent of a husband or partner [7]. Developing HIV prevention options that women can use therefore remains a global concern, given the soaring rates of HIV infection among women. Pre-exposure prophylaxis (PrEP), in which HIV uninfected persons with ongoing HIV risk use antiretroviral medications as chemoprophylaxis against sexual HIV acquisition, is a promising new HIV prevention strategy [8–11].

2. HIV prevention biomedical interventions

2.1. Microbicides

2.1.1. CAPRISA 004

Tenofovir gel was the first ARV-based microbicide to be tested in an effectiveness trial. CAPRISA 004 was a phase 2B microbicide study that tested peri-coitally applied 1% TDF vaginal gel among 889 South African women conducted from May 2007 to March 2010. The trial found a 39% (95% CI, 6–60%; p = 0.017) lower HIV infection rate in women using 1% tenofovir gel as compared to the women using placebo gel when used in a coitally dependent regimen [12]. Tenofovir gel was shown to be safe when used up to 12 h before sex and again within 12 h after sex (BAT), for a maximum of two doses in 24 h. The drug was found to be 54% effective among women who were the highest adherers (gel adherence > 80%). Participants who adhered to the dosing regimen in more than 80% of sex acts were the least likely to acquire HIV (54% lower risk of infection).

2.1.2. FACTS 001

FACTS 001 was a phase III safety and effectiveness double-blind, randomised, placebo-controlled trial of pericoital tenofovir 1% gel for HIV prevention in 18–30 year Women at nine sites in South Africa [17]. The study evaluated the safety and effectiveness of pericoital TFV 1% gel when using the BAT-24 regimen (before and after sex; no more than 2 doses in 24 h) among women at nine sites in South Africa. A total of 2059 women were randomized to tenofovir 1% gel or to placebo and instructed women to apply the gel 12 h before and within 12 h after sex, the same schedule used in CAPRISA 004. The study was conducted between Oct 2011 and Aug 2014. In 3036 person-years of observation accrued, 123 HIV infections occurred (HIV incidence: 4.0/100 women years); 61 in the TFV arm and 62 in the placebo group (incidence rate ratio [IRR], 1.0; 95% CI: 0.7–1.4). In a nested case-cohort sub-study (n = 214) that examined TFV drug levels in quarterly cervicovaginal lavage (CVL) samples in HIV seroconverters vs controls, high TFV in CVL was significantly associated with a reduction in HIV acquisition (HR, 0.52; 95% CI, 0.27–0.99; $p = 0.04$).

Considering all adherence data, the FACTS 001 team calculated that women used gel for an average of 50–60% of sex acts. Majority of participants were not able to achieve sufficiently high levels of gel coverage required for protection which underscores the need for a range of HIV prevention options for young women which may be easier to integrate into their lives.

2.2. Oral PrEP

2.2.1. Partner's PrEP

The Partners PrEP Study was a three-arm phase III, randomized, double-blind, placebo-controlled, 3-arm trial of daily oral TDF & FTC/TDF PrEP for the prevention of HIV acquisition by HIV seronegative partner in heterosexual HIV serodiscordant partnerships. It was one of the two land marker studies that provided evidence to support US Food and Drug Administration approval for FTC-TDF PrEP. The study demonstrated PrEP HIV protective effectiveness against HIV infection of 67% (95% CI 44–81%, $p < 0.0001$) for TDF and 75% (95% CI 55–87%, $p < 0.0001$) for FTC/TDF [13] compared to person receiving placebo. The HIV protection effects of TDF and FTC/TDF were in women and men. For TDF, efficacy among women was 71% and was 63% among men; for FTC/TDF, efficacy was 66% in women and 84% in men—all were statistically significant. In a follow-on open-label demonstration project of integrated delivery of ART and PrEP for prevention in HIV sero-discordant couples, the investigators observed virtual elimination of incident HIV [13].

2.2.2. FEM-PrEP Study

The FEM-PrEP Study was a phase 3, randomized, placebo-controlled, trial that assessed of the effectiveness of daily oral FTC/TDF for HIV prevention among HIV-uninfected women 18–35 years in Kenya, South Africa and Tanzania [14]. The trial was stopped early by Independent Data Monitoring Committee due to futility at the time of study stop. No significant safety concerns were noted. Adherence by self-report and pill counts was high, but plasma drug levels revealed that only 15–26% of samples from seroconverters had TDF detected and only 26–38% of non-seroconverting controls. Thus, the investigators concluded that PrEP adherence was too low to assess PrEP's HIV protection. Less than 40% of the HIV-uninfected women in the TDF–FTC group had evidence of recent pill use at visits that were matched to the HIV-infection window for women with seroconversion.

2.2.3. TDF2 study

The TDF2 study was a phase 2B study that assessed the safety, adherence and efficacy of daily oral FTC/TDF in 1200 (45.7% women) HIV-uninfected heterosexual male and female participants aged 18–39 years conducted in Botswana [15]. After a 1563 person-years of observation (median, 1.1 years; maximum, 3.7 years), FTC/TDF PrEP resulted in a 62.6% reduction in HIV acquisition for participants assigned to FTC/TDF compared to placebo (HR, 0.37; CI, 21.5–83.4, p = 0.013). As treated analysis provided protective efficacy of 77.9% (95% CI, 41.2–93.6; p = 0.01) for FTC/TDF versus placebo, overall, and 75.4% (23.7, 94.4; p = 0.02) for women. No significant safety concerns were noted, though participants randomized to the FTC/TDF arm did experience more nausea, vomiting and dizziness than those randomized to placebo.

2.2.4. *MTN-003/Vaginal and Oral Interventions to Control the Epidemic (VOICE)*

Was a phase 2B safety and effectiveness study of tenofovir 1% gel, tenofovir disoproxil fumarate tablet and emtricitabine/tenofovir disoproxil fumarate tablet for the prevention of HIV infection in women [16]. The primary aim of the VOICE trial was to estimate the safety and effectiveness of daily treatment with vaginal TFV gel, as compared with placebo gel, and of oral TDF and oral TDF-FTC, as compared with oral placebo, in preventing sexually acquired HIV-1 infection in women.

A total of 5029 were enrolled in the study were followed up monthly and assessed for HIV seroconversion. A total of 312 HIV-1 infections occurred; the incidence of HIV-1 infection was 5.7 per 100 person-years. In the modified intention-to-treat analysis, the effectiveness was −49.0% with TDF (hazard ratio for infection, 1.49; 95% confidence interval [CI], 0.97–2.29), −4.4% with TDF-FTC (hazard ratio, 1.04; 95% CI, 0.73–1.49), and 14.5% with TFV gel (hazard ratio, 0.85; 95% CI, 0.61–1.21). Adherence to study product among those in the active arms was generally very low. TFV was detectable in 30%, 29%, and 25% of random plasma samples from participants in the TDF, TDF-FTC, and TFV gel arms of the study, and an inverse correlation was demonstrable between detection of TFV in plasma and characteristics predictive of HIV-1 acquisition.

2.2.5. *Partner's demonstration project*

OLE projects have been called for as part of the pathway to scale-up of PrEP. Previous studies like the Partner's PrEP that assessed effectiveness of oral truvada and tenofovir for HIV prevention among sero-discordant couples in Kenya and Uganda have shown that when participants are given the active product through open-label access projects, even those with previous poor adherence during the clinical trial are now more likely to use product when they know they are now using the active product [13]. From a protection level of about 73% in the partner's PrEP, researchers have reported substantially reduced HIV risk of up to 95% when used with high adherence [17], **Figure 1**.

2.3. Vaginal rings

2.3.1. *MTN-020— A Study to Prevent HIV Infection with a Ring with Extended ring (ASPIRE)*

Intravaginal rings offer a strategy to deliver antiretroviral PrEP medications with lesser opportunities for adherence challenges than for daily oral pills or vaginal gels [18]. ASPIRE was a phase III study conducted among 2629 sexually active HIV-negative women ages 18–45 at 15 clinical research sites in Malawi, Uganda, South Africa and Zimbabwe to determine whether a vaginal ring containing the ARV drug dapivirine is a safe and effective method for protecting against the sexual transmission of HIV when used by women for a month at a time. The study found HIV risk was reduced by 27% overall—for women group assigned to use the dapivirine ring compared placebo ring group—and 37% in a planned second analysis that excluded data from two sites with less than ideal retention and adherence. Notably high protection (56%) was observed in women >21 years, who also appeared to use the ring most consistently, **Figure 2** [10].

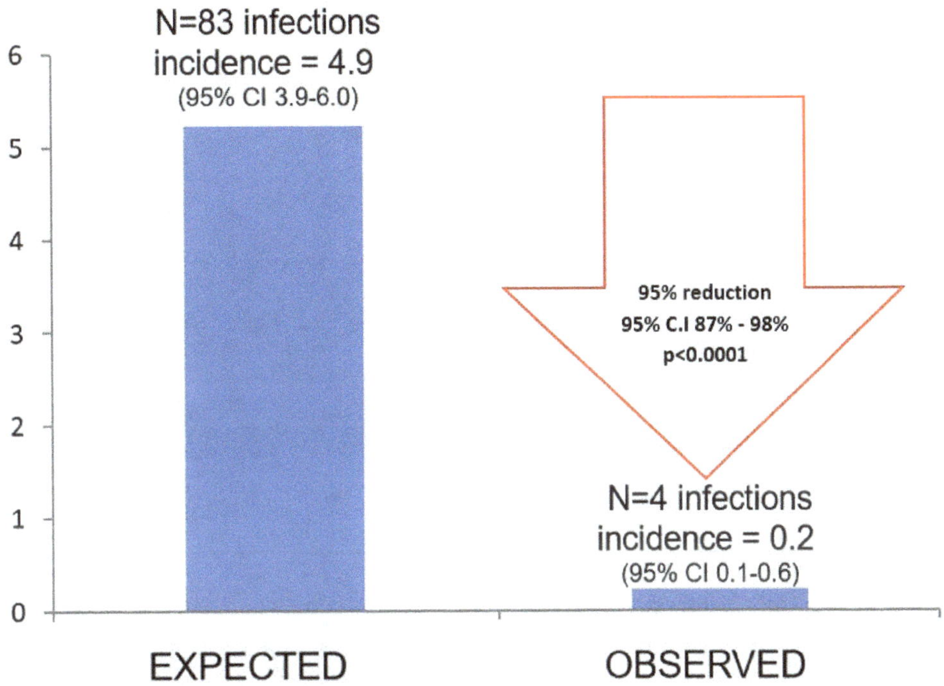

Figure 1. HIV incidence in Partner's PrEP demonstration project [17].

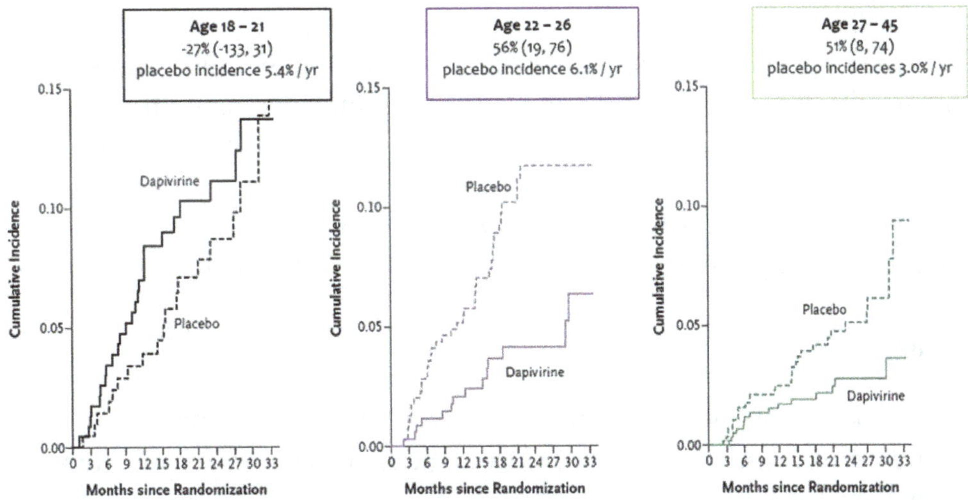

Figure 2. Age and HIV-1 protection in ASPIRE [10].

A summary of the outcomes of recent HIV prevention trials among women is provided in **Table 1**.

Study	Study population	Sample size	Results
CAPRISA 004 *South Africa* (Tenofovir Gel)	Women	889	39% [CI = 6–60] effectiveness of coitally-dependent vaginal TFV gel
iPrEx *Brazil, Ecuador, Peru, South Africa, Thailand, US* (Oral Truvada)	Gay men, other MSM, transgender women	2499	44% [CI = 15–63] effectiveness of daily oral FTC/TDF
TDF2 Study *Botswana* (Oral Tenofovir)	Men and women	1200	62% [CI = 22–83] effectiveness of daily oral FTC/TDF
Partners PrEP Study *Kenya, Uganda* (Oral Truvada/Tenofovir)	Serodiscordant couples	4758	67% [CI = 44–81] efficacy daily oral TDF 75% [CI = 55–87] efficacy daily oral FTC/TDF
FEM-PrEP *Kenya, S Africa, Tanzania* (Oral Truvada)	Women	1950	Futility of daily oral FTC/TDF 6% [CI = −52 to 41]
ASPIRE *Uganda, Malawi, South Africa, Zimbabwe*	Women	2629	27% [CI= 1–46] effectiveness of dapivirine vaginal ring

Table 1. Outcomes of recent HIV prevention trials involving women.

2.3.2. MTN-025—HIV open-label prevention extension (HOPE)

HOPE is an open-label study of vaginal ring for preventing HIV among former ASPIRE participants. Women who took part in ASPIRE, a trial that found a vaginal ring containing an antiretroviral (ARV) drug called dapivirine was safe and helped protect against HIV, are now being offered the opportunity to use the ring as part of a new study called HOPE. HOPE builds on the results of ASPIRE by gathering additional information on the ring's safety, how women use the ring knowing that it can help reduce their risk of HIV and the relationship between adherence and HIV protection. Women who participated in a similar study called the RING study by the international partnership for microbicides (IPM) are being followed up under the dapivirine ring extended access and monitoring (DREAM OLE) protocol.

2.4. Discussion

High HIV incidence among young women in Africa [1] highlights the need for female-controlled HIV prevention. Social, structural and economic disparities perpetuate vulnerabilities of women. The lower social and economic power of women makes it difficult for them to negotiate safe sex [18]. In stable partnerships, condom use is low, and women are often unaware of their partner's HIV status [19]. Therefore, a need exists for HIV prevention methods that women can initiate themselves. Scaling up of proven biomedical technologies for women at high risk is therefore a high priority. Daily oral tenofovir-based PrEP, dapivirine vaginal ring and antiretroviral treatment as prevention are some of the promising biomedical technologies for prevention options for women.

Multiple studies of PrEP have shown that oral ARVs, when used consistently, reduce the risk of HIV infection in people who are at high risk by up to 92% including among women [5]. Currently, FTC-TDF is the medication with a label indication as PrEP against HIV acquisition recommended by the World Health Organization (WHO) and the United States Centers of Diseases Control and Prevention [20, 21]. Consequently, recent landmark approvals in sub-Saharan Africa, including South Africa [22] and Kenya [23], and commitment from large-scale funding partners (including PEPFAR) are leading to accelerated roll-out of TDF-based PrEP for high-risk populations. TDF alone or TDF with lamivudine are other as an alternative to suggested by WHO [24]. Importantly, other new oral PrEP drugs (e.g. maraviroc) are currently being evaluated [25]. Although some PrEP trials in African women did not show effectiveness against HIV [14, 16, 26], follow-on analyses from those two studies have consistently provided strong evidence of very low adherence to PrEP in those studies [16, 27].

Prevention technologies such as vaginal ring containing ARV provide tremendous promise for the HIV prevention field as they provide HIV prevention options that fit in women's lives. The recent demonstration of moderate HIV protection conferred by monthly vaginal ring containing medication dapivirine is a step in right direction. An important feature of the dapivirine ring is its high level of safety [28]. This excellent safety profile also suggests that minimal medical monitoring would be needed, potentially making it both a practical and cost-effective option in under-resourced settings. The next step is to ensure that the vaginal ring is safe for all women at risk of HIV acquisition including pregnant and breastfeeding women.

For HIV uninfected women in known serodiscorant partnership, initiation and sustained use of ART by their infected male patterns are another highly effective prevention options for couples [5]. Women who want to conceive or with HIV positive partners who have not yet initiated ART, PrEP as bridge to ART prevention strategy is an attractive and highly effective HIV option. In PrEP as a bridge to ART strategy, PrEP is offered to HIV-uninfected person as a 'bridge' to ART in the discordant partnership—that is, until ART initiation by the HIV-infected partner and for the first 6 months after ART is started or viral suppression. This strategy demonstrated nearly elimination of HIV transmission within serodiscordant couples in Uganda and Kenya [29].

A robust pipeline of new PrEP drugs and formulations is not only important for advancing demonstrated success of products but also for addressing limitations of current biomedical technologies with the ultimate goal of prevention options that fit women's needs to ensure they will be used at scale. The current pipeline of ARV-based prevention products includes oral pills (miravorac), vaginal rings (tenofovir), vaginal and rectal gels, vaginal films, long-acting injectable ARVs (rilpivirine, cabotegravir) and multipurpose technologies that could combine ARV to reduce women's risk of HIV and STIs while providing effective contraception.

3. Summary

Oral PrEP trials have demonstrated a decrease in HIV infection rates of between 44 and 77%. But it is now proven that with good adherence, Truvada, a once-a-day pill can reduce HIV infection rates by at least 92%. Because of high level of effectiveness, oral PrEP has been licensed for high-risk populations in the US, Canada, Kenya and South Africa. Efforts to have the dapivirine vaginal ring licensed for HIV prevention among women are currently underway. The process is an important one that takes time. It's anticipated that regulatory approvals could be received by 2018 in some countries in Africa. Results of the ASPIRE and RING studies are a boost to efforts focused on developing and evaluating next generation products, such a 3-month ring (just four rings would provide a woman a full year of protection), and combination rings that can provide protection against HIV, other STIs and unintended pregnancy. A vaginal ring could offer an important option as part of combination strategies or as a stand-alone method for women unable or not willing to use other strategies like medical male circumcision, condoms and oral PrEP.

Author details

Flavia Matovu Kiweewa[1,2,*], Kenneth K. Mugwanya[1,3] and Francis Kiweewa[1,4]

*Address all correspondence to: fmatovu@mujhu.org

1 Makerere University School of Public Health, Makerere University College of Health Sciences, Kampala, Uganda

2 University of Witwatersrand, Johannesburg, South Africa

3 University of Washington, Seattle, United States

4 Makerere University-Walter Reed Project, Kampala, Uganda

References

[1] UNAIDS. Report on the global AIDS epidemic 2015.

[2] Seidman D, Weber S, Aaron E, Cohan D, Grant R. The FACTS about women and pre-exposure prophylaxis. The Lancet HIV. 2015;2(6):e228.

[3] Gray RH, Kigozi G, Serwadda D, Makumbi F, Watya S, Nalugoda F, et al. Male circumcision for HIV prevention in men in Rakai, Uganda: a randomised trial. The Lancet. 2007;369(9562):657–66.

[4] Weiss HA, Halperin D, Bailey RC, Hayes RJ, Schmid G, Hankins CA. Male circumcision for HIV prevention: from evidence to action? AIDS. 2008;22(5):567–74.

[5] Cohen MS, McCauley M, Gamble TR. HIV treatment as prevention and HPTN 052. Current Opinion in HIV and AIDS. 2012;7(2):99.

[6] Patterson TL, Shaw WS, Semple SJ. Reducing the sexual risk behaviors of HIV+ individuals: outcome of a randomized controlled trial. Annals of Behavioral Medicine. 2003;25(2):137–45.

[7] Wawer MJ, Sewankambo NK, Serwadda D, Quinn TC, Kiwanuka N, Li C, et al. Control of sexually transmitted diseases for AIDS prevention in Uganda: a randomised community trial. The Lancet. 1999;353(9152):525–35.

[8] Elias CJ, Coggins C. Female-controlled methods to prevent sexual transmission of HIV. AIDS (London, England). 1996;10:S43–51.

[9] Jiang J, Yang X, Ye L, Zhou B, Ning C, Huang J, et al. Pre-exposure prophylaxis for the prevention of HIV infection in high risk populations: a meta-analysis of randomized controlled trials. PLoS One. 2014;9(2):e87674.

[10] Baeten JM, Grant R. Use of antiretrovirals for HIV prevention: what do we know and what don't we know? Current HIV/AIDS Reports. 2013;10(2):142–51.

[11] Control CfD, Prevention. Update to Interim Guidance for Preexposure Prophylaxis (PrEP) for the Prevention of HIV Infection: PrEP for injecting drug users. MMWR Morbidity and Mortality Weekly Report. 2013;62(23):463.

[12] Karim QA, Karim SSA, Frohlich JA, Grobler AC, Baxter C, Mansoor LE, et al. Effectiveness and safety of tenofovir gel, an antiretroviral microbicide, for the prevention of HIV infection in women. Science. 2010;329(5996):1168–74.

[13] Baeten JM, Heffron R, Kidoguchi L, Mugo NR, Katabira E, Bukusi EA, et al. Integrated delivery of antiretroviral treatment and pre-exposure prophylaxis to HIV-1–serodiscordant couples: a prospective implementation study in Kenya and Uganda. PLoS Medicine. 2016;13(8):e1002099.

[14] Van Damme L, Corneli A, Ahmed K, Agot K, Lombaard J, Kapiga S, et al. Preexposure prophylaxis for HIV infection among African women. New England Journal of Medicine. 2012;367(5):411–22.

[15] Thigpen MC, Kebaabetswe PM, Paxton LA, Smith DK, Rose CE, Segolodi TM, et al. Antiretroviral preexposure prophylaxis for heterosexual HIV transmission in Botswana. New England Journal of Medicine. 2012;367(5):423–34.

[16] Marrazzo JM, Ramjee G, Richardson BA, Gomez K, Mgodi N, Nair G, et al. Tenofovir-based preexposure prophylaxis for HIV infection among African women. New England Journal of Medicine. 2015;372(6):509–18.

[17] Baeten J, Heffron R, Kidoguchi L, Mugo N, Bukusi E, Katabira E, editors. Near elimination of HIV transmission in a demonstration project of PrEP and ART. Conference on Retroviruses and Opportunistic Infections (CROI); 2015.

[18] Langen TT. Gender power imbalance on women\'s capacity to negotiate self-protection against HIV/AIDS in Botswana and South Africa. African Health Sciences. 2005;5(3):188–97.

[19] Wagner GJ, Holloway I, Ghosh-Dastidar B, Ryan G, Kityo C, Mugyenyi P. Factors associated with condom use among HIV clients in stable relationships with partners at varying risk for HIV in Uganda. AIDS and Behavior. 2010;14(5):1055–65.

[20] Centers for Disease Control and Prevenion. Preexposure prophylaxis for the prevention of HIV infection in the United States-2014: A clinical practice guideline. [Accessed on February 9, 2017];2014 :1–67. http://www.cdc.gov/hiv/pdf/prepguidelines2014.pdf.

[21] World Health Organization. Guideline on when to start antiretroviral therapy and on pre-exposure prophylaxis for HIV. http://apps.who.int/iris/bitstream/10665/186275/1/9789241509565_eng.pdf. Accessed May 10, 2016.

[22] Bekker L-G, Rebe K, Venter F, Maartens G, Moorhouse M, Conradie F, et al. Southern African guidelines on the safe use of pre-exposure prophylaxis in persons at risk of acquiring HIV-1 infection. Southern African Journal of HIV Medicine. 2016;17(1):1–11.

[23] http://emtct-iatt.org/wp-content/uploads/2016/09/Guidelines-on-Use-of-Antiretroviral-Drugs-for-Treating-and-Preventing-HI....pdf Guidelines on Use of Antiretroviral Drugs for Treating and Preventing HIV Infection in Kenya 2016 Edition Accessed October 2016.

[24] World Health Organization. Consolidated guidelines on the use of antiretroviral drugs for treating and preventing HIV infection—recommendations for a public health approach, second edition, 2016. Geneva, Switzerland: World Health Organization, 2016. http://www.who.int/hiv/pub/arv/arv-2016/en/.

[25] Abraham BK, Gulick R. Next generation oral PrEP: beyond tenofovir. Current Opinion in HIV and AIDS. 2012;7(6):600.

[26] Rees H, Delany-Moretlwe S, Lombard C, editors. FACTS 001: a multi-centred phase III randomised, double-blind, placebo-controlled tiral of periocoital tenofovir 1% gel for HIV prevention in Women. Conference on Retroviruses and Opportunistic Infections; 2015.

[27] Corneli AL, Deese J, Wang M, Taylor D, Ahmed K, Agot K, et al. FEM-PrEP: adherence patterns and factors associated with adherence to a daily oral study product for pre-exposure prophylaxis. JAIDS Journal of Acquired Immune Deficiency Syndromes. 2014;66(3):324–31.

[28] Baeten, Jared M., et al. "Antiretroviral prophylaxis for HIV prevention in heterosexual men and women." *New England Journal of Medicine* 367.5 (2012): 399-410.

[29] Heffron R, Pintye J, Matthews LT, Weber S, Mugo N. PrEP as peri-conception HIV prevention for women and men. Current HIV/AIDS Reports. 2016;13:131–9.

4

Exercise Therapy for Acquired Immune Deficiency Syndrome (AIDS) Patients

Jeanne M. Grace

Abstract

Background: Highly active antiretroviral therapy (HAART) has reduced mortality and morbidity in HIV-infected patients and transformed HIV infection from an acute to a chronic disease, not only increasing the life expectancy but also adding to the potential side effects associated with drug therapy. Exercise has been fused as an important adjuvant therapy and can play a valuable role in the management of health in HIV/AIDS patients.

Methods: EBSCOhost, Science Citation Index, CINAHL database, PsycINFO, Cochrane Database of Systematic Reviews, Physiotherapy Evidence Database, and SPORTDiscus were searched between 1996 and May 2016. Searches of published and unpublished abstracts were conducted, as well as a hand search of reference lists and tables of contents of relevant journals and books were conducted. A total of 60 studies met the inclusion criteria.

Results: Most studies failed to indicate the optimum type (mode), intensity, frequency, and duration of aerobic excercise (AE), progressive resistive exercise (PRE), and a combination of AE and PRE (CARE) prescribed to HIV-infected individuals in relation to the different clinical stages of the disease.

Conclusion: The findings provide information that clarifies the optimal mode, duration, frequency, and intensity of AE, PRE, and CARE prescribed to the different clinical stages of HIV patients. The exercises recommended have the potential to benefit HIV patients and should be adopted by clinical exercise therapists.

Keywords: aerobic exercise, CD4 count, highly active antiretroviral therapy, immunodeficiency, progressive resistive exercise

1. Introduction

Medical advances in the treatment of the HIV disease with highly active antiretroviral therapy (HAART) converted HIV infection into a chronic condition that has been related to several comorbidities [1], disability, impairment in daily activities, and decreased exercise capacity [2, 3]. Increased longevity in the HAART era has dramatically reduced mortality and morbidity of HIV-infected patients [4, 5]. Although HAART has dramatically reduced the prevalence of the wasting syndrome and immunosuppression in HIV patients [6], HAART is associated with anthropometric and metabolic conditions including insulin resistance, dyslipidemia, and abnormal distribution of body fat [5, 7, 8].

Exercise is a key management strategy employed by rehabilitation health professionals for health promotion and rehabilitation of patients with HIV/AIDS [9, 10]. Exercise has the potential to ameliorate a range of side effects associated with HIV infection, as well as the cardiometabolic and morphological complications (i.e., mitochondrial dysfunction, inflammation, and oxidative stress) that may accompany HAART. A large body of scientific evidence suggests that exercise can delay the progression of the disease, improve quality of life [11, 12], improve aerobic capacity [3, 9, 13], improve functional ability [14], have beneficial effects on insulin resistance and diabetes [15], improve oxidative stress [13, 16], improve muscle strength [9, 17], improve lipid profile [13, 18], and reduce the risk of cardiovascular disease [1, 19] in people with HIV infection. Of importance is that exercise is generally regarded as safe and there is no evidence to suggest that regular exercise will suppress immune function in asymptomatic and symptomatic individuals with HIV/AIDS [10, 20]. Exercise training, however, apparently confers no beneficial effect on HIV status and viral load [20, 21].

Exercise studies in HIV/AIDS patients indicate that aerobic exercise (AE) [19, 20] and progressive resistive exercise (PRE) [22] improve various health indices in HIV-infected patients with a combination of aerobic and progressive resistive exercise (CARE) more effective than applying only one component [10]. CARE has recently been employed and recommended by the American College of Sports Medicine [23].

2. HIV disease stages and classification

It is of critical importance to recognize HIV disease stages and classification systems not only for tracking and monitoring the HIV epidemic but also for providing clinicians and patients with important information about the clinical management of the disease. Clinical exercise therapists should therefore consider the HIV disease stages as well as the varying needs during each stage in order to adjust the exercise prescription (Ex Rx) accordingly. Two major classification systems currently are in use: The World Health Organization Clinical Staging and Disease Classification System and the US Centres for Disease Control and Prevention (CDC) classification system [24]. The WHO Clinical Staging and Disease Classification System are used in resource-constrained settings without access to CD4 cell count measurements or other diagnostic and laboratory testing methods whereas the CDC disease staging system assesses the severity of HIV disease by CD4 cell counts and by the presence of specific HIV-related conditions. The CDC disease staging system should be used because it incorporates the CD4 cell count categories; knowledge of which is important for the clinical exercise therapist because this may dictate changes in Ex Rx.

The CDC categorization of HIV/AIDS is based on the lowest documented CD4 cell count and on previously diagnosed HIV-related conditions (**Table 1**).

CD4 cell count categories	Clinical categories		
	A Asymptomatic, acute HIV, or PGL	B* Symptomatic conditions, not A or C	C# AIDS-indicator conditions
(1) ≥500 cells/μL	A1	B1	C1
(2) 200–499cells/μL	A2	B2	C2
(3) <200 cells/μL	A3	B3	C3

Abbreviations: PGL = persistent generalized lymphadenopathy

* Category B Symptomatic Conditions - Consult the AIDS Education and Training Centre [24].

Category C AIDS-Indicator Conditions - Consult the AIDS Education and Training Centre [24].

Note: Reprinted with permission from AETC.

Table 1. CDC classification system for HIV-infected adults and adolescents [24].

For example, if a patient had a condition that once met the criteria for category B but now is asymptomatic, the patient would remain in category B. Additionally, categorization is based on specific conditions, as indicated by the AIDS Education and Training Centre [24]. Patients in categories A3, B3, and C1-C3 are considered to have AIDS [24]. The AIDS Education and Training Centre (AETC) can be referred to for a detailed account of the symptomatic conditions for the different clinical categories [24].

3. Pre-exercise evaluation/testing

HIV/AIDS individuals should be screened for the presence, signs, symptoms, and/or risk factors suggestive of cardiovascular, pulmonary, or metabolic diseases, as well as other conditions (e.g., orthopedic limitations, pregnancy) that require special attention to (i) aid in the development of a safe and effective Ex Rx and (ii) optimize safety during exercise testing [23]. Regardless of stage of disease progression, all HIV-infected individuals should consult with their physician and obtain medical clearance prior to participating in an exercise program. Once cleared to exercise, it is recommended that the patient consult a clinical exercise therapist for advice and guidelines on an exercise program tailored to the individual's physical function, health status, exercise response, and stated goals.

	Time point/Frequency								
Lab test	**Entry into Care**	**ART Initiation or Modification**	**2 to 8 Weeks Every 6 Months**	**After ART Initiation or Modification**	**Every 3 to 6 Months**	**Every 12 Months**	**Treatment Failure**	**Clinically Indicated**	**If ART Initiation is Delayed[b]**
CD4 Count	√	√		√ During first 2 years of ART or if viremia develops while patient on ART or CD4 count <300 cells/mm^3		√ After 2 years on ART with consistently suppressed viral load: CD4 Count 300–500 cells/mm^3: •Every 12 months CD4 Count >500 cells/mm^3: •CD4 monitoring is optional	√	√	Every 3-6 month
Fasting lipid profile[c]	√	√			√ If abnormal at last measurement	√ If abnormal at last measurement		√	√ If normal at baseline, annually
Fasting Glucose or Hemoglobin A1C	√	√		√ If abnormal at last measurement		√ If abnormal at last measurement		√	√ If normal at baseline, annually

[a] If ART initiation occurs soon after HIV diagnosis and entry into care, repeat baseline laboratory testing is not necessary.

[b] ART is indicated for all HIV-infected individuals and should be started as soon as possible. However, if ART initiation is delayed, patients should be retained in care, with periodic monitoring as noted above.

[c] Consult the National Lipid Association's recommendations for management of patients with dyslipidaemia

Table 2. Laboratory monitoring schedule for HIV-infected patients before and after initiation of antiretroviral therapy[a] [37].

A comprehensive pre-exercise test evaluation for HIV-infected individuals includes (i) medical history, (ii) physical examination, and (iii) HIV-related laboratory tests. The physician should provide medical information (e.g., stage of disease, CD4 count, HAART, and other medications used, history of symptoms, and recent illness), whereas the clinical exercise therapist can acquire exercise-related medical information by using the Canadian Physician Clearance Form (ePARmed-X+) [25] as a positive response is expected when using the Canadian Activity Readiness Questionnaire for Everyone (PAR-Q+) [26]. The PARmed-X+ is a form developed for use by physicians and clinical exercise therapists to assist in addressing medical concerns regarding physical activity participation that were identified by the PAR-Q+.

Health-related quality of life (HRQOL) has emerged as an important topic in the treatment of HIV infection, with HIV-infected patients generally demonstrating a HRQOL that is lower than that of the general population [11, 27]. Clinical exercise therapists should use the Multidimensional Quality of Life Questionnaire for Persons with HIV (MQOLHIV) to monitor HRQOL for patients living with HIV disease [28]. HRQOL has become increasingly important with the goals of therapy now, including improvement of HRQOL, in addition to reduction of symptoms, virus suppression, and extension of survival. Repeated assessment can be used to track changes in functional status over time; monitor, assess, and optimize treatment effects and enhance communication between patient and provider with the potential to improve the health care process and overall survival [28]. With physical training regarded as a non-pharmacological treatment, use of HRQOL will be helpful to monitor and improve adherence [29] because the development of side effects can worsen HRQOL and lead to treatment non-adherence [30].

Regardless of the disease status of HIV-infected individuals, it is important to assess their current fitness level prior to developing an exercise program [31]. Despite the lower functional capacities of HIV-infected individuals [11], the standard physical fitness tests applicable to the apparently healthy populations can be applied [31]. BP and ECG are monitored during exercise testing due to the increased prevalence of cardiovascular impairments and cardiac dysfunction [23].

Components of the physical examination conducted by the clinical exercise therapist should include the following:

1. Body composition: It includes body weight, body mass index (BMI), skin fold measurement of subcutaneous fat (fat percentage), standard circumference sites (thigh, calf, arm, chest, waist, and hip), waist-to-hip ratio (WHR) [21, 23], muscle mass, lean body mass [32], and self-reported body shape changes [33]. Perceived body image can be measured with the Body Image Scale (BIS) that is a 12-item, disease-specific, valid and reliable tool that measures perceived body image along five dimensions (comfort, competence, appearance, predictability, and existential self). Each item utilizes a five point visual analogue scale and scores range from 12 to 60 (higher scores reflect poorer body image) [34].
2. Physical capacity: The modified Bruce protocol or submaximal YMCA cycle ergometer test is used to determine cardiorespiratory fitness [23]. For assessing muscular strength, six-repetition maximum (6 RM) or 10 RM protocol may be more appropriate because the

affected population is generally untrained [31]. A grip strength dynamometer can be used to determine the maximum isometric strength of the hand and forearm muscles [17].

3. Neuromuscular function: Gait analysis and balance test (e.g., Stork stand) should be conducted because peripheral neuropathy, which can be a consequence of fast hyperlactatemia at rest which many people living with HIV/AIDS present, is a common symptom of HIV infection [31, 35].

4. Functional capacity: The Lower Extremity Functional Scale (LEFS) can be used as a measure of patients' initial function, ongoing progress, and outcome, as well as used to set functional goals [36].

3.1. Laboratory tests

To assist the clinical exercise therapist, it is recommended that a physician conduct the following laboratory tests for HIV-infected individuals:

1. Cardiometabolic: It is fasting blood lipids (total cholesterol, LDL-C, HDL-C, and triglycerides), fasting glucose or hemoglobin A1c (HbA1C), and CD4 cell count when diagnosed with HIV as well as prior to the start of HAART [10, 21]. **Table 2** indicates the laboratory monitoring schedule for HIV-infected patients before and after initiation of antiretroviral therapy[a] [37].

2. Bone mineral density (BMD): The literature recommends that for all HIV-infected postmenopausal women and men aged > 50 years, BMD should be tested and, if the results of the test do not warrant medical treatment, the test should be repeated every 2–5 years, depending on the proximity to thresholds for therapy [38].

3. Electrocardiography: Due to the increased risk of heart disease, a resting 12-lead electrocardiogram is recommended [31].

4. Special considerations prior to prescribing an exercise program

Clinical exercise therapists should consider various factors (e.g., clinical/treatment characteristics) when prescribing an exercise program for HIV-infected individuals. HIV-infected individuals adapt readily to exercise training and therefore can the general FITT principle of Ex Rx for apparently healthy adults applied to those carrying HIV [23, 39]. Additional drug-related physical, psychological, and physiological side effects including lethargy, nausea, vomiting, diarrhea, headaches, fever, muscle pain, occasional dizziness, peripheral neuropathy, fatigue, anemia, mitochondrial toxicity, depression, and myopathy must be considered [37]. In particular, the following symptoms, adverse effects, and comorbidity should be taken into account:

4.1. HIV/AIDS wasting syndrome

It is a syndrome of unintentional weight loss that occurs with advanced HIV infection. It is defined as an involuntary weight loss of greater than 10% from baseline body weight during the previous 12 months or a 5% loss of weight during the previous 6 months [40].

4.2. Lipodystrophy

It is as an all-encompassing term used to describe a metabolic complication of fat loss, fat gain, or a combination of fat loss and gain, which is associated with some antiretroviral (ARV) therapies given to HIV-infected individuals [41]. *Lipoatrophy* is the loss of subcutaneous fat, particularly evident in the face, buttocks, and limbs. *Lipohypertrophy* is the accumulation of visceral and central fat in the abdomen, dorsocervical region ("buffalo hump"), or breasts. *Fat redistribution* is an all-encompassing term used to describe lipohypertrophy, lipoatrophy, and/or mixed syndrome in HIV-infected individuals [42, 43].

4.3. Dyslipidemia

HAART is associated with hypercholesterolemia, increases in LDL-C, hypertriglyceridemia, and lowered HDL-C [2, 44].

4.4. Diabetes

HAART adversely affects insulin sensitivity and glucose tolerance [45, 46]. Clinical exercise therapists should also distinguish between the three subgroups of patients with diabetes: those with pre-existing diabetes who contract HIV; those who have diabetes at onset of HIV infection; and others who develop hyperglycemia after commencing HAART. These subgroups need to be managed differently. Pre-existing type 2 diabetes mellitus may continue to be managed, after diagnosis of HIV, with the same drug therapy that was being used prior to detection of HIV [46]. It is important to counsel these patients about a possible deterioration in metabolic function, and the chances of drug interactions between oral antidiabetic drugs and HAART. Patients diagnosed with diabetes and HIV together may be treated according to guidelines for uninfected individuals. Patients developing diabetes after HAART may benefit from insulin, because it is a safe and effective method of treatment [46].

4.5. BMD

Initiation of ART is associated with a 2–6% decrease in BMD over the first 2 years [47]. HIV-infected individuals receiving protease-inhibitor-based HAART (up to 30%) are more likely to display significant bone demineralization [48].

4.6. Cardiometabolic disease (CMD) risk

The incidence of CMD increases in HIV-infected individuals, and HAART is associated with an increase in both peripheral and coronary artery disease [49, 50]. Risk factors such as hyperlipidemia [44], oxidative stress [51], impaired glucose tolerance, and increased insulin resistance [45], accumulation of visceral fat [52], inflammation secondary to HIV [53], and the effects of some antiretroviral drugs all contribute to the risk of developing CMD [54].

5. Program prescription

Exercise training is well established as an important non-pharmacological therapy for HIV-infected individuals and one of the key approached being explored to deal with the complications and symptoms of HIV/AIDS [9, 55]. The primary goals (depending on the stage of the disease) for prescribing exercise to HIV-infected patients are to improve HRQOL, physical, and physiological, functional, and neuromuscular function capacity, decrease the risk of CMD, and promote long-term exercise compliance. It is therefore advised to include both short- and long-term individualized goals based on the subjective and objective findings in the patient's assessment. In addition to the symptoms, adverse effects, and comorbidity considerations mentioned previously, clinical exercise therapists should take into account the individual's: (i) physical function; (ii) functional limitations and likes/dislikes; (iii) health status; (iv) availability of equipment and time available to train; (v) exercise dose response (desired goal, type of exercise, and intensity, duration, and frequency of training); and (vi) coordination among members of the multidisciplinary team [10, 23]. HIV/AIDS is a progressive disease; therefore, clinical exercise therapists should frequently reassess the patient's physical, physiological, functional, and neuromuscular capacity (at least every 6–8 weeks) to determine whether the exercise program is still meeting the individual needs and goals of the patient. As mentioned earlier, HIV-infected individuals adapt readily to exercise training, and therefore, the general FITT principle of Ex Rx for apparently healthy adults can be applied to those carrying HIV [23, 39]. An Ex Rx is the process whereby the recommended exercise regimen is designed in a systematic and individualized manner in terms of the Frequency (How Often?), Intensity (How Hard?), Time (How Long?), and Type/Mode (What Kind?), or the FITT principle of Ex Rx [56].

5.1. Frequency

Frequency refers to how often an individual engages in an activity, usually the number of days per week [56]. Most HIV studies have used a three times weekly intervention for both the aerobic exercise (AE) and progressive resistive exercise (PRE) component [12, 13, 57] with success three/four times per week [31], a few studies have reported positive results twice weekly [39, 58]. **Table 3** indicates the specific frequency of the AE and PRE component according to the different clinical categories with the corresponding CD4 cell count for each category [55]; for example, HIV-infected individuals in clinical category A1 (asymptomatic, acute HIV, or persistent generalized lymphadenopathy with ≥500 cells/μL) (**Table 1**) and clinical category A2 (asymptomatic, acute HIV, or persistent generalized lymphadenopathy with 200–499 cells/μL) (**Table 1**) can perform PRE three times per week and aerobic AE five times per week whereas clinical category C HIV-infected individuals (AIDS indicator conditions with <200 cells/μL) (**Table 1**) can perform PRE twice per week and AE three times per week (**Table 3**) [55]. There should be a rest day between the PRE sessions and, if time constraints are present, separate resistive programs into upper and lower body workouts.

It is recommended to complete flexibility exercises during the warm-up and cool-down of an exercise session. Neuromuscular exercises can be performed two to three times per week by those HIV-infected individuals who are severely debilitated from the disease, typically those from the Centres for disease control clinical categories A3, B3, and C1-C3 (**Table 1**).

5.2. Intensity

Intensity is the level of exertion experienced during the activity. Individuals can monitor their rate of perceived exertion (RPE) with Borg's RPE scale that subjectively rates exercise intensity from 6 to 20 with 6 corresponding to "no exertion at all" and 20 corresponding to "maximal exertion" [59]. A person can also use a definitive scale by tracking heart rate. For the aerobic component, a 40–60% exercise intensity of VO_2R (difference between VO_{2max} and resting VO_2) or heart rate reserve (HRR) [31] or 50–85% of HR_{max} [10] is recommended to HIV-positive individuals.

The recommended exercise intensity for the PRE component is 50–90% of one-repetition maximum (1RM) [12]; 60% of 1RM [23] with an intensity of 35–50% of 6–10RM for patients from the Centres for disease control clinical categories A3, B3, and C1–C3 (**Table 3**) [55]. The specific intensities of the PRE component according to the different clinical categories with the corresponding CD4 cell count for each category are displayed in (**Table 3**) [55].

Clinical Category	Physical Fitness classifications[a]	Frequency[b]		Intensity[c]			Time		Type (mode)
		Kcal. wk^{-1}	d. wk^{-1}	HRR/$\dot{V}O_2R$	% HR_{max}	Perception of effort[d]	Total Weekly Duration per day (min)	Total Weekly Duration per week (min)	
A (Asymptomatic, acute HIV, or PGL)	Average–good	>2,000	5 **(AE)** 3 **(PRE)**	65%–80% **(AE)**; 65%–85% of 1RM or 2–3 sets of 10–15 reps **(PRE)**	80%–91% **(AE)**	Moderate–hard	30–90 **(AE + PRE)**	200–300	**AE**: Cycle, walk, jog, row **PRE**: Target major muscle groups using weights, cables/pulleys/resistance bands, bodyweight and plyometrics
B (Symptomatic conditions not A or C)	Fair–average	1,500–2,000	3–5 **(AE)** 2–3 **(PRE)**	55%–70% **(AE)**; 55%–85% of 1RM or 2 sets of 10–12 reps **(PRE)**	74%–84% **(AE)**	Moderate	30–90 **(AE + PRE)**	200–300	**AE**: Cycle, walk, row **PRE**: Target major muscle groups using weights, cables/pulleys/resistance bands, bodyweight
C (AIDS – Indicator conditions)	Poor	500–1,000	3 **(AE)** 2 **(PRE)**	30%–45% **(AE)**; 35%–50% of (6–10RM) or 1–2 sets of 8–10 reps **(PRE)**	57%–67% **(AE)**	Light–moderate	20–30 **(AE + PRE)**	60–150	**AE**: Cycle, walk, hydrotherapy **PRE**: Target major muscle groups using cables/pulleys/resistance bands, bodyweight

Kcal–kilocalories; $\dot{V}O_2R$–oxygen uptake reserve; HRR–heart rate reserve; $\%HR_{max}$–% age–predicted maximal heart rate; AE–aerobic exercise; PRE–progressive resistive exercise; PGL–persistent generalized lymphadenopathy.

[a] Fitness classification based on normative fitness data categorized by $\dot{V}O_{2max}$.

[b] Maximum frequency (d.wk^{-1}) of combined AE and PRE for clinical category A = 5; B = 5; C= 3.

[c] The various methods to quantify exercise intensity in this table may not necessarily be equivalent to each other.

[d] Perception of effort using the rating of perceive exertion (RPE) [23] or talk test [23].

Include 5 to 10 minutes of pre-exercise warm-up and cool-down exercises.

Table 3. Recommended FITT framework for the frequency, intensity, time, and type of aerobic exercise (AE) and progressive resistive exercise (PRE) for different HIV clinical categories [55].

5.3. Time

Time refers to the duration of an exercise session [56] and depends on the intensity as well as the goal of the exercise. AE performed at a higher intensity performed for a shorter duration produces the same results as exercise done at a moderate intensity for a longer duration. A duration of 45 min for the AE component [12] or 30–60 min [23] including a 5–10 min warm-up and cool-down is recommended. The duration of the AE component for patients from the Centres for disease control clinical categories A3, B3, and C1-C3 is 20–30 min (**Table 3**) [55].

The recommended duration of the PRE component is 30–90 min with a volume of three sets of eight reps [12], two sets of eight to ten repetitions [31], or 30 min to complete two to three sets of 10–12 exercises [23]. One to two sets of eight to ten repetitions are recommended for patients from the Centres for disease control clinical categories A3, B3, and C1–C3 (**Table 3**) [55].

The duration of the flexibility component is 5–10 min with a volume of three sets of 20–30 s. Similarly, the duration of the neuromuscular component is 5–10 min with the volume determined by the specific neuromuscular exercise.

5.4. Types (modes) of exercise

Types of activity include aerobic, balance, flexibility, and resistance (or strength) training which help patients achieve different health goals [56]. In HIV-infected individuals, the appropriate exercise mode depends on the patient's functional impairments, preference, and safety issues regarding the stage of the disease [12, 60].

5.4.1. AE

Aerobic exercise is safe to perform (even at high intensities) and may lead to significant improvements in selected outcomes of cardiovascular fitness, body composition, and psychological status in HIV-infected individuals [19]. Individual studies have shown an improvement in VO_{2max} and other measures of fitness [10, 13], improvement in body composition (decreases in fat percentage, increases in leg muscle area and abdominal fat loss), [13, 21] reduced anxiety, stress, and depressive mood [22], improvement in QOL [11], as well as improvement in lipid profile [8] and glucose tolerance [21]. Crossover effects have also been reported whereby aerobic exercise may lead to improved strength [3, 19]. Type or mode of AE to improve the cardiovascular system includes running, walking, swimming, aerobics classes, circuit training, and cycling [55].

5.4.2. PRE

Progressive resistive exercise is safe and effective in medically stable adults living with HIV [22, 32]. PRE can increase body weight and peripheral girth, and reverse muscular atrophy [61]. Training effects include an increase in strength [17, 61], improvements in body composition (increasing BMI and lean body mass) [17, 62], and improvements in psychological status and

QOL [10], insulin sensitivity [63], and lipid profile [64]. PRE that stresses the muscular system includes weights, cables/pulleys/resistance bands, body weight, and plyometrics [31, 55].

5.4.3. Combined aerobic and resistive exercise (CARE)

The combination of the two exercise modalities, AE and PRE, is recommended by the American College of Sports Medicine [23] and seems not only to be safe but well tolerated by HIV-infected individuals. A combination of aerobic and progressive resistive exercise (CARE) appears to be more effective than applying only one component [10]. Research studies have shown an improvement in VO_{2max} and other measures of fitness [3, 10, 13], functional capacity [10, 14], improvement in body composition (decreases in fat percentage, increases in abdominal fat loss, BMI, and lean body mass) [8, 13, 57], increases in viral load and cell counts for TCD4+/TCD8 [13], improvement in QOL [8, 9, 11] and mood state [61], as well as improvement in lipid profile [13] and glucose tolerance [21].

6. Special considerations during exercise training

For asymptomatic HIV-infected individuals, the ACSM's guidelines regarding contraindications for exercise applicable to healthy individuals should apply as there are no current guidelines for individuals with HIV/AIDS [23].

It is important that HIV-infected individuals report increased feelings of tiredness or exhaustion (minor increases in feelings of fatigue should not be a reason for exercise discontinuation), lower gastrointestinal distress (especially diarrhea), shortness of breath, or a sense of increased effort in performing activities of daily living [31].

Dizziness, swollen joints, or vomiting preclude exercise participation [23].

The exercise sessions of symptomatic individuals with HIV/AIDS or those diagnosed with comorbidities should be supervised [23].

7. Conclusion

Evidence-based research indicates that AE, PRE, and a combination thereof by HIV-infected individuals are safe and positively influences the cardiometabolic and morphological complications that may accompany HAART as well as a range of side effects associated with the HIV disease itself. The current exercise guidelines available in the literature are generalized and they do not consider the specific clinical stages with significant gaps in knowledge as to the minimal and optimal duration, frequency, mode, and intensity of exercise needed to produce beneficial changes in HIV patients. Most of the studies referred to have not approached the exercise program from a dose-response perspective or from the perspective of validating commonly used exercise prescriptions for HIV-infected individuals. The research provides information that clarifies the optimal mode, duration, frequency, and intensity of AE and PRE prescribed to the different clinical stages of HIV patients. Clinical exercise therapists should adopt the recommended guidelines that will benefit HIV patients.

Author details

Jeanne M. Grace

Address all correspondence to: Gracej@ukzn.ac.za

Discipline of Biokinetics, Exercise and Leisure Sciences, College of Health Sciences, University of Kwazulu Natal, Westville, Durban, South Africa

References

[1] Neto MG, Zwirtes R, Brites C. A literature review on cardiovascular risk in human immunodeficiency virus-infected patients: implications for clinical management. The Brazilian Journal of Infectious Diseases. 2013;17: 691–700. doi:10.1016/j.bjid.2013.05.004

[2] Giannarelli C, Klein RS, Badimon JJ. Cardiovascular implications of HIV-induced dyslipidemia. Atherosclerosis. 2011;219: 384–389. doi:10.1016/j.atherosclerosis.2011.06.003

[3] O'Brien KK, Tynan AM, Nixon SA, Glazier RH. Effectiveness of aerobic exercise for adults living with HIV: systematic review and meta-analysis using the Cochrane Collaboration protocol. BMC Infectious Diseases, 2016;16: 182. doi:10.1186/s12879-016-1478-2

[4] Peters BS, Conway K. Therapy for HIV past, present, and future. Advances in Dental Research. 2011;23: 23–27. doi:10.1177/0022034511399082

[5] Blanco F, San Román J, Vispo E, Lopez M, Salto A, Abad V, Soriano V. Management of metabolic complications and cardiovascular risk in HIV-infected patients. AIDS Rev. 2010;2: 231–241. PMID: 21179187

[6] Anuurad E, Semrad A, Berglund L. Human immunodeficiency virus and highly active antiretroviral therapy-associated metabolic disorders and risk factors for cardiovascular disease. Metabolic Syndrome and Related Disorders. 2009;7: 401–409. doi:10.1089/met.2008.0096

[7] Garg A. Lipodystrophies: genetic and acquired body fat disorders. The Journal of Clinical Endocrinology & Metabolism. 2011;96: 3313–3325. doi:10.1210/jc.2011-1159#sthash.i21n4Idx.dpuf

[8] Ogalha C, Luz E, Sampaio E, Souza R, Zarife A, Neto MG, Netto E, Brites C. A randomized, clinical trial to evaluate the impact of regular physical activity on the quality of life, body morphology and metabolic parameters of patients with AIDS in Salvador, Brazil. JAIDS Journal of Acquired Immune Deficiency Syndromes. 2011;57: S179–S185. doi:10.1097/QAI.0b013e31821e9bca

[9] Gomes-Neto MG, Conceição CS, Carvalho VO, Brites C. Effects of combined aerobic and resistance exercise on exercise capacity, muscle strength and quality of life in HIV-infected patients: a systematic review and meta-analysis. PloS One. 2015;10: e0138066. doi:10.1371/journal.pone.0138066

[10] Gomes-Neto M, Conceicao CS, Carvalho VO, Brites C. A systematic review of the effects of different types of therapeutic exercise on physiologic and functional measurements in patients with HIV/AIDS. Clinics. 2013;68: 1157–1167. doi:10.6061/clinics/2013(08)16

[11] Mbada CE, Onayemi O, Ogunmoyole Y, Johnson OE, Akosile CO. Health-related quality of life and physical functioning in people living with HIV/AIDS: a case–control design. Health and Quality of Life Outcomes. 2013;11: 1–8. doi: 10.1186/1477-7525-11-106

[12] Gomes Neto M, Ogalha C, Andrade AM, Brites C. A systematic review of effects of concurrent strength and endurance training on the health-related quality of life and cardiopulmonary status in patients with HIV/AIDS. BioMed Research International. 2013;3: 1–8. doi:10.1155/2013/319524

[13] Garcia A, Fraga GA, Vieira Jr RC, Silva CM, Trombeta JC, Navalta JW, Prestes J, Voltarelli FA. Effects of combined exercise training on immunological, physical and biochemical parameters in individuals with HIV/AIDS. Journal of Sports Sciences. 2014;32: 785–792. doi:10.1080/02640414.2013.858177

[14] Mendes EL, Andaki AC, Amorim PR, Natali AJ, Brito CJ, Paula SO. Physical training for HIV positive individuals submitted to HAART: effects on anthropometric and functional parameters. Revista Brasileira de Medicina do Esporte. 2013;19: 16–21. doi: 10.1590/S1517-86922013000100003

[15] Bevilacqua M, Dominguez LJ, Barbagallo M. Insulin Resistance and the cardiometabolic syndrome in HIV infection. Journal of The Cardiometabolic Syndrome. 2009;4: 40–43. doi:10.1111/j.1559-4572.2008.00027.x

[16] Deresz LF, Lazzarotto AR, Manfroi WC, Gaya A, Sprinz E, Oliveira ÁR, Dall'Ago P. Oxidative stress and physical exercise in HIV positive individuals. Revista Brasileira de Medicina do Esporte. 2007;13: 275–279. doi:10.1590/S1517-86922007000400013

[17] Kietrys D, Galantino ML. Can progressive resistive exercise improve weight, limb girth, and strength of individuals with HIV disease? Physical Therapy. 2014;94: 329–333. 10.2522/ptj.20120466

[18] Stradling C, Chen YF, Russell T, Connock M, Thomas GN, Taheri S. The effects of dietary intervention on HIV dyslipidaemia: a systematic review and meta-analysis. PloS One. 2012;7: e38121. doi:10.1371/journal.pone.0038121

[19] O'Brien K, Nixon S, Tynan AM, Glazier R. Aerobic exercise interventions for adults living with HIV/AIDS. Cochrane Database Systematic Review. 2010;8: 1–7. doi: 10.1002/14651858.CD001796.pub3

[20] Hand GA, Lyerly GW, Jaggers JR, Dudgeon WD. Impact of aerobic and resistance exercise on the health of HIV-infected persons. American Journal of Lifestyle Medicine. 2009;3: 489–499. doi:10.1177/1559827609342198

[21] Fillipas S, Cherry CL, Cicuttini F, Smirneos L, Holland AE. The effects of exercise training on metabolic and morphological outcomes for people living with HIV: a systematic review of randomised controlled trials. HIV clinical trials. 2010;11: 270–282. doi:10.1310/hct1105-270

[22] O'Brien K, Tynan AM, Nixon S, Glazier RH. Effects of progressive resistive exercise in adults living with HIV/AIDS: systematic review and meta-analysis of randomized trials. AIDS care. 2008;20: 631–653. doi:10.1080/09540120701661708

[23] Thompson PD, Arena R, Riebe D, Pescatello LS. American College of Sports Medicine. ACSM's guidelines for exercise testing and prescription. 9th Ed. Philadelphia: Lippincott Williams & Wilkins; 2013. 445 p. doi:10.1249/JSR.0b013e31829a68cf

[24] AETC. AIDS Education and Training Centre Guide for HIV/AIDS Clinical Care. [Internet]. 2014. Available from: http://aidsetc.org/guide/hiv-classification-cdc-and-who-staging-system [Accessed 2016-04-21]

[25] ePARmed-X+. ePARmed-X+ Physician Clearance Follow-Up. [Internet]. 2015. Available from: http://eparmedx.com/wp-content/uploads/2013/03/ePARmedX-Physician-Clearance-Form-2014.pdf [Accessed 2016-04-21]

[26] The Physical Activity Readiness Questionnaire for Everyone. [Internet]. 2015. Available from: http://eparmedx.com/wp-content/uploads/2013/03/PARQplusJan2015.pdf [Accessed 2016-04-20]

[27] Imam MH, Flora MS, Moni MA, Shameem RK, Haque MA, Mamun SA. Health related Quality of Life with HIV/AIDS in different stages of HIV infection. Mymensingh medical journal: MMJ. 2012;21: 509–515. PMID: 22828552

[28] Clayson DJ, Wild DJ, Quarterman P, Duprat-Lomon I, Kubin M, Coons SJ. A comparative review of health-related quality-of-life measures for use in HIV/AIDS clinical trials. Pharmacoeconomics. 2006;24: 751–765. PMID: 16898846

[29] Burgoyne RW, Tan DH. Prolongation and quality of life for HIV-infected adults treated with highly active antiretroviral therapy (HAART): a balancing act. Journal of antimicrobial chemotherapy. 2008;61: 469–473. doi:10.1093/jac/dkm499

[30] Gordon LL, Gharibian D, Chong K, Chun H. Comparison of HIV virologic failure rates between patients with variable adherence to three antiretroviral regimen types. AIDS patient care and STDs. 2015;29: 384–388. doi:10.1089/apc.2014.0165

[31] Durstine JL. American college of sports medicine's exercise management for persons with chronic diseases and disabilities. 3rd Ed.Champaign: Human Kinetics; 2009. 439 p. doi:10:0736074333

[32] Sakkas GK, Mulligan K, DaSilva M, Doyle JW, Khatami H, Schleich T, Kent-Braun JA, Schambelan M. Creatine fails to augment the benefits from resistance training in patients with HIV infection: a randomized, double-blind, placebo-controlled study. PLoS One. 2009;4: e4605. doi:10.1371/journal.pone.0004605

[33] Hsue PY, Squires K, Bolger AF, Capili B, Mensah GA, Temesgen Z, Wanke CA, Wohl DA. Screening and assessment of coronary heart disease in HIV-infected patients. Circulation. 2008;118: e41–47. doi:10.1161/CIRCULATIONAHA.107.189626

[34] Law M, Friis - Møller N, Weber R, Reiss P, Thiebaut R, Kirk O, D'Arminio Monforte A, Pradier C, Morfeldt L, Calvo G, El - Sadr W. Modelling the 3-year risk of myocardial infarction among participants in the Data Collection on Adverse Events of Anti - HIV Drugs (DAD) study. HIV medicine. 2003;4: 1–10. doi:10.1046/j.1468-1293.2003.00138.x

[35] Prentice WE, Kaminski TW. Rehabilitation techniques for sports medicine and athletic training. 5th Ed. New York, NY: McGraw-hill; 2004. 850 p. doi:10.0073376612

[36] Binkley JM, Stratford PW, Lott SA, Riddle DL. The Lower Extremity Functional Scale (LEFS): scale development, measurement properties, and clinical application. Physical Therapy. 1999;79: 371–383. PMID: 10201543

[37] Aidsinfo. HIV/AIDS drug side effects [Internet] 2016. Available from: https://aidsinfo.nih.gov/contentfiles/lvguidelines/adultandadolescentgl.pdf [Accessed 2016-04-27]

[38] Aberg JA, Kaplan JE, Libman H, Emmanuel P, Anderson JR, Stone VE, Oleske JM, Currier JS, Gallant JE. Primary care guidelines for the management of persons infected with human immunodeficiency virus: 2009 update by the HIV medicine Association of the Infectious Diseases Society of America. Clinical infectious Diseases. 2009;49: 651–681. doi:10.1086/605292

[39] Hand GA, Phillips KD, Dudgeon WD, William Lyerly G, Larry Durstine J, Burgess SE. Moderate intensity exercise training reverses functional aerobic impairment in HIV-infected individuals. AIDS Care. 2008;20: 1066–1074. doi:10.1080/09540120701796900

[40] Selik RM, Mokotoff ED, Branson B, Owen SM, Whitmore S, Hall HI. Revised surveillance case definition for HIV infection—United States, 2014. MMWR Recommendations and Reports. 2014;63: 1–10. ISSN: 1057-5987

[41] Finkelstein JL, Gala P, Rochford R, Glesby MJ, Mehta S. HIV/AIDS and lipodystrophy: Implications for clinical management in resource-limited settings. Journal of the International AIDS Society. 2015;18: 19033. doi:10.7448/IAS.18.1.19033

[42] Mercier S, Gueye NF, Cournil A, Fontbonne A, Copin N, Ndiaye I, Dupuy AM, Cames C, Sow PS, Ndoye I, Delaporte E. Lipodystrophy and metabolic disorders in HIV-1-infected adults on 4-to 9-year antiretroviral therapy in Senegal: a case-control study. Journal of Acquired Immune Deficiency Syndromes. 2009;51: 224–230. doi:10.1097/qai.0b013e31819c16f4

[43] van Griensven J, De Naeyer L, Mushi T, Ubarijoro S, Gashumba D, Gazille C, Zachariah R. High prevalence of lipoatrophy among patients on stavudine-containing first-line antiretroviral therapy regimens in Rwanda. Transactions of the Royal Society of Tropical Medicine and Hygiene. 2007;101: 793–798. doi:10.1016/j.trstmh.2007.02.020

[44] Husain NE, Ahmed MH. Managing dyslipidemia in HIV/AIDS patients: challenges and solutions. HIV/AIDS (Auckland, NZ). 2015;7: 1–10. doi:10.2147/HIV.S46028

[45] Gianotti N, Visco F, Galli L, Barda B, Piatti P, Salpietro S, Bigoloni A, Vinci C, Nozza S, Gallotta G, Lazzarin A. Detecting impaired glucose tolerance or type 2 diabetes mellitus by means of an oral glucose tolerance test in HIV-infected patients. HIV Medicine. 2011;12: 109–117. doi:10.1111/j.1468-1293.2010.00860.x

[46] Kalra S, Kalra B, Agrawal N, Unnikrishnan AG. Understanding diabetes in patients with HIV/AIDS. Diabetology & Metabolic Syndrome. 2011;3: 1–7. doi: 10.1186/1758-5996-3-2

[47] McComsey GA, Tebas P, Shane E, Yin MT, Overton ET, Huang JS, Aldrovandi GM, Cardoso SW, Santana JL, Brown TT. Bone disease in HIV infection: a practical review and recommendations for HIV care providers. Clinical Infectious Diseases. 2010;51: 937–946. doi:10.1086/656412

[48] Harris VW, Brown TT. Bone loss in the HIV-infected patient: evidence, clinical implications, and treatment strategies. Journal of Infectious Diseases. 2012;205: S391-S398. doi:10.1093/infdis/jis199

[49] Zhou DT, Kodogo V, Chokuona KF, Gomo E, Oektedalen O, Stray-Pedersen B. Dyslipidemia and cardiovascular disease risk profiles of patients attending an HIV treatment clinic in Harare, Zimbabwe. HIV/AIDS (Auckland, NZ). 2015;7: 145–155. doi:10.2147/HIV.S78523.

[50] Capili B, Anastasi JK, Ogedegbe O. HIV and general cardiovascular risk. Journal of the Association of Nurses in AIDS Care. 2011;22: 362–375. doi:10.1016/j.jana.2010.12.002

[51] Masiá M, Padilla S, Fernández M, Rodríguez C, Moreno A, Oteo JA, Antela A, Moreno S, del Amo J, Gutiérrez F, CoRIS B. Oxidative stress predicts all-cause mortality in HIV-infected patients. PloS One. 2016;11: e0153456. doi:10.1371/journal.pone.0153456

[52] Snopková S, Matýsková M, Povolná K, Polák P, Husa P. HIV lipodystrophy. Vnitrni Lekarstvi. 2010;56: 1217–1222. PMID: 1261108

[53] Kip AE, Balasegaram M, Beijnen JH, Schellens JH, de Vries PJ, Dorlo TP. Systematic review of biomarkers to monitor therapeutic response in leishmaniasis. Antimicrobial agents and chemotherapy. 2015;59: 1–44. doi:10.1128/AAC.04298-14

[54] Sued O, Figueroa MI, Cahn P. Clinical challenges in HIV/AIDS: Hints for advancing prevention and patient management strategies. Advanced Drug Delivery Reviews. 2016;103: 5-19. doi:10.1016/j.addr.2016.04.016

[55] Grace JM, Semple SJ, Combrink S. Exercise therapy for human immunodeficiency virus/AIDS patients: Guidelines for clinical exercise therapists. Journal of Exercise Science & Fitness. 2015;13: 49–56. doi:10.1016/j.jesf.2014.10.003

[56] Oberg E. Physical activity prescription: our best medicine. Integrative Medicine. 2007;6: 18–22.

[57] Ley C, Leach L, Barrio MR, Bassett S. Effects of an exercise programme with people living with HIV: research in a disadvantaged setting. African Journal of AIDS Research. 2014;13: 313–319. doi:10.2989/16085906.2014.961937

[58] Fillipas S, Oldmeadow LB, Bailey MJ, Cherry CL. A six-month, supervised, aerobic and resistance exercise program improves self-efficacy in people with human immunodeficiency virus: a randomised controlled trial. Australian Journal of Physiotherapy. 2006;52: 185–910. doi:10.1016/S0004-9514(06)70027-7

[59] Borg G. Borg's perceived exertion and pain scales. Campaign: Human Kinetics; 1998. 104 p. Accession Number: 1998-07179-000

[60] Baar K. Training for endurance and strength: lessons from cell signaling. Medicine and Science in Sports and Exercise. 2006;38: 1939–1944. doi: 10.1249/01.mss0000233799.62153.19

[61] Shephard RJ. Physical impairment in HIV infections and AIDS: responses to resistance and aerobic training. The Journal of Sports Medicine and Physical Fitness. 2015;55: 1013–1028. PMID: 24947921

[62] Keithley JK, Swanson B. HIV-associated wasting. Journal of The Association of Nurses in AIDS Care. 2013;24: S103-S111. doi:10.1016/j.jana.2012.06.013

[63] Broholm C, Mathur N, Hvid T, Grøndahl TS, Frøsig C, Pedersen BK, Lindegaard B. Insulin signaling in skeletal muscle of HIV-infected patients in response to endurance and strength training. Physiological Reports. 2013;1: e00060. doi:10.1002/phy2.60.

[64] Zanetti HR, Cruz LG, Lourenço CL, Ribeiro GC, Leite MA, Neves FF, Silva-Vergara ML, Mendes EL. Nonlinear resistance training enhances the lipid profile and reduces inflammation marker in people living with HIV: a randomized clinical trial. Journal of Physical Activity and Health. 2016;2: 1543–5474. PMID: 26901242

5

HIV-Associated Vasculopathy

Ashraf Alqaqa

Abstract

HIV vasculopathy is a wide range of clinical spectrum related to HIV infection. Increasing longevity of HIV-infected individuals secondary to antiretroviral therapy advancements has resulted in increasing the number of patients with HIV-related vasculopathy. Clinicians need to be aware of the different types of HIV vasculopathy to be able to diagnose and manage the pathology and improve patient care.

Keywords: HIV vasculopathy, vascular disease, carotid disease, aortic aneurysm, peripheral arterial disease, cerebral vasculopathy

1. Introduction

Human immunodeficiency virus (HIV) reduces the immunity of a body, making it vulnerable to opportunistic diseases. HIV was first reported in the USA in 1981, in young homosexual men. The young men were said to have severe opportunistic infections [1]. Two years later the virus was labeled as HIV and acquired immune deficiency syndrome (AIDS), if advanced [2]. A patient is diagnosed with AIDS when their immune system is significantly low, and their CD4 count is <200 cells/μl. The areas most affected with HIV/AIDS-infected persons are the Sub-Saharan regions of Africa. More than 72% of the world's population with HIV live in Africa. According to the 2007 report on HIV/AIDS, the world's total population living with this infection is about 33 million [3]. The burden of the worldwide epidemic of HIV infection continues to increase, especially in the developing world. Third World countries experience a vast financial burden of managing and treating HIV-infected and affected persons with scarce resources. The new advancement of potent antiretroviral therapies has, however, made it possible for more patients to live longer, allowing healthcare providers to witness new clinical manifestations of the chronic HIV infection.

There have been major improvements in novel clinical management in a bid to manage HIV [2]. For instance in 1987, HIV was for the first time linked to vasculopathy, impulsive arteriovenous fistula and arterial occlusive disease or aneurysmal infection [4]. The prevalence of symptomatic vasculitis in HIV patients is about 1% according to recent studies [5]. The chief objective of this review will be to describe the HIV-associated vasculopathies in various parts of the body.

Pathogenecity of HIV, which is associated with vasculopathy, is rather complex and hence not fully comprehended. The complexity is a result of several factors such as inflammatory and immunological response to HIV infections. These factors lead to deleterious and dynamic effects on the endothelial and smooth muscle cells of the blood vessels.

HIV infection results in several interleukins and tumor necrosis factor-α (TNF-α) in response to production of viral proteins by the virus. The HIV-transactivator of transcription protein (*tat*) and viral envelope glycoprotein component (gp120) are believed to induce and mediate the inflammatory responses to vessels. This inflammation consequently results in the production of cytokines and adhesion molecules that interfere with endothelial function. In essence, the viral protein accesses the smooth muscle component of the media layer through CD4 surface receptor. Ultimately, this results into abnormal proliferation of the smooth muscle, and abnormal activation of the coagulation cascade [6–10].

Histological studies show an infiltration of the large vessels surrounded by different inflammatory cells including neutrophils, lymphocytes, monocytes and plasma cells in HIV-infected persons. The infiltration of those cells results in obliterate endarteritis, which is an occlusion of the vessels supplying the vasa vasorum, and leads to ischemia, and necrotic changes of the vessel wall are induced [7–11]. Studies of the biopsy and culture of those aneurysms, however, fail to reveal infectious pathogens.

A murine AIDS model has helped investigate pathogenesis of acquired AIDS. In this model the murine leukemia virus (MuLV) is injected into mice. The mice characteristically develop hypergammaglobulinemia, splenomegaly, lymphadenopathy, T-cell and B-cell functional abnormality. The mice also become highly susceptible to opportunistic infections. The murine AIDS and human AIDS have a lot of similarities regarding immune function alterations. Further clinical progression based on this model and vessel wall animal models has suggested a link between endothelial dysfunction and vasculopathy. It has been found that aortas from infected mice have increased concentrations of ICAM-1 and VCAM-1. Moreover, decrease in their contractile responses and impairment in the endothelium-dependent relaxation are observed.

Pathological findings, conversely, have indicated the thinning of the media layer as a result of the viral infection. In addition, they have indicated a direct viral invasion of the aortic fibroblasts at the level of the adventitia. It has therefore been postulated that an autoimmune destructive process can happen as a result of the similarity in the DNA sequence of the viral glycoprotein and a component of the matrix of the vessel wall. Important to note is that, no strong evidence has been found to support this theory.

It has been postulated that an autoimmune destructive process is possible where there is a DNA sequence of the viral glycoprotein, and a component of the matrix of the vessel wall. This, however, is not fully agreeable as there is lack of strong evidence to support the theory [8–12].

To diagnose HIV-associated vasculopathy, other causes of arterial occlusions and aneurysms have to be eliminated. These are mycotic aneurysms caused by syphilis and tuberculosis. Second, arterial occlusions caused by Takayasu's arteritis, vasculitis, and systemic lupus erythematosus (SLE) and Behcet's disease. Finally, elimination of antiphospholipid antibody syndrome-related aneurysms which make close differentials [13–15].

Recent studies indicate that various symptoms of HIV disease have been affecting almost all body organs. For example, studies in radiological, clinical and postmortem indicated cerebral, cardiac, renal and peripheral vascular pathologies in HIV-infected persons. This chapter will look at different HIV-associated vasculopathies affecting the main organ systems in a body.

2. HIV-associated large vessel aneurysm

The large arteries' condition in HIV-infected persons is not very researched, as it is a rare occurrence. Its pathology is different from atherosclerosis and mycotic aneurysm. It is considered a distinct clinical and pathological entity. It is non-infective vasculopathy, where the microbiological cultures of blood, aneurysm wall and thrombus are negative. Furthermore, the patients with atherosclerotic aneurismal disease are older in comparison to patients with aneurysms related to HIV. HIV-related aneurysm is commonly found in young patients in their 30s [10–14].

While the condition stands to affect any large artery, aneurysms typically affect superficial femoral, carotid and popliteal artery. Aneurysms are not uncommonly found to be multiple and have primarily pseudoaneurysm-like focal saccular transformations. Medical practitioners are therefore advised to screen patients for multiplicity using ultrasound or CT scan with contrast. Leukocytoclastic vasculitis of the vasa vasorum and periadventitial vessels is an important mechanism which weakens the wall of the vessel, and leads to focal disruption of the wall at the position of transmural necrosis. This mainly causes the false impression of aneurysm [9, 10, 13, 14]. The symptoms associated with the aneurysm depend on its location and size. It might be that compressive symptoms in an adjacent organ or structure result in life-threatening hemodynamic instability in case of a rupture. Thromboembolic and venous thrombosis are also likely complications of the aneurysm which have often been reported.

Majority of HIV-infected persons with associated aneurysm have advanced immunosuppressed state. This is usually indicated by abnormally reversed CD4:CD8 ratio. Such patients illustrate an abnormally low CD4 count (a median of about 400 cells/μl only). In addition, if such patients have high globulin level, they exhibit low serum albumin consistently [9–13].

While deciding the management approach of HIV-infected persons with asymptomatic aneurysm, it's important to take into consideration their clinical condition and nutrition status. With this in mind, symptomatic aneurysm lesions should be treated according to the standard guidelines, rules and open surgery standard therapy. The use of endovascular therapy has also gained popularity over the past years. HIV-infected patients should be optimized according to standard practice such as an earlier intervention. Conservative treatment on the other hand would be the best option for patients with advanced HIV/ AIDS. Low albumin (<35 g/l) and CD4 count are both indicators of poor operative outcome. Clinical management should, however, maintain a consistency in administering antiretroviral therapy regardless of CD4 level. This is because such prevalence is indicator of an advanced phase of the condition [8–11, 13, 14].

3. Cerebral vasculopathy

Cerebral vasculopathy in HIV-infected patients is infrequently observed. The disease is believed to be under-diagnosed in most cases according to recent reports. HIV vasculopathy of the central nervous system affects small- to medium-sized blood vessels. The HIV-associated aneurysmal disease is frequently of a fusiform type, and occurs in young adults. This type of aneurysm affects carotids and extracranial vessels mainly. On the other hand, the intracranial aneurysm is a rare discovery and is often observed in children. Some reports have linked the low CD4 counts to increased chances of intracerebral vasculopathy occurrence [11, 12, 15, 16].

The primary pathogenesis of intracerebral vasculopathy is not known. However, various studies have shown that postmortem histological examination indicates damage of the interior elastic lamina and fibrosis. This histological examination has also shown interference of the media along with intimal hyperplasia. The resulting aneurysmal and occlusive patterns of this disease tend to lead to ischemic and/or hemorrhagic complications [10–14].

The pathogenesis of HIV-associated cerebral aneurysms has also been postulated to be a result of immune response to the HIV protein. This occurs, according to various researches, inside the endothelial cell. It has been suggested that the use of antiretroviral therapy may exacerbate the vasculopathy because it can lead to immune reconstitution inflammatory syndrome (IRIS) [15, 16].

A similar theory suggested that an abnormal and significant change in the vascular response to blood flow, which occurs due to changes in circulating cytokines and growth factors, can lead to vascular remodeling. These changes are thought to play a main role in aneurismal dilatation. The production of cytokines and growth factors is believed to be caused by opportunistic infections, which involve the blood vessel endothelial wall, allowing it to abnormally increase. Such repeated infections contribute to an amplified production of elastase, which increases the thickness and fragmentation of the internal elastic lamina. Such changes in the lamina are associated with development of fusiform aneurysms. Because of this suggested association, patients with cerebral aneurysm should be investigated for underlying opportunistic infections [11–13].

4. Carotid disease in HIV patients

Carotid intima-media thickness (IMT) measurement by B-mode high-resolution ultrasound is a noninvasive method of assessing atherosclerosis. It is also a strong predictor of cardiovascular events. IMT is considered in HIV persons to evaluate cardiovascular risk.

The prevalence of carotid atherosclerosis in HIV population varies, and correlates with Framingham risk score (FRS). The higher the FRS, the higher the prevalence. The prevalence is estimated to be 26.6% in the very low-risk group and 76.5% in high-risk group. The carotid IMT of individuals with HIV infection was, on average, 0.04 mm thicker (95% confidence interval; and 0.02–0.06 mm, $p < 0.001$) than that of individuals without HIV infection. Carotid plaque also has been found to be 1.5-fold more frequent in HIV patients in comparison to non-infected persons.

It is believed that the traditional CVD risk factors, in addition to HIV infection factors, play a role in this pathology. However, the role of ART is still not clearly confirmed. There are several studies that have suggested the use of ART as a significant and an independent risk associated with carotid atherosclerosis in HIV-infected patients. Moreover, it has been found that there is a moderate independent association between HIV immunological marker and increased carotid IMT and plaque presence [16, 17].

5. HIV-associated vascular thrombosis

Even though women comprise the highest population of HIV-infected persons in Africa, their male counterparts are said to be more likely to have primary arterial thrombosis. In addition, they are likely to present with late advanced limb ischemia. The pathophysiology of this disease is not well comprehended. Several causes of primary HIV infection-associated thrombosis have been documented. The levels of total proteins and the von Willebrand factor have been found to be increased in such patients. This suggested that endothelial cell dysfunction may play a role, as a predisposing factor for primary thrombosis. Hypercoagulable states associated with the HIV infection, including antiphospholipid antibody syndrome, deficiencies in free protein S, protein C, and antithrombin III, could predispose patients to arterial thrombosis [18, 19].

What is unique about HIV-associated vascular thrombosis is the normality of the arterial tree proximal to the thrombosed arteries by duplex ultrasonography, angiography and macroscopic appearance. Second is the thrombosis of all distal vessels with no demonstrable runoff. Duplex ultrasonography also showed hyperechoic 'spotting' in the arterial wall, the 'string of pearls sign', which has also been observed in patients with HIV-associated arterial aneurysms. Both endothelial dysfunction and coagulation abnormality of the HIV patients were found to correlate with the state of immunosuppression [19, 20].

When managing HIV-associated occlusive vasculopathy, the vascular surgical rules should be followed. Patients having less CD4 count should not be excluded from surgical intervention, since surgical findings show that its success does not depend on CD4 levels. The treatment for primary arterial thrombosis includes surgical thrombectomy with or without thrombolysis. The use of corticosteroid post thrombectomy has been considered previously, although it did not decrease the rethrombosis rate. The treatment modality available unfortunately did not significantly alter the level of amputation. The rate of limb salvage in such cases is about 27%. According to therapy researches, it is clear that therapies do not address the underlying ongoing processes. It's important to note that such studies are only but a few; they are sporadic and reflect individual experiences [19–24].

Venous thrombosis is reported as a complication in HIV-infected patients. It is believed to be a result of disturbance of coagulation process. It is estimated that deep vein thrombosis in HIV-infected patients of up to 5% is attributable to a process of thrombophilia. In addition, protein anticardiolipin antibodies and protein C deficiency have been reported in such patients [25–29].

6. HIV-associated peripheral arterial disease

Peripheral arterial disease is a significant clinical management issue in HIV-infected patients. The disease creates a risk of cardiovascular disease, and is associated with increased morbidity and mortality rate. HIV-infected individuals are believed to have higher prevalence and more severe forms of PAD. Measuring ankle-brachial index (ABI) is the initial noninvasive test to diagnose PAD. It usually correlates to obstructive disease and more than 50% stenosis by angiography in the lower extremity arterial system, if abnormal. Moreover, post-exercise ABI measurement could be used to uncover milder diseases.

Low ABI and high ABI readings have been linked to atherosclerosis and increased cardiovascular events. The exact prevalence of PAD in HIV population is still under-studied and not clearly defined. The studies are not numerous and the existing ones show contradicting results. However, the prevalence is believed to be higher than in normal population and in the range of 9.8–13.9%. High ABI prevalence in HIV patients has risen and is estimated to be in the range of 13.3–19.7%. However, none of the classical vascular risk factors were associated with ABI measurements.

Post-exercise ABI measurement change is suggestive of PAD in HIV-infected patients. It has been reported to range from 10.9% to 26.5%, depending on the criteria used. The exercise test was performed to symptomatic versus asymptomatic HIV-patients. Interestingly, the post-exercise changes in ABI are not associated with traditional atherosclerosis risk factors such as diabetes mellitus, hypertensive disorder and dyslipidemia. Screening for subclinical PAD using post-exercise measurement is encouraged in HIV-infected patients, even when they do not depict symptoms of PAD. PAD has a frequent occurrence in young HIV population and coexists with critical limb ischemia. In HIV-infected patients, there is growing evidence suggesting a high prevalence of PAD and a higher risk of developing severe and accelerated atherosclerosis. PAD in HIV patients is six-fold more than in HIV-negative patients [30–33].

The antiretroviral protease inhibitor induces dyslipidemia, making HIV infection a risk factor for atherosclerosis. HIV causes direct injury to the arterial wall, resulting in the initiation of the inflammatory process. Such inflammations contribute to the development of premature atherosclerosis. Endothelial dysfunction in HIV-infected patients is associated with increasing levels of soluble adhesion molecules, cytokines and procoagulant proteins. The effect of the HIV-associated proteins gp(120)on endothelium have been suggested to cause endothelial dysfunction [25–28, 32, 33]. In addition, PAD in HIV-infected patients can occur even in undetectable viral levels or in absence of severely suppressed immune system. This can be explained by the chronic inflammatory state in HIV patients. PAD, in addition, does not correlate to Framingham risk score in the HIV-infected population [34].

7. HIV and atherosclerotic coronary artery disease

HIV-infected patients live longer since the introduction of ART. It is believed that the risk of atherosclerosis in HIV patients is increased because of associated metabolic disturbances. The coronary disease in such infected individuals is considered distinctive. It is usually more diffuse and is associated with circumferential-intimal thickening, atherosclerotic plaques and abnormal proliferation of the smooth muscle. The muscles with luminal protrusions share several similarities with cardiac transplant vasculopathy [34–38]. Reports have suggested that the most common initial presentation of the HIV patient with CAD is acute myocardial infarction and its mortality can go as high as 24%. In addition, more than 40% test positive to triple vessel disease [39–41].

Coronary artery disease (CAD) is commonly observed in patients who are on ART. During a study conducted on this, HIV-infected patients who were not using ART showed a slight risk of ischemic heart disease. The risk was slightly higher in HIV-infected persons who were on ART. However, during the post-ART period there was a significant increase in the risk of ischemic cardiac disease in the HIV-infected population. The 3-year risk for myocardial infarction was 3.6-fold higher in patients on ART in comparison to those who were not [34, 38–43].

There are numerous metabolic changes that are associated with ART (protease inhibitor in particular). They include impaired glucose metabolism and lipodystrophy as a result of increased insulin insensitivity, and they tend to accelerate the atherosclerosis process. The data regarding nucleoside reverse transcriptase inhibitors, as a risk for CAD, are not very clear. In a D.A.D study, abacavir and didanosine were found to be associated with increased risk of myocardial infarction. Consequently, abacavir has been linked to higher cardiovascular events in first 6 months of the infection. Conversely, other studies could not establish a similar relationship, especially after controlling the traditional cardiovascular risk factors. Furthermore, no link was established in non-nucleoside reverse transcriptase inhibitors and integrase inhibitors as an association with cardiovascular events [20, 44–47].

On one hand, HIV infection has been postulated to independently increase the risk of premature CAD. The mechanism by which the virus can accelerate atherosclerosis is multifactorial and complex. This mechanism involves the activation of inflammatory cells, which changes the immune response in HIV patients. This leads to exposure to a variety of xenoantigens from HIV infection and other viral and bacterial infections. These infections result in the ignition of a continuous inflammatory condition that speeds up atherosclerosis [21, 30, 34].

Endothelial dysfunction is an early marker of atherosclerosis. Endothelial dysfunction has been found in young HIV-infected individuals and has been attributed to increased viral load. HIV affects directly the endothelium function and results in increased levels of prothrombotic plasma markers such as von Willebrand factor, b2 microglobulin and thrombomodulin. In addition, it leads to increased levels of the circulating inflammatory molecules, interleukin 6 and D-dimer.

Prevention of CAD is a cornerstone in clinically managing HIV-infected patients. Careful cardiac screening of individuals who are receiving ART is important. Patients with a history in cardiovascular risk factors stand to benefit from such screening as they are at a higher risk.

Identification of asymptomatic atherosclerotic diseases of the coronaries would help to maximize patients' therapy. By the use of risk stratification tests such as coronary artery calcium score, high sensitivity C-reactive protein and carotid intima-medial thickness, HIV patients with higher risk of cardiovascular events can be identified. This will protect such patients from aggressive risk factors through modification and preventive measures.

Interruption of chronic ART therapy is highly discouraged as it could lead to increase in cardiovascular-associated morbidity and mortality. The SMART study has shown that the risk of cardiovascular morbidity and mortality has increased significantly. This is in patients who were assigned to a CD4 cell count guided therapy arm, as compared to their counter parts with continuous therapy arm. However, no studies or theories support an association of CD4 count and CAD [34, 43].

The conventional cardiovascular risk factors are found to be higher in HIV patients. Patients with smoking habits particularly, experience increased risk of atherosclerosis and increase the prothrombotic state [38, 39]. Controlling and modifying the risk factors and comorbidities is important in managing atherosclerosis. The fasting lipids should be checked before starting ART, and followed up to adjust therapy according to the lipids' value changes. If statin therapy is needed to treat high low-density lipoprotein (LDL) levels, the dose to be used should be identified carefully. This is because the risk of statin drug interaction and possible rhabdomyolysis is higher in HIV patients. PI, ritonavir and some antimicrobial agents inhibit specific cytochrome P450 enzymes, which are important in metabolizing several statins. This is because such agents could increase the toxicity of those drugs. Pravastatin (20–40 mg), low-dose atorvastatin (10 mg) and rosuvastatin (5–10 mg) have been suggested as safe if used with protease inhibitors. Ezetimibe can also be added to statin therapy to achieve target levels of LDL. Fibrates are used to control hypertriglyceridemia, if the concentration is above 500 mg/dL.

8. Pulmonary arterial hypertension

HIV-related pulmonary arterial hypertension (PHT) is estimated to occur in 0.5% of the HIV population. It is usually present with nonspecific symptoms such as dyspnea on exertion, lower extremity edema and fatigue. PHT is considered a poor prognostic finding and it is said to lead to right ventricular dysfunction, therefore significantly increasing the mortality rate.

The pathogenesis of HIV-related PHT is complex and still not very well understood. Factors that are believed to participate in the pathogenesis are related to the viral infection in patients. It is believed that the HIV virus stimulates an immune response, which leads to the release of different cytokines and growth factors. This may include the potent vasoconstrictors, endothelin-1, interleukin 6, tumor necrosis factor and platelet-derived growth factor. These immunological responses result in endothelial damage, intimal fibrosis, and stimulate the proliferation of the smooth muscle and fibroblast of the arterioles. Eventually, the pathological structural changes lead to the formation of plexiform lesion. The lesion is quite similar to those found in PaHTN caused by other factors. More recent evidence suggests that the patient's immunologic response, virus HIV-negative factor (Nef), HIV-transactivator of transcription (Tat) accessory proteins and human herpes virus-8 coinfection, may play an important role to cascade events.

Its prognosis is poor and the reported mortality rate is said to be high. PaHTN in HIV population is an independent predictor of mortality with 1-year survival rate reported to range from 51% to 88%. The severity of HIV infection and CD4 cell count has no apparent correlation with this complication. The effect of highly active antiretroviral therapy regimens on the clinical course is still not well defined and is presently being investigated. However, it has been suggested that long-duration treatment with HAART might reduce mortality rate. Currently the treatment of HIV-PaHTN is similar to that of idiopathic pulmonary arterial hypertension patients. There have been reports of the use of diuretics, anticoagulation, phosphodiesterase V inhibitors and calcium channel blockers to treat HIV-PaHTN. HAART prostacyclin analogs (e.g.epoprostenol and endothelin) and receptor inhibitors (such as bosentan) were found to be effective in reducing the pulmonary arterial pressure in HIV patients. Heart-lung transplantation is the last treatment option in this subgroup of patients [21, 22, 34].

9. Conclusion

HIV-associated vascular diseases is not a common occurrence, even though it is considered to be of significant clinical importance. A comprehensive screening for possible etiology such as co-infections, lymphoproliferative disease, and autoimmune disorders, before other pathological attributions to HIV infection is important for appropriate patients' management. HIV-associated vascular disease can be manifested either as aneurysms or occlusive forms. The two forms of diseases can lead to hemorrhagic or ischemic life-threatening complications, respectively.

Author details

Ashraf Alqaqa

Address all correspondence to: ayqs@yahoo.com

Tennova Healthcare, Tennessee, USA

References

[1] Friedman-Kien, A., et al. Kaposis sarcoma and Pneumocystis pneumonia among homosexual men—New York City and California. *MMWR. Morbidity and Mortality Weekly Report*, 1981. **30**(25): 305–308.

[2] Barre-Sinoussi, F., et al. Isolation of T-lymphotropic retrovirus from a patient at risk for acquired immune deficiency syndrome (AIDS). *Revista de investigación clínica*, 2004. **56**(2): 126–129.

[3] Organization, W.H. *Unaids report on the global aids epidemic*. Geneva: UNAIDS and World Health Organization, 2010.

[4] Bayley, A. Surgical pathology of HIV infection: lessons from Africa. *British Journal of Surgery*, 1990. **77**(8): 863–868.

[5] Joshi, V.V., et al. Arteriopathy in children with acquired immune deficiency syndrome. *Fetal and Pediatric Pathology*, 1987. **7**(3): 261–275.

[6] Nair, R., et al. Arterial aneurysms in patients infected with human immunodeficiency virus: a distinct clinicopathology entity? *Journal of Vascular Surgery*, 1999. **29**(4): 600–607.

[7] Chetty, R. Vasculitides associated with HIV infection. *Journal of Clinical Pathology*, 2001. **54**(4): 275–278.

[8] Botes, K., and Van Marle, J. Surgical intervention for HIV related vascular disease. *European Journal of Vascular and Endovascular Surgery*, 2007. **34**(4): 390–396.

[9] Chetty, R., Batitang, S., and Nair, R. Large artery vasculopathy in HIV-positive patients: another vasculitic enigma. *Human Pathology*, 2000. **31**(3): 374–379.

[10] Nair, R., et al. Occlusive arterial disease in HIV-infected patients: a preliminary report. *European Journal of Vascular and Endovascular Surgery*, 2000a. **20**(4): 353–357.

[11] Nair, R., et al. Clinical profile of HIV-related aneurysms. *European Journal of Vascular and Endovascular Surgery*, 2000b. **20**(3): 235–240.

[12] Mulaudzi, T. HIV-associated vasculopathy. *Continuing Medical Education*, 2009. **27**(7): 320–322.

[13] Bulsara, K.R., Raja, A., and Owen, J. HIV and cerebral aneurysms. *Neurosurgical Review*, 2005. **28**(2): 92–95.

[14] Tipping, B., et al. Stroke caused by human immunodeficiency virus–associated intracranial large-vessel aneurysmal vasculopathy. *Archives of Neurology*, 2006. **63**(11): 1640–1642.

[15] Kossorotoff, M., et al. Cerebral vasculopathy with aneurysm formation in HIV-infected young adults. *Neurology*, 2006. **66**(7): 1121–1122.

[16] Periard, D., Cavassini, M., Taffé, P., Chevalley, M., Senn, L., Chapuis-Taillard, C., de Vallière, S., Hayoz, D., Tarr, P.E., Swiss HIV Cohort Study. High prevalence of peripheral arterial disease in HIV-infected persons. *Clinical Infectious Diseases*, 2008. **46**(5): 761–767.

[17] Benjamin, L.A., Bryer, A., Emsley, H.C., Khoo, S., Solomon, T., Connor, M.D. HIV infection and stroke: current perspectives and future directions. *The Lancet Neurology*, 2012. **11**(10): 878–890.

[18] Woolgar, J., et al. Colour doppler and grey scale ultrasound features of HIV-related vascular aneurysms. *The British Journal of Radiology*, 2002. **75**(899): 884–888.

[19] Committee, W., Cardio-and cerebrovascular events in HIV-infected persons. *AIDS*, 2004. **18**(13): 1811–1817.

[20] Law, M., et al. Modelling the 3-year risk of myocardial infarction among participants in the data collection on adverse events of anti-HIV drugs (DAD) study. *HIV Medicine*, 2003. **4**(1): 1–10.

[21] Dubé, M.P., et al. Effects of HIV infection and antiretroviral therapy on the heart and vasculature. *Circulation*, 2008. **118**(2): e36–e40.

[22] Khunnawat, C., et al. Cardiovascular manifestations in human immunodeficiency virus-infected patients. *The American Journal of Cardiology*, 2008. **102**(5): 635–642.

[23] Friis-Moller, N., et al. Class of antiretroviral drugs and the risk of myocardial infarction. *The New England Journal of Medicine*, 2007. **356**(17): 1723–1735.

[24] Mehta, N.J., and Khan, I.A. HIV-associated coronary artery disease. *Angiology*, 2003. **54**(3): 269–275.

[25] Shingadia, D., et al. Takayasu's arteritis in a human immunodeficiency virus—infected adolescent. *Clinical Infectious Diseases*, 1999. **29**(2): 458–459.

[26] Hsue, P.Y., et al. Progression of atherosclerosis as assessed by carotid intima-media thickness in patients with HIV infection. *Circulation*, 2004. **109**(13): 1603–1608.

[27] Calza, L., Manfredi, R., and Chiodo, F. Statins and fibrates for the treatment of hyperlipidaemia in HIV-infected patients receiving HAART. *AIDS*, 2003. **17**(6): 851–859.

[28] Boccara, F., Teiger, E., and Cohen, A. Stent implantation for acute left main coronary artery occlusion in an HIV-infected patient on protease inhibitors. *The Journal of Invasive Cardiology*, 2002. **14**(6): 343–346.

[29] Boccara, F., et al. Clinical characteristics and mid-term prognosis of acute coronary syndrome in HIV-infected patients on antiretroviral therapy. *HIV Medicine*, 2005. **6**(4): 240–244.

[30] Tabib, A., et al. Accelerated coronary atherosclerosis and arteriosclerosis in young human-immunodeficiency-virus-positive patients. *Coronary Artery Disease*, 2000. **11**(1): 41–46.

[31] Rickerts, V., et al. Incidence of myocardial infarctions in HIV-infected patients between 1983 and 1998: the Frankfurt HIV-cohort study. *European Journal of Medical Research*, 2000. **5**(8): 329–333.

[32] Klein, D., et al. Do protease inhibitors increase the risk for coronary heart disease in patients with HIV-1 infection? *Journal of Acquired Immune Deficiency Syndromes (1999)*, 2002. **30**(5): 471–477.

[33] Friis-Moller, N., et al. Combination antiretroviral therapy and the risk of myocardial infarction. *New England Journal of Medicine*, 2003. **349**(21): 1993–2003.

[34] Alqaqa, A., et al. Cardiac sequelae of human immunodeficiency virus disease. *The American Journal of the Medical Sciences*. 2014. **348**(1): 82–86. doi:10.1097/MAJ.0000000000000258. Review.

[35] Hsue, P.Y., et al. Clinical features of acute coronary syndromes in patients with human immunodeficiency virus infection. *Circulation*, 2004. **109**(3): 316–319.

[36] Matetzky, S., et al. Acute myocardial infarction in human immunodeficiency virus–infected patients. *Archives of Internal Medicine*, 2003. **163**(4): 457–460.

[37] Escaut, L., et al. Coronary artery disease in HIV infected patients. *Intensive Care Medicine*, 2003. **29**(6): 969–973.

[38] Boccara, F., et al. Percutaneous coronary intervention in HIV infected patients: immediate results and long term prognosis. *Heart*, 2006. **92**(4): 543–544.

[39] Blyth, D., et al. An experience with cardiopulmonary bypass in HIV-infected patients. *Cardiovascular Journal of South Africa: Official Journal for Southern Africa Cardiac Society [and] South African Society of Cardiac Practitioners*, 2005. **17**(4): 178–185.

[40] Trachiotis, G.D., et al. Cardiac surgery in patients infected with the human immunodeficiency virus. *The Annals of Thoracic Surgery*, 2003. **76**(4): 1114–1118.

[41] Castillo, J.G., et al. Cardiovascular surgery in patients with HIV: epidemiology, current indications, and long-term outcome. *Revista Española de Cardiología (English Edition)*, 2008. **61**(5): 480–486.

[42] Mulaudzi, T., et al. Thrombectomy in HIV related peripheral arterial thrombosis: a preliminary report. *European Journal of Vascular and Endovascular Surgery*, 2005. **30**(1): 102–106.

[43] Boccara, F., et al. Coronary artery bypass graft in HIV-infected patients: a multicenter case control study. *Current HIV Research*, 2008. **6**(1): 59–64.

[44] Sagcan, A., et al. Spontaneous bilateral perirenal hematoma as a complication of polyarteritis nodosa in a patient with human immunodeficiency virus infection. *Rheumatology International*, 2002. **21**(6): 239–242.

[45] Yonou, H., et al. Simultaneous bilateral perirenal hematomas developing spontaneously in a patient with polyarteritis nodosa. *The Journal of Urology*, 1999. **162**(2): 483.

[46] Qaqa, A.Y., et al. Epidemiologic aspects of abnormal ankle brachial index in the HIV infected population. *International Angiology*. 2012. **31**(3): 227–233. Erratum in: *International Angiology*, 2013. **32**(2): 260.

[47] Qaqa, A.Y., et al. The role of postexercise measurements in the diagnosis of peripheral arterial disease in HIV-infected patients. *Angiology*, 2011. **62**(1): 10–14.

6

Molecular Mechanisms Controlling HIV Transcription and Latency – Implications for Therapeutic Viral Reactivation

Michael D. Röling, Mateusz Stoszko and Tokameh Mahmoudi

Abstract

Persistence of transcriptionally silent replication competent HIV-1 is a major barrier to clearance of the virus from patients; current combinatorial antiretroviral therapies are successful in abrogating active viral replication, but are unable to eradicate latent HIV-1. A "shock and kill" strategy has been proposed as a curative approach in which latent virus is activated and infected cells are removed by immune clearance, while new rounds of infection are prevented by antiretroviral therapy. Much effort has been put toward understanding the molecular mechanisms maintaining HIV latency and the nature of reservoirs, to provide novel therapeutic targets. This has led to the development of latency reversal agents (LRAs), some of which are undergoing clinical trials. Targeting multiple mechanisms underlying HIV latency via a combination of LRAs is likely to result in more potent activation of the latent reservoir. Therefore, novel as well as synergistic combinations of therapeutic molecules are required to accomplish more potent latency reversal.

Keywords: HIV-1 latency, Latency reversal agents (LRAs), Combinatorial antiretroviral

1. Introduction

Human immunodeficiency virus-1 (HIV-1) is a lentivirus, a subgroup of Retroviridae. Like all retroviruses, HIV-1 virions consist of an RNA genome with viral proteins encapsulated in a viral envelope. The viral proteins execute key steps to establish a productive infection by stably integrating into the host genome. Unlike most retroviruses, HIV-1 can also directly infect nondividing cells. HIV-1 preferably infects a subset of T-lymphocytes (CD4+ T-cells) that play a crucial role in the immune response. HIV-1 infection causes exhaustion and ultimately depletion of the host immune system, a syndrome termed acquired immuno-deficiency syndrome (AIDS). HIV-1 came into prominence with the outbreak of the AIDS epidemic in the 1980s. Major steps have been taken toward treating this viral infection. In particular, combinatorial antiretroviral therapy (cART) successfully abrogated HIV-1 replication. Thus, for compliant patients with access to c-ART, HIV infection has become a chronic rather than a lethal disease. However, cessation of antiretroviral therapy results in viral rebound in infected patients, even after years of cART. This is because in a small fraction of infected cells, HIV persists in a latent but replication-competent state. Latent HIV is unaffected by cART, but infection can rebound upon cART interruption. Therefore, HIV latency is the main challenge in developing a curative therapy for HIV.

The quest for an HIV-1 cure involves the development of either a sterilizing or a functional cure. A sterilizing cure would require complete removal of replication competent viral genetic material from the infected patient and thus the stable depletion of latently HIV-infected cells. A functional cure, on the other hand, requires the patient's immune system to suppress HIV-1 replication life-long in the absence of cART without disease progression, loss of CD4+ T cells and HIV transmission. The functional cure does not aim to eradicate the virus entirely from the patient. Both the sterilizing and functional cure strategies are currently the subject of major research efforts.

2. Clinical picture of HIV

The AIDS epidemic in the 1980s led to the identification of HIV as the causative agent. AIDS is a condition in which depletion of CD4+ T-cells overtime leads to the loss of the host immune system's ability to fight infections and cancers, eventually leading to death. As HIV was identified as the causative agent, cure efforts focused on disrupting the viral lifecycle. In the early 1990s, the first antiretroviral therapies – monotherapies – had limited success as they resulted in rebound of viremia due to the appearance of resistant viral strains. Resistant HIV required novel therapeutic strategies. Therefore, a combination of anti-retrovirals, targeting distinct steps of the viral life cycle was developed, so-called combinatorial antiretroviral therapy (cART). cART has proven to be extremely successful in lowering the amount of viral RNA in plasma below the limits of detection by standard laboratory techniques. Unfortunately, the therapy does not eradicate the virus as cessation of medication causes re-emergence of viral replication [1–3]. Thus, a fraction of the virus escapes the effects of cART. The source for this recurring viral replication is a small pool of latently infected cells that harbor integrated proviruses which, while silent, are not recognized by either the immune system nor are they subject to cART. Moreover, HIV can persist in the presence of cART in certain anatomical sites if drug penetrance is incomplete.

According to the World Health Organization (WHO), the number of HIV-infected individuals worldwide in late 2014 was estimated to be approximately 37 million [4]. The vast majority of infected people live in sub-Saharan Africa, where access to appropriate diagnostic centers and cART is limited. Estimates put new infections at 5,600 a day in 2014.

2.1. HIV-1 replication cycle and state-of-the-art antiretroviral therapy

HIV-1, as all viruses, is a parasite of the host cell and hijacks key cellular processes to establish a productive infection. To produce new virions, the virus goes through a viral replication cycle. HIV's replication cycle consists of entering the cell by docking at the cell surface receptor CD4 and co-receptors CCR5/CXCR5 and fusing to the cell, un-packaging of the genome, reverse transcription of the viral RNA genome into double-stranded DNA, which is the main component of the pre-integration complex, followed by integration of the double-stranded DNA genome into the host genome, transcription of the provirus, translation of viral proteins, and ultimately virion biogenesis followed by budding from host cell and maturation. Modern cART targets most steps in the HIV viral replication cycle (Figure 1). There are currently 28 approved agents for the treatment of HIV infection [5]. They fall into six mechanistic major classes, which act at different stages in the HIV replication cycle:

1. Fusion inhibitors: enfuvirtide (ENF, T-20), the only currently available fusion inhibitor, binds to the gp41 receptor site, preventing the fusion of the virus with the target cell.

2. C-C chemokine receptor type 5 (CCR5) antagonists: maraviroc (MVC) is currently the only available CCR5 antagonist. This drug is an entry inhibitor, specifically blocking the human chemokine receptor CCR5.

3. Nucleoside (nucleotide) reverse transcriptase inhibitors (NRTIs) block the addition of nucleosides to the DNA chain during reverse transcription of RNA.

4. Non-nucleoside reverse transcriptase inhibitors (NNRTIs) bind to and inhibit the enzyme reverse transcriptase (RT), preventing conversion of viral RNA to DNA during infection.

5. Integrase inhibitors (INIs): raltegravir (RAL), elvitegravir (EVG) and dolutegravir (DTG) are the only currently available drugs in this class. They target the HIV enzyme integrase (IN) that is required for insertion of viral genetic material into human DNA.

6. Protease inhibitors (PIs) bind to the catalytic site of HIV aspartic protease, blocking the processing of viral proteins (eg. Saquinavir).

These antivirals comprise the various current cART regimens that are used in the clinic. cART has proven to be extremely successful in suppressing viral replication in compliant patients. In fact, it has been argued that the theoretical potential of cART has already been reached [6]. Therefore, in the developed world with access to medication, HIV has become a chronic and not a lethal disease.

2.2. The burden of lifelong cART

Implementation of cART has provided long-term suppression of viral replication, improving the life expectancy and life quality of infected patients. Unfortunately, the economic burden of cART is debilitating. According to the Centers for Disease Control and Prevention (CDC), lifetime costs of treating HIV infection is estimated to be $379,668 per infected individual in the United States [7].

Moreover, patients on cART overtime can experience several side effects of cART such as: cardiovascular diseases (e.g., myocardial infarction); non-AIDS cancers (e.g., anal cancer, liver cancer, Hodgkin's disease); liver, kidney, and bone disease as well as neurologic complications, such as dementia [8]. Interestingly, most of these conditions are associated with the ageing process. Hence, it is thought, that HIV infection controlled by cART accelerates ageing. And importantly, HIV persists in a latent state that is not targeted by cART, rendering cART a therapeutic management of the disease as opposed to a curative treatment. Thus, there is much need to develop a curative therapy for HIV.

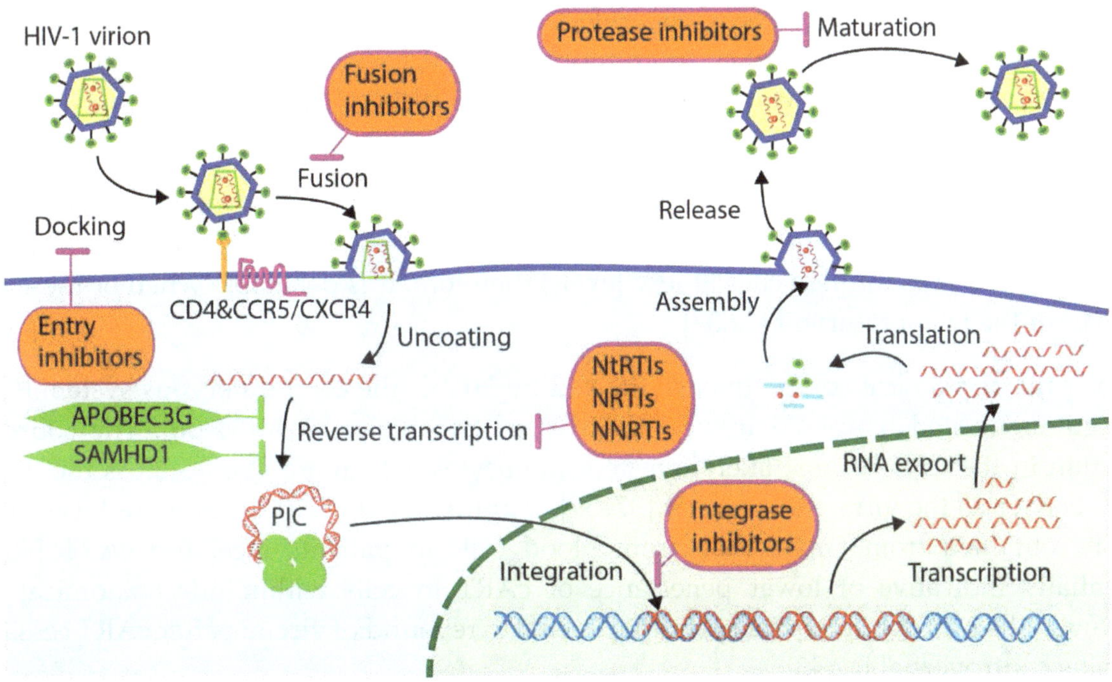

Figure 1. The viral replication cycle can be targeted pharmacologically at different stages

2.3. Clinical latency

The first step in finding a cure for HIV-1 infection is to identify the main source of cells that carry silenced, replication-competent HIV-1. Therefore, it is critical to define which cells or anatomical compartments constitute a reservoir of latent but replication-competent HIV-infected cells.

HIV-1 infects cells expressing the cell surface CD4 receptor and either of the co-receptors CCR5 or CXCR4. These cells include T helper cells, monocytes, macrophages, and dendritic cells. *In vivo,* HIV infects mostly activated CD4+ T-cells as quiescent and resting CD4+ T-cells are less permissive to infection due to low expression of CD4 and CCR5, and minimal metabolism [9–12]. The low metabolism is characterized by low levels of available dNTPs for reverse transcription and lack of energy sources [13–17]. Additionally, the cortical actin barrier in resting cells is thought to inhibit virus entry, reverse transcription and nuclear import [18,19]. However, the biggest pool of latently infected cells comprises resting memory CD4+ T-cells.

It is thought that these latent infections are predominantly generated while activated infected cells revert back to a resting memory state [20–22]. During this process, as the genome of the (partially) activated cell condenses and is silenced in transition to a memory state, so does the HIV genome [14,15]. There is also evidence for direct infection of resting cells by HIV, resulting in the generation of a latent infection [23]. Studying these cells in patients is challenging as the frequency of latently infected cells in suppressed patients is very low, estimated to be 1 latent cell per 1 million of uninfected cells [24,25]. Due to the long half-life of a latently infected resting memory CD4+ T-cells (estimated at 44 months), cART would take over 70 years in order to eradicate HIV from the infected patient [6,26,27].

Naive T-cells are also found to be latently infected; however, the frequency of such cells is even smaller than resting memory cells [28]. Interestingly, the naive T-cell reservoir may increase over time in suppressed individuals due to high proliferation of these cells compared to resting memory cells [29].

HIV is found also in cells of monocyte/macrophage lineage such as macrophages in brain and lung sections of infected individuals on anti-retroviral therapy [30,31]. However, proviral transcription occurs in these cells at low levels; therefore, it is debatable whether these cells are part of the latent reservoir [32,33].

Among the anatomical compartments affected by HIV-1, the central nervous system (CNS) and gut-associated lymphoid tissues (GALT) are two major sites [34–36]. The source of infection in the CNS is most likely infected monocytes, which are able to cross the blood–brain barrier as the virus itself cannot [37–39]. Approximately 5-10 times more HIV-1 RNA can be obtained from GALT than from blood cells in patients receiving cART [40,41], potentially indicative of lower penetrance of cART in cells within this anatomical site. However, the contribution of these compartments to rebound of viremia after cART cessation remains controversial [42,43].

2.4. Clinical proof-of-concepts for HIV-1 eradication

Thus far, only one patient, the so-called Berlin patient, was cured from HIV-1 after receiving treatment for acute myeloid leukemia [44,45]. HIV eradication in this patient was accomplished after several rounds of radio- and chemotherapy, total body irradiation, and two hematopoietic stem cell (HSC) transplantations from a donor bearing homozygous thirty-two base pair deletion in the CCR5 co-receptor gene (CCR5Δ32) were performed. The mutant CCR5 impedes viral entry of R5 tropic viruses in the first phase of the infection [46–49]. It is estimated that between 1% and 15% of the European Caucasian population harbor this mutation, while it occurs less frequently in African and Asian populations [47, 48]. In this patient, cART was ceased a day before the first transplant and after 7 years, no viremia or other indications of viral replication have been detectable [52].

Following the success of the case of the "Berlin patient", two HIV-1-positive patients, the "Boston patients", received HSCs transplants after developing Hodgkin's lymphoma [53]. Both patients carried heterozygous CCR5Δ32 mutation. While still under cART regimen, no viral production was observed which led to cessation of therapy. Unfortunately, after several months, strong viral rebound occurred in these patients. Follow-up analysis pointed to the likely presence of a small refractory source of cells, which is thought to have seeded the viral rebound; phylogenic studies revealed that only a few latent proviruses contributed to the viral rebound [53]. Several other similar studies have been conducted with infected patients suffering from either leukemias or lymphomas who received autologous or allogenic HSC transplantation alongside cART as a strategy to deplete the latent pool of cells. However, in most of these studies, viral rebound was detected following therapy interruption [54].

In another case, the Mississippi baby, an infant presumably infected *in utero*, received cART 30 h after birth. As newborns do not have resting memory CD4+ T-cells, it was reasoned that cART will prevent establishment of the latent reservoir – the main impediment in eradication strategies. One month after therapy, viremia reached undetectable levels and cART was stopped after 18 months. Unfortunately, 2 years post therapy interruption, rebound of viremia was detected (52, http://www.niaid.nih.gov/news/newsreleases/2014/pages/mississippibaby-hiv.aspx).

The immune system of rare "elite controllers" maintains low HIV-1 plasma levels, without the need of medication for many years. Although the capability of these patient to control viral replication is not completely understood, their circulating myeloid dendritic cells and CD8+ T-cells are more effective in depletion of infected CD4 T-cells [56–61]. Interestingly, the ARNS VISCONTI cohort showed that cessation of long-term cART, started during the acute phase of HIV-1 infection, resulted in post-treatment control (PST) of infection. Fourteen of the studied individuals were able to keep or even further reduce the viral reservoir. Furthermore, these individuals were able to maintain long-lasting, low level of viremia [62]. Recently, a perinatally infected baby displayed more than 11 years of HIV-1 remission. At 3 months of age, plasma HIV-RNA reached 2.1 x 10^6 copies/ml, and cART was administered for about 5–6 years. At 6.8 years of age, no HIV-1 RNA was detectable and cART was discontinued. After more than 12 years, plasma viremia still remains undetectable [63]. Therefore, this case provides the first evidence that early initiated, long-term cART can result in stable and durable HIV-1 remission.

Data from the Berlin and Boston patients provided a rationale for the creation of HIV-resistant cells. Since the CCR5Δ32 homozygous mutation is not lethal and not associated with abnormal immune functions [52], many approaches to silence the CCR5 gene have been or are under investigation [64–67]. These studies all employ genome editing technologies such as transcription activator-like effector nuclease (TALEN), clustered regularly interspaced short palindromic repeats (CRISPRs) or zinc-finger nucleases (ZNFs), which target the genome with high specificity and introduce deletions in the sequence of interest, in this case in the DNA sequence of CCR5 or/and CXCR4 co-receptors [64,65,68]. The rationale for this approach is based on the notion that cells bearing mutated CCR5 protein are not permissive to infection with R5 HIV-1 viruses, while cells with a mutated CXCR4 are resistant to C4 viruses. The double knock-out of both CCR5 and CXCR4 would allow resistance to infection regardless of viral tropism. However, the safety of such an approach remains to be elucidated. Uninfected HSCs isolated from infected individuals are engineered with either technology and then transfused back into patients. The ZNF approach targeting CCR5 has shown some promising results, although the sizes of cohorts used have been small. Gene-modified cells persisted in patients over 9 months, and cells seemed to expand and undergo trafficking to other tissues [66]. An increase in CD4+ T-cell counts was observed in all individuals. Importantly HIV-1 DNA in the blood decreased. The encouraging outcome of this study has resulted in phase II clinical trials.

Another gene therapy-based approach is the introduction of HIV-1 expression-dependent suicide genes encoding either toxic or pro-apoptotic proteins such as members of the Bcl-2 protein family. Constructs that are responsive to Tat and Rev viral proteins were tested [69]. While obtaining encouraging results, activity of such suicide genes only affects cells that are actively producing viruses, thus the latent pool of cells would still be unaffected.

Despite many attempts at HIV-1 cure, thus far only two cases, the "Berlin patient" and the early treated infant have resulted in eradication [44,45,63]. Due to safety and economic issues associated with transplantation and gene therapy approaches, broad use of such a therapeutic approach is not feasible for HIV cure. Moreover, the gene therapy approach provides a functional rather than sterilizing cure. Nevertheless, all these studies provided valuable insights into the biology of the latent reservoirs. They constitute a proof-of-concept for HIV-1 cure. Moreover, it seems that immediate initiation of cART contributes to restricting the establishment of the latent pool.

These studies highlight the need for more robust, cheaper, and feasible treatments in order to achieve HIV-1 eradication among all infected individuals. In 2004, the concept of so-called "shock and kill" or "kick and kill" therapy was proposed [70–72]. The aim is to specifically reactivate proviruses in latently infected cells ("shock") and eliminate the infected cells via viral cytophatic effects or/and render the cells susceptible to immune clearance ("kill"). New rounds of infection would be prevented by cART. "Shock and kill" therapy relies on the identification of potent and specific latency reversal agents (LRAs) alongside induction of an effective immune response against the reactivated latent pool of cells. The LRAs currently under investigation do not result in sufficient reactivation of latent HIV *in vivo*. Therefore, novel molecules that specifically reactivate latent HIV-1 are urgently needed.

3. Model systems and assays to detect and study HIV-1

To study the complex nature of HIV-1 latency, reliable model systems are required that recapitulate the nature and dynamics of the latent reservoir in vivo. Several cell lines of lymphocytic or monocytic lineage, primary-cell models, as well as animal models, are used to study HIV latency [73].

3.1. Cell lines

Immortalized cell lines of T-cell and monocytic origin are cost-effective and easy to use in the study of latent HIV. They allow fast read-outs in large scale for mechanistic molecular characterization of HIV gene expression. Therefore, cell lines are an attractive platform for screening and mechanistic characterization of LRAs. To generate a latent cell line, cells must first be latently infected with a HIV derived virus. Several different HIV derived viruses are used ranging from full length to minimal virus and can make use of a wide range of reporter constructs (e.g. GFP or luciferase). The viral Tat/TAR axis is of vital importance for the transcriptional regulation of HIV and can be included or excluded from the viral construct used. Latent infection of relevant cell lines derived from T-cells or monocytic lineage, depending on reservoir of interest generate cell lines that can be used to study the molecular mechanisms of HIV latency [74–78].

Ach-2 and U1 cells are characterized by low expression of HIV-1, which can be strongly upregulated upon TNFα or mitogens stimulation [74,79]. However, in these cell lines, latency results from mutations in Tat protein (U1 cell-line) or in RNA stem loop TAR (Ach-2) [76,77]. Therefore, these cell lines do not represent complexity of latency found *in vivo*, however, they do allow Tat/TAR-independent HIV-1 reactivation investigation.

A more appropriate system to study latency are J-Lat cell lines derived from Jurkat cells of T-lymphocytic origin [78, 80,81]. These cells have integrated replication-competent full-length or minimal proviral constructs with an intact promoter and Tat-TAR axis, a *GFP* reporter gene replaces the *Nef* sequence in full-length proviruses or is located downstream of *Tat* in minimal proviruses [78].

These cell lines have been extremely useful to delineate the molecular requirements of HIV transcription activation and silencing. Although useful for molecular analysis and screening platforms, the cell line model systems of HIV latency also present some limitations; first, clonal cell lines are derived from a single integration event, and therefore do not reflect the diverse distribution of integration sites in the host chromatin [82,83]. Consistently, results vary depending on the cell lines used, indicating possible clonal cell line effects [84]. Due to the above mentioned limitations and the considerable difference between cell line models and primary cells in terms of proliferative capacity, genomic stability and mechanisms involved in establishing and maintaining latency, generally latency models based on primary cells are preferable.

3.2. Primary cells

To more closely resemble infection *in vivo* and validate putative LRAs more accurately, several primary cell models have been developed. Depending on the cell status at infection, these models can be divided into two groups.

The first group relies on purification of CD4+ T-cells from healthy donors, that are then activated and subsequently infected. Depending on the method, CD4+T-cells are purified and stimulated with a-CD3/IL-2 [85], a-CD3/aCD-28 [86], a-CD3/aCD-28/IL-2 [87], or Ag-MDDC (antigen-loaded monocyte-derived dendritic cells; [88]), and infected with virus. Productively infected cells die due to virus-induced apoptosis or become latent by reverting back to a resting state. To limit infection to only one replication cycle, replication-defective viruses or antiretroviral drugs are also used. The rationale for these systems rely on the notion that a portion of activated, infected CD4+ T-cells transition to a quiescent state, shutting down general transcription and slowing down metabolism, resulting in latency [6,25,28,89–91]. Depending on the method used, different populations of latently infected cells are generated for use in reactivation studies. In the methods suggested by Sahu and Marini central memory T (T_{CM}) cells remain in culture, in Yang's protocol mainly effector memory T (T_{EM}) cells are produced, in Bosque and Planelles's method cells phenotype resembles central memory-like (T_{CM}). The main disadvantage of these methods is the time needed to obtain results, which varies from 1 to 4 months. Furthermore, they are labor-intensive and technically challenging.

The second group uses direct infection of resting memory CD4+ T-cells, which immediately after integration become latent. Cells are infected after purification and can be used after several days for reactivation studies [90, 91]. Stimulation of CCR7, CXCR3, or CCR6 receptors increases the susceptibility of resting memory CD4+ T-cells to infection without T-cell activation. In the methods of Swiggard and Lassen, central memory T (T_{CM}) and effector memory T (T_{EM}) cells are the source of latent HIV-1; in Saleh's method naïve resting memory T-cells, in addition to T_{CM} and T_{EM} cells, constitute the latent pool. The main advantage of these methods is the time needed to evaluate the potency of putative LRA, as results can be obtained within one week.

Depending on the protocol used, the amounts of cells that become latent differ from as little as 1% to up to 40%. In models where cells are activated, on average more latently infected cells are generated. Using these models, we can quantify the level of reactivation of HIV-1 in a reliable manner by measuring the production of the viral protein p24 by enzyme-linked immunosorbent assay (ELISA) or quantification of viral transcription by quantitative RT-PCR, or by detection of GFP/luciferase in case of reporter-based constructs.

A novel detection method distinguishes uninfected, productively infected, and latently infected cells using a dual reporter system. A modified HIV-1 derived genome containing GFP as a reporter of viral transcriptional activity and mCherry under an EF1a promoter as a reporter of infection (latent or productive) allows easy isolation of the different cell populations [23].

Ultimately, the golden standard for testing activity of LRAs are primary cells from infected individuals under cART obtained by leukophoresis, a process in which white blood cells are specifically isolated while other blood components are reverted back to the patients' circulatory system. The isolated cells are uninfected, latently infected, and infected with defective viruses. Large amounts of CD4+ T-cells are required and isolated from patients for testing LRAs.

The development of primary cell models greatly improved the quest for LRAs, yet results differ between each model system [84]. No *in vitro* models completely recapitulate the full range of latent cells *in vivo*; instead, only a small sub-fraction of latently infected cells is represented. Hence, the validation process of putative LRAs requires testing on cells derived from infected individuals [93].

3.3. Animal models of HIV-1 infection

The number of animal models available to study latency is limited. The toxicity of putative LRAs can be assessed with use of mouse and non-human primate (NHP) models [94]. Two mouse models have been developed and used in HIV latency studies: the humanized SCID

(SCID-hu) mouse, transplanted with human thymus and liver fragments, and the humanized blood, liver, and thymus (BLT) mouse which has a human immune system with full mucosal immunity [95–97]. Unfortunately, SCID-hu mice do not express human proteins involved in the viral replication cycle; therefore, the study of HIV-1 in these mice is restricted to events taking place within organs of human origin in this model. In addition, HIV-1 is not responsive to cART in these animals. BLT mice are a better model of HIV-1 infection, as they produce resting memory CD4+ T-cells of human origin. However, some components of cART do not repress replication in BLT mice [34].

NHP models employ the Simian immunodeficiency virus (SIV) infection in rhesus and pig tailed macaques to recapitulate HIV-1 infection in humans [98,99]. NHP models allow the monitoring of the spread of infection. Moreover, infection in this model can be controlled by antiretroviral therapy. NHP models are helpful in studying the first stages of latency establishment, as investigating this part of HIV-1 infection is extremely challenging in patients, as the pool of latently infected cells is established early during infection [100]. One caveat to the use of SIV-based NHP models of HIV latency is that the viral 5′LTR or promoter of SIV is considerably different in sequence from HIV-1 [101] and therefore latent SIV response to LRAs, which is a direct consequence of promoter-mediated transcription activation may vary substantially from latent HIV-1. In addition, animal models are far more expensive than cell-based systems. Nor do they fully reflect human infection or metabolism. Finally, ethical concerns are inherent to the use of NHP models of HIV latency.

3.4. Detection of the latent reservoir

The study of latent HIV infection requires accurate measurement of the size of the latent reservoir and the extent of reactivation following LRA treatment. Depending on the experimental aim, different detection methods can be employed. These methods generally rely on PCR, protein quantification, or reporter detection.

The quantitative viral outgrowth assay (QVOA) is a well-established method to estimate the latent pool. The assay relies on the use of serial dilutions of cells obtained from an infected individual in co-culture with uninfected cells that are permissive to infection. Viral proteins are detected by ELISA. Unfortunately, QVOA is time-consuming, costly, and might generate false-negative results as not all replication-competent proviruses are reactivated, and thus not detected [83].

The HIV reservoir can be approximated by detecting the number of viral DNA copies present in the cells. The recently introduced digital droplet PCR (ddPCR) improves on classic and nested qRT-PCR by simultaneously amplifying thousands of nanoliter reactions in combination with very sensitive detection system based on flow cytometry [94,102,103]. ddPCR is therefore superior to nested qRT-PCR in its ability to resolve rare events such as latent HIV-1. Although PCR based methods provide increased sensitivity for the detection of viral genetic material, these approaches also detect defective proviruses, which results in false-positive results.

Another recent PCR-based method for reservoir detection evades false positive results from defective proviruses. The *Tat/rev* induced limiting diluting assay (TILDA) relies on PCR amplification of multiply spliced RNA (msRNA) of *tat/rev* transcripts that are present in productively infected cells and absent in latent infection [104]. Small amounts of cells isolated from patients are divided into two equal parts and distributed in limiting dilution. One half is left unstimulated while the other is activated with PMA/Ionomycin. After 12 hours, cells are lysed and subjected to ultrasensitive nested RT-PCR. By employing statistical modeling, the frequency of cells that are expressing msRNA in both groups is estimated and based on the unstimulated group a threshold of activation can be set. Using the TILDA assay, the size of the reservoir is estimated at 24 cells per million, which is more than measured by QVOA but less than measured by PCR methods [24,83,104]. The assay more accurately estimates the true size of the latent reservoir, is highly sensitive, reproducible, fast, relatively inexpensive, and requires only 10 mL of patients' blood. However, a limitation on the TILDA assay is that it detects the presence of viral transcripts but not the production or release of infectious viral particles; therefore, it may still overestimate the true size of the reservoir, yet to a smaller extent than other PCR-based methods. Additionally, signal detection relies on amplification of highly variable region of the HIV-1 DNA; therefore, detection of all subspecies of HIV-1 might be challenging and require extra optimization steps.

Unfortunately, all current methods to detect latent HIV-1 have limitations. First, the pool of latently infected cells in patients is extremely low, resulting in a high noise-to-signal ratio. Furthermore, defective or hyper-mutated proviruses are detectable by PCR-based techniques, yet irrelevant for eradication strategies. Moreover, not all replication-competent proviruses are inducible in the first round of treatment, yet get reactivated upon subsequent rounds of stimulation [83]. Thus, assays to measure latency reversal are overestimating – in the case of PCR-based methods – or underestimating – in the case of QVOA – the latent pool. This poses a main problem in measuring efficiency of the reactivation of HIV-1. A captivating approach employing the use of a biomarker (e.g., gene), which responds to treatment in the same way as HIV-1, would allow more easily quantifiable assessments as to whether latent HIV in patient cells would be responsive to a particular treatment.

4. Molecular mechanisms of latency

Although replication-competent, latent HIV is transcriptionally silenced but susceptible to reactivation upon certain stimuli. Following integration into the host genome, transcription from the HIV genome is controlled by key cellular host factors, and subject to host cell gene regulation similar to endogenous genes. Since viral transcription initiation, elongation, and termination are tightly regulated by host proteins, HIV is also widely used as a model system to study gene regulation.

4.1. Host antiretroviral mechanisms thwart infection

Host defense mechanisms impede HIV-1 infection. Upon entering the cell, HIV's RNA genome is reverse transcribed into double-stranded DNA (dsDNA). This process requires freely available deoxynucleotide triphosphates (dNTPs). By limiting the pool of freely available dNTPs, the nucleotide scavenger SAMHD1 restricts viral replication in non-cycling myeloid cells and quiescent CD4+ T-cells [105–108]. Additionally, SAMHD1 has 3′–5′ exoribonucleases (RNAse) activity that specifically cleaves single-stranded RNA [109,110]. Interestingly, Vpx, encoded by HIV-2 and Simian immunodeficiency virus, is an accessory protein packaged into the virion, which induces SAMHD1 degradation [111].

Additionally, APOBEC3G limits viral replication by catalyzing the deamination of cytidine to uridine in the viral single-stranded DNA (ssDNA) genome during reverse transcription [112]. Interestingly, APOBEC3G is inactive in memory CD4+T-cells, which helps to explain why this cell type is more permissive to HIV-1 infection. Therefore, activated CD4+ T-cells are the main target cell type of HIV infection and of the main source of the latent reservoir.

4.2. Integration of HIV into the host genome required by host factors

The reverse-transcribed viral DNA genome is incorporated in the pre-integration complex (PIC). The PIC is imported into the nucleus. Host factors identified so far that affect viral integration are lens epithelium-derived growth factor (LEDGF/p75/PSIP1) and hepatoma-derived growth factor related protein 2 (HRP- 2/ HDGFRP2), through an integrase binding domain. In the absence of LEDGF, provirus integration is decreased 10-fold and HIV's pattern of integration is altered [113–115]. Simultaneous LEDGF and HRP-2 knockdown further decreases viral replication [116]. Nevertheless, knockdown of both factors does not completely abolish HIV-1 integration, indicating that IN alone and/or in cooperation with other host factors can still integrate the viral genome [117]. PIC nuclear import stimulates export to the cytoplasm of INI-1 and PML, disrupting this effect greatly improves integration efficiency [118–120]. Upon knockdown of transportin-3/TNPO3 and nuclear pore protein RanBP2/Nup35 HIV-1 integrates randomly [121]. Therefore, nuclear import affects the site of integration with a preference for open chromatin.

4.3. Pre-integration vs post-integration latency

Two states of latency can be defined based on the integration state of HIV: pre-integration latency and post-integration latency. Defects in integration or in a prior phase of the viral replication cycle (e.g., incomplete reverse transcription) might result in unintegrated viral DNA. The half-life of the linear pre-integration complex is approximately 1 day [122]. The linear unintegrated viral DNA can also be circularized, resulting in slightly extended half-life of the virus [123]. In quiescent cells, the pre-integrated virus can reside near the centromere for weeks [124]. Unintegrated virus can replicate, albeit very inefficiently [125]. The half-life of both forms of unintegrated virus is too short and replication inefficient to serve as the source required for the long-term persistence of latent HIV making pre-integration latency less clinically relevant.

Post-integration latency occurs when the HIV virus is stably integrated into the host genome, but a productive infection is not achieved. The site of integration and the abundance of transcription factors are crucial for determining whether an infection will be latent or productive. The site of integration will determine the chromatin environment (such as histone modifications), relative position to other genes (intronic insertion vs gene desert) and position within the nucleus of the provirus.

4.4. Integration biases

The site of integration greatly determines the transcriptional activity of the provirus. HIV preferentially integrates into active genes both in patient material and transformed cell lines [82,126–128]. Moreover, HIV-1 integrates in regions of genome that are in close proximity to nuclear envelope [129]. Latent integrations are in or close to alphoid repeat elements in heterochromatin, whereas productive integrations avoid insertion in or near heterochromatin [78]. Integration is associated with transcription-inducing histone modifications (i.e., H3 & H4 acetylation and H3K4 methylation) but not transcription-inhibiting modifications (i.e., H3K27 trimethylation and DNA CpG methylation) [130]. A comparison of integration sites in resting and activated CD4+ T-cells showed that in both cell types HIV integrates in active genes. However, in activated cells, insertions were enriched for gene dense, CpG island-rich and high G/C-content regions [131]. Latency in infected Jurkat cell lines correlated with integrations in gene deserts, centromeric heterochromatin, and highly expressed cellular genes [128]. Within the nucleus, HIV-1 is located mostly in decondensed chromatin at the nuclear periphery, while it disfavors heterochromatic regions [132]. Interestingly, latent proviruses were found to interact with a pericentromeric region of chromosome 12 in quiescent cells [133]. In a study of viremic progressors and viremic controllers, integration was enriched into, or in close proximity to, Alu repeats, local hotspots, and silent regions of the genome [134]. In addition, close proximity of the provirus to PML bodies is associated with latency, an association that is lost upon reactivation [135].

4.5. Integration relative to host genes affects transcriptional state of the provirus

Sense and antisense integration relative to host genes can greatly affect the transcriptional state of HIV. Integration in sense orientation can lead to promoter occlusion, whereas integration in antisense orientation can lead to collision of the transcriptional machinery. Promoter occlusion occurs when the transcriptional machinery is depleted from the viral promoter by a dominant host promoter that is transcribed and negatively affects proviral expression.

Indeed, chimeric transcripts of the host gene and in sense viral integrations were observed [136,137]. Additionally, Han et al. compared the effect of sense and antisense insertions of HIV relative to the active HPRT gene [138]. In this setting, sense integration enhanced viral expression whereas antisense integration (transcriptional collision) led to suppression. Sense integrations were shown to be modestly preferred in latent cells, a preference that was not present in productively infected cells [139]. Transcriptional interference and transcriptional collision are examples of host genes interference with viral expression. On the other hand, reactivation of HIV may lead to suppression of host gene expression [136]. Indeed, in a cell model with a latent integration into the HMBOX1 gene, the host gene was repressed upon viral reactivation [140].

4.6. Viral transcription starts at the 5'LTR

The provirus is flanked by a 5′ and 3′ long terminal repeats (LTRs). While transcription can be initiated from both LTRs, the 5′ LTR is dominant and serves as the HIV promoter, although 3′ transcription is activated when the 5′ LTR is defective [141]. Transcriptional interference has been proposed as the mechanism by which the 5′ LTR exerts its dominance over the 3′ [142]. Interestingly, low-level antisense transcription takes place at the 3′ LTR, a mechanism by which latency can be maintained [143–147]. Sense transcription results in at least 40 coding transcripts due to alternative splicing of the HIV-1 genome [148]. Finally, both LTRs also act as a source of negative sense transcription, which could potentially affect the expression of neighboring genes [149,150].

4.7. The 5′ LTR contains numerous putative transcription factor binding sites

HIV-1 encodes a potent trans-activating protein – Tat – that drives viral expression during productive infection. However, initially, before sufficient levels of Tat are expressed, the provirus relies on host factors to initiate transcription. The 5′ LTR contains three regions – U3, R, and U5 (Figure 2) [151]. The R region, immediately next to the transcription start site (TSS), contains the trans-activation response (TAR) element, an important regulator of HIV expression. The U3 region contains the core promoter (nucleotides –78 to –1 upstream of TSS), a core enhancer (nucleotides –105 to –79), and a modulator region (nucleotides –454 to –104) [152,153]. The core promoter contains three Sp1 binding sites in tandem, a TATA box, and an initiator element at the transcription start site. The core enhancer contains two NF-kB-binding sites. The modulator region – so-called because early experiments with deletion upstream of the LTR caused increased activity of the LTR – was shown by later experiments to contain binding sites for both repressive and activating factors including nuclear factor of activated T-cells NFAT, STAT5, NF-kB p65/p50 heterodimers, lymphocyte enhancer factor (LEF-1), CCAAT/enhancer binding protein (C/EBP) factors, AP-1, and activating transcription factor/ cyclic AMP response element binding (ATF/CREB) factors (Figure 2) [152,154–162]. It is well established that these transcription factors have binding sites within HIV-1 sequence. Moreover, they are strong activators of HIV-1 transcription of which NF-κB is considered the most critical [163–166]. In addition to the presence of these sites, bioinformatic tools indicate that this region of the HIV LTR contains a tightly clustered distribution of multiple transcription factor consensus binding elements [167].

4.8. Positive host factors bind to the 5′ LTR

Initial transcription of HIV-1 is entirely dependent on host factors. Nuclear factor kappa-light-chain-enhancer of activated B cells (NF-kB) is a hetero dimer comprised of p50 and p65 subunits involved in T-cell activation. NF-kB acts as a transcription factor and is a potent activator of HIV-1 transcription initiation and elongation. It interacts and functions cooperatively with numerous proteins. Independent of Tat, NF-kB can reactivate HIV to high expression levels [168]. Mutated NF-kB-binding sites on the LTR inhibit basal transcription and Tat transactivation [169]. NF-kB, Sp1, and other factors (LEF-1, Ets1, and TFE-3) bind to sites near NF-kB sites and synergistically activate HIV transcription, even in the presence of repressive

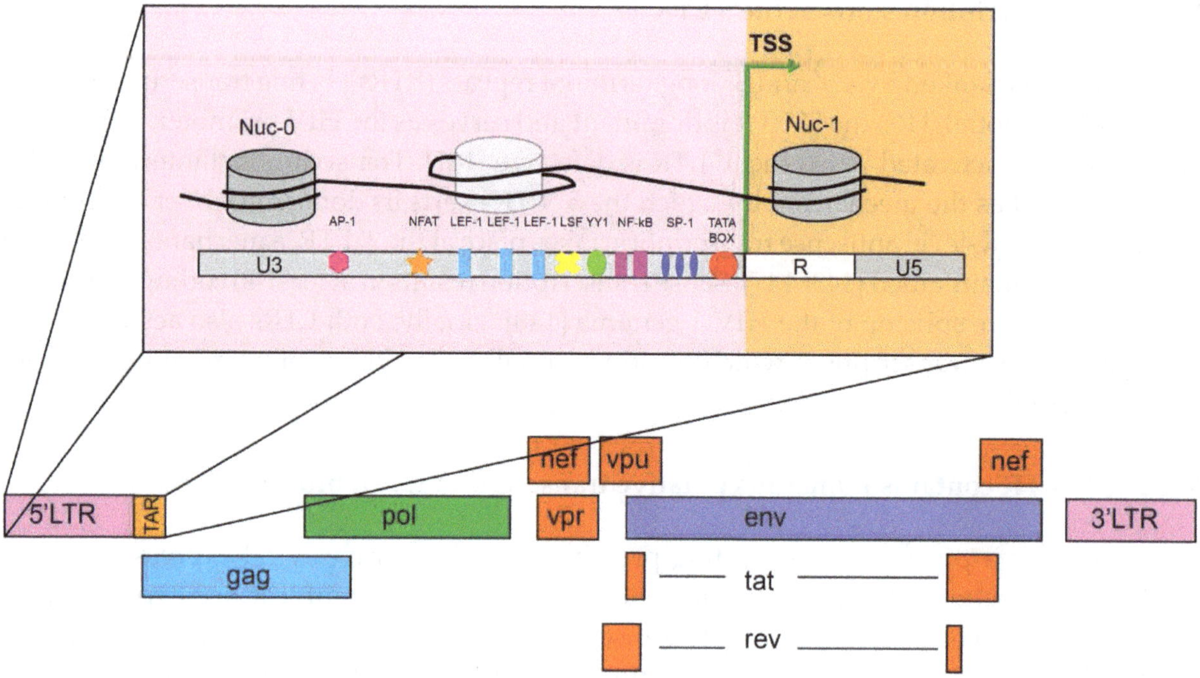

Figure 2. The genome of HIV-1

chromatin structures [170,171]. NF-kB and AP-1, a heterodimer of proteins from the c-Fos, c-Jun, ATF, and JDP families, cooperatively trans-activated LTR activity through the ERK1/ERK2 mitogen-activated protein kinase (MAPK) pathway [161]. Acetylation of Lys310 in NF-kB p65 subunit is an activating mark that is removed by NAD+-dependent protein deacetylases SIRT1 and SIRT2 [172]. Tat positively affects NF-kB by inhibiting SIRT1 and stimulating degradation of IkB, a protein that sequesters NF-kB in the cytoplasm [169,173]. The viral nucleocapsid (NC) protein enhances NF-kB-mediated activity by interacting with the LTR [174]. p65 recruits THIIH which is part of the preinitiation complex and its subunit CDK7 with kinase activity activates CDK9, resulting in increased HIV transcription [175,176]. The cell surface receptor OX40, bound by its ligand gp34, activates transcription from 5′ LTR, in a manner dependent on the presence of NF-kB-binding sites on the LTR [177]. The transcription factor E2F-1, a regulator of S-phase gene expression, inhibits LTR transcription through the recruitment of p50 at the NF-kB-binding sites on the LTR [178].

Members of the SV40-promoter (Sp) specific transcription factor family regulate LTR activity. Sp1 and Sp4 are activators of HIV-1 [179]. Expression of Sp transcription factors changes during monocytic maturation, suggesting differences in susceptibility to LTR activation during differentiation [180].

Nuclear factor of activated T-cells (NFAT) can induce LTR activity in T-cells [155]. NFAT recruits HATs through CBP/p300, which results in reactivation of HIV-1 transcription [181]. The Janus kinase (JAK)/signal transducers and activators of transcription (STAT5) can stimulate or inhibit HIV transcription. STAT5 binds to its binding sites in the U3 enhancer region on the LTR where it promotes transcription [156]. In response to a broad range of cytokines (e.g., IL-2, IL-7, IL-15) and granulocyte-macrophage colony-stimulating factor (GM-

CSF) JAK-mediated phosphorylation of a C-terminal tyrosine residue activates STAT5A and STAT5B. Homodimers or heterodimers of activated STAT5A and STAT5B translocate to the nucleus to stimulate HIV expression [182,183]. Interestingly, STAT5Δ, an isoform of STAT5 truncated on the C-terminus, acts as a repressor of LTR activity [184]. Indeed, in the promonocytic cell line U1 high levels of STAT5Δ are present. Upon stimulation with GM-CSF, STAT5Δ blocks RNAPII from binding to LTR U3 region, inhibiting activity of HIV promoter [185]. STAT5Δ promotes p50 homodimers binding to the LTR, contributing to latency maintenance [186].

In monocytes and macrophages, CCAAT/enhancer binding protein (C/EBP) factors are crucial for activation of HIV-1 [160,187–189]. C/EBP, a member of the bZIP superfamily, contains a DNA-binding domain and a leucine zipper for homo- and heterodimerizations. Similar to Sp-1, levels of C/EBP vary during myeloid development [190]. Interestingly, the HIV-1 LTR contains several C/EBP binding sites [159].

Some studies employing mutagenesis of binding sites for activator protein-1 (AP-1) within proviral genome showed that AP-1 transcription factor is the crucial activator of proviral transcription, as proviruses with altered AP-1-binding sites were less prone to reactivation even if treated with strong activator such as phorbol 12-myristate 13-acetate – PMA [191]. Furthermore, the latent pool was bigger in cells infected with a virus carrying a deletion in AP-1 sites, implicating that the AP-1 protein is necessary for successful provirus transcription [192]. Heterodimeric protein AP-1 is formed upon phosphorylation od c-Jun N-terminal kinase (JNK) in JNK/MAPK pathway [193]. It is well established that activation of TLR signaling induces nuclear localization of NF-kB and AP-1 mediated via JNK pathway [194–196].

In addition to the already mentioned host factors, the potent viral trans-activating protein Tat and to a lesser extent the multifunctional viral protein, viral protein R (Vpr), positively affect viral transcription. Productive infection requires the presence of Tat. Exogenous expression of Tat rescues HIV from latency [197]. A defective Tat mutant (C22G) is incapable of full-length viral expression [198]. Additionally, the Tat mutant (H13L) is more prone to establish latency [197]. Tat recruits the positive transcription elongation factor b (P-TEFb), which shifts RNAPII promoter proximal pausing to transcriptional elongation leading to a productive infection [199,200]. P-TEFb consists of CDK9, a serine/threonine kinase, and CyclinT1. The N-terminal cystein-rich region of Tat (Cy22-Cy37) binds to CycT1 through Zn2+-mediated interactions [201–203].

Vpr is a multifunctional HIV-1 protein that plays a role in nuclear import of the PIC and cell cycle arrest in proliferating cells. Vpr also activates LTR activity through multiple mechanisms. Vpr recruits p300 to the 5′ LTR increasing acetylation, resulting in HIV-1 transcription [204]. Moreover, Vpr interacts with Sp1 and TFIIB, part of the transcription initiation complex, stimulating proviral transcription [204–206].

4.9. Repressive host factors at the 5′ LTR

Not all host transcription factors have an activating effect on LTR activity (Figure 3). YY1 and LSF recognize binding sequences in the LTR and repress transcription through epigenetic modification [207]. C-promoter binding factor-1 (CBF-1) also represses HIV through epigenetic silencing [208,209]. c-Myc recruits an epigenetic silencing factor to repress HIV-1 [210].

Transcription factors initiate LTR activity, but full-length transcripts are not produced because transcription elongation is inhibited. DRB sensitivity-inducing factor (DSIF), a heterodimer composed of hSpt4 and hSpt5 proteins, induces capping of RNA from newly initiated transcription complexes [211]. The subunit hSpt5 interacts directly with nascent RNA as it appears from the RNAPII exit site and recruits negative elongation factor (NELF) (Figure 3) [212–214]. Escape of transcripts from the promoter proximal pause site is prevented by NELF, which induces termination of transcription over several hundred bases [215]. Moreover, the binding sequence of NELF subunit E recognizes a homologous sequence on TAR, increasing association of NELF with the LTR, which results in transcription silencing. Indeed, experiments where NELF is knocked down show higher basal HIV transcription and reactivation from latency [216–218].

A novel, RNA interference independent, mechanism mediated by microprocessor and termination factors causes transcriptional silencing and chromatin remodeling at the HIV-1 promoter [219]. Microprocessor binds to TAR, which is then cleaved by Drosha into two RNAs, a 5′-end and 3′-end product. The 5′ is further processed in an Rrp6-dependent manner into a transcription repressing RNA species. The 3′ RNA recruits termination factor Xrn2 and Setx, which induces RNAPII pausing and premature termination of transcription [219].

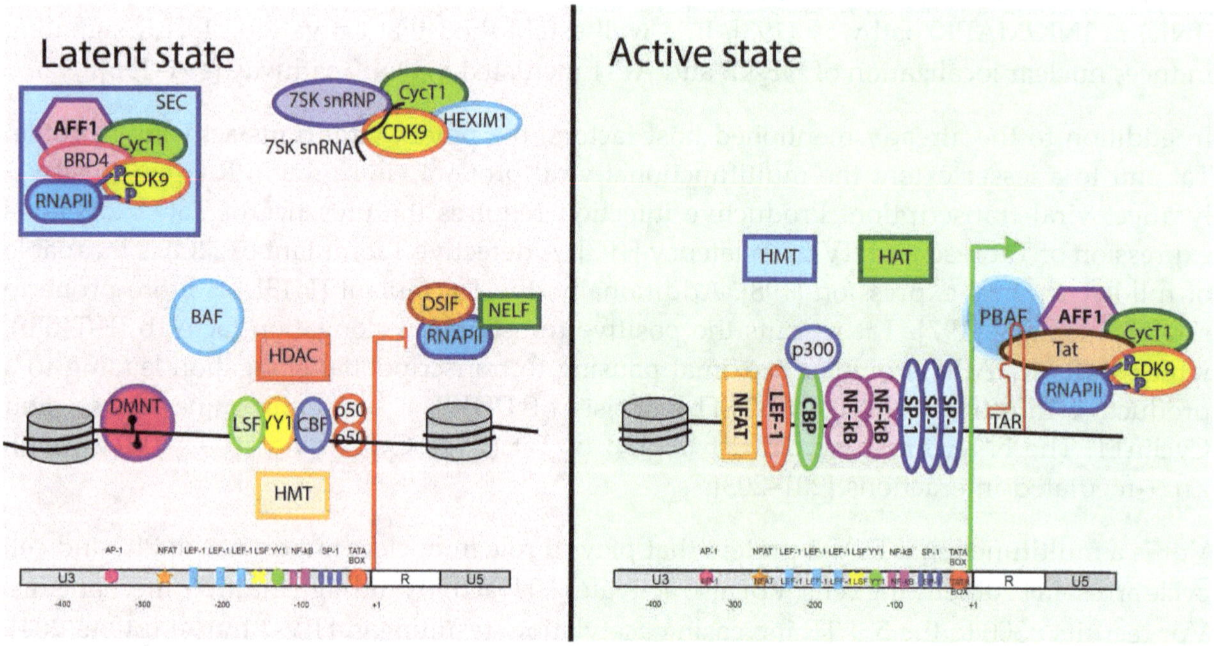

Figure 3. Molecular mechanisms in latent and productive HIV-1 infection

4.10. Host factors induce transcriptional initiation, but not elongation

While some host transcription factors recruit RNAPII, in the absence of Tat, transcription elongation does not occur resulting in the generation of short abortive transcripts by promoter proximal pausing [220,221]. These ~60nt transcripts include TAR, which has a stem-loop structure and binds near the HIV 5′LTR, inhibiting RNA-polymerase. TAR directly binds Tat, which recruits transcriptional elongation complex to the LTR [222].

4.11. Tat-dependent transcription leads to productive infection

If cells become activated or due to leaky transcription, Tat can be produced. Tat binding to P-TEFb induces significant conformational changes in P-TEFb, allowing Tat and CycT1 to cooperatively recognize and stably bind TAR [200,223].

Tat-P-TEFb phosphorylates NELF-E resulting in the dissociation of NELF from TAR and the paused RNAPII complex [214,216,218,224]. CDK9 phosphorylates RNAPII at the carboxyl terminal domain (CTD) at Ser2 and Ser5 residues of the 52 heptad repeats, which regulates progression to the elongation phase of transcription [225–227]. The phosphorylation status determines regular and alternative RNA splicing and the 3′ end recruitment of polyadenylation factors [228,229]. Ser2 phosphorylation of the RNAPII CTD recruits splicing-associated c-Ski-interacting protein, SKIP, and stimulates elongation transcription and alternative splicing of the Tat-specific splice site through interactions with U5snRNP proteins and tri-snRNP110K [230].

Phosphorylation of hSpt5, a subunit of DSIF, by CDK9 converts it into a positive elongation factor that prevents nascent RNA from breaking of from the transcription complex prematurely and inhibits pausing of RNAPII at arrest sites [231,232]. By removing several blocks Tat-P-TEFb induces transcriptional elongation as well as co-transcriptional processing. During active transcription elongation, increased recruitment of RNAPII to TSS maintains a stable level of RNAPII at the promoter proximal region [218]. Throughout transcription, Tat-P-TEFb remains associated with the elongating transcription machinery [231,233,234].

4.12. P-TEFb can be recruited in active and inactive form in the nucleus by Tat

In activated T-cells, inactive P-TEFb predominantly resides in the 7SK small nuclear ribonucleoprotein (snRNP) complex (Figure 3) [235–237]. The 7SK snRNP complex consists of 7SK snRNA, HEXIM1 (or its homolog HEXIM2), the La-related protein 7 (LARP7), and the 7SK-specific 5′ methylphosphate capping enzyme (MePCE). The snRNA functions as a scaffold: it binds two units of P-TEFb and one HEXIM1/2 homo-/heterodimers [238,239]. MePCE and LARP7 protect the 7SK RNA from nuclease degradation, MePCE binds the 5′ end, LARP7 the polyuridine 3′ end [240–242]. Tat disrupts the interaction between pTEFb and HEXIM1/7SK snRNA and recruits P-TEFb to 5′ LTR, resulting in active transcription [226].

BRD4 can also recruit P-TEFb from 7SK snRNP [241,243], to promote transcription. Due to similarities in their C-terminal P-TEFb interacting domains [244], Tat and BRD4 compete for P-TEFb [245,246]. In a latent model, knockdown of BRD4 results in Tat-dependent reactivation of HIV-1 [247].

Bromodomain and extra-terminal domain family of proteins (BET) play an important role in repression of the HIV-1 transcription. BET proteins are responsible for the recruitment of P-

TEFb to transcribed genes [246,248]. BRD4 competes with viral protein Tat for binding site on pTEFb, and it represses HIV-1 transcription [245,246]. Knockdown of BRD2 indicates this protein contributes to the maintenance of latency. These results are consistent with the notion that BRD2 is binding to remodeling factors such as HDACs [249,250].

P-TEFb can be recruited to transcription complexes by other factors. CTIP2 recruits P-TEFb by binding HEXIM1 and negatively regulates the complex by repressing the CDK9 kinase activity of P-TEFb [251]. Phosphorylation of HEXIM1 at Tyr271 and Tyr 274 decreases retention of P-TEFb in the 7SK RNP [252]. Additionally, through the binding of nascent RNA, SRSF2 and P-TEFb are released from the 7SK complex and induce transcription elongation in a manner similar to TAR/Tat-mediated recruitment of P-TEFb [253].

4.13. P-TEFb is a subunit of the super elongation complex

P-TEFb is required for activation of HIV transcription but does not explain the maximum observed viral expression; therefore, additional factors are necessary [254,255]. P-TEFb is an integral part of the super elongation complex (SEC) (Figure 3), which is a potent activator of transcriptional elongation of host genes [234,256]. It is composed of one of two scaffold proteins, AF4/FMR2 proteins AFF1 or AFF4. Translocations of AFF1 and AFF4 resulting in fusion proteins are commonly found in mixed lineage leukemia (MLL) [257–259]. The resultant fusion proteins cause aberrant recruitment of SEC to MML-specific genes [260]. AFF1 and AFF4 recruit many other proteins to the SEC [261], such as ELL family of elongation stimulatory factors ELL1 and ELL2, which inhibit RNAPII pausing and synergistically improve Tat-transactivation with P-TEFb [256]. Moreover, knockdown of ELL2 strongly suppresses viral expression. [203,210,230,252]. Tat and AFF4 inhibit the polyubiquitination-mediated degradation of ELL2, increasing available levels of SEC. [256,262].

4.14. Tat can be extensively post-translationally modified – "Tat code"

Modifications on numerous amino residues of Tat regulate the interaction with a wide variety of host proteins. In comparison to the histone code which is used to explain the multiple modification on histone tails and their function, a "Tat-code" has been proposed [34]. Tat is phosphorylated on Ser16 and Ser 46 by CDK2, modifications which result in transcription inhibition [263]. Acetylation of Lys28 increases affinity for P-TEFb binding and is removed by HDAC6 [264–266]. Tat dissociates from TAR and binds acetyltransferase PCAF which acetylates Tat at Lys50 and Lys51 [264,265,267–270]. Acetylated Lys50 allows recruitment of the PBAF (SWI/SNF B) chromatin remodeling complex to the LTR [267,271–273]. SIRT1 deacetylates Tat at Lys50 as part of a late phase of transcriptional regulation, striping Tat of acetyl groups allowing its reuse in subsequent rounds of transcriptional cycles [274]. Mono-methyl-transferase Set7/9 and LSD1, respectively, methylate and demethylate Lys51. Demethylated Lys51 of Tat enhances HIV-1 transcription [275,276]. Hdm2 polyubiquitinates Lys71, activating Tat [277].

4.15. Nucleosome positioning at the 5′ LTR controls viral expression

Regardless of integration position, the latent 5′ LTR typically contains two nucleosomes, Nuc-0 and Nuc-1, at fixed positions [278]. Nuc-1 blocks transcription elongation as it is positioned just downstream of the TSS. Nuc-1 is displaced upon virus reactivation [278–280]. Nucleosomes can be altered by chromatin remodeling complexes. A third unstable or loosely positioned nucleosome is located in between nuc-0 and nuc-1 [281] (Figures 2 and 3A).

BCL11B, together with the chromatin remodeling complex NuRD, strongly represses HIV-1 transcription [282]. BCL11B is specifically expressed in T-cells and neurons. Interestingly, the NuRD complex consists of several proteins with histone deacetylase activities – i.e., HDAC1 and HDAC2 [283,284].

The ATP-dependent chromatin remodeler BAF (SWI/SNF-A) was discovered by our group to be essential to both the establishment and maintenance of HIV latency (Figure 3). The BAF complex utilizes energy from ATP to push Nuc-1 from an energetically favorable position upstream of the TSS to a suboptimal region, downstream of TSS, resulting in a transcriptional block [281]. siRNA depletion of the BAF complex de-repressed proviral transcription. Furthermore, in siRNA-mediated BAF knockdown, latency establishment occurred less frequently than in the presence of the functional complex. The PIC through LEDGF interacts with INI-1 a subunit of BAF, allowing nucleosomes to be deposited at the provirus, contributing to latency establishment [118].

4.16. Epigenetic modifications regulate latency

Epigenetic modifications of nucleosomes such as histone-acetylation and -methylation and of DNA such as DNA-methylation play an important role in regulating the proviral transcription. Nucleosomes are the basic units of organization of chromatin and consist of a combination of histone subunits. Histones have an amino acids tail that can be extensively modified. Two broadly studied modifications that regulate expression effects are histone-acetylation and histone-methylation

Histone-acetylation by histone acetyl transferases (HATs) induces chromatin loosening, while histone deacetylases (HDACs) reverse the effect by removing the acetyl group (Figure 3). HATs such as p300/CREB-binding protein (p300/CBP) and p300/CBP-associated factor (P/CAF) can be recruited to activate the HIV LTR [158,285]. HDAC1, HDAC2, HDAC3, and HDAC6 repress HIV [286–289]. Numerous host factors recruit HDACs to the LTR. A negative regulator of P-TEFb, CTIP2 in cooperation with COUP-TF and Sp1 also recruits HDAC1 and HDAC2 to the HIV LTR in microglial cells [290,291]. Host factors LSF and YY1 co-operatively bind to the LTR, where YY1 recruits HDAC1 to deacetylate Nuc-1[207]. CBF-1 and c-Myc also repress HIV through the recruitment of HDAC1 [208–210].

Methylation of histones by histone methyltransferases (HMT) can act as an activating or repressing mark depending on the histone tail residue modified (e.g., methylation of lysine 4 on histone 3 (H3K4) is activating whereas H3K9, H3K27, and H4K20 methylation is repressive). HMTs modify specific histone residues, e.g., EZH2 (H3K27me3), SUV39H1 (H3K9me3), G9a (H3K9me2), and G9a like protein, GLP (H3K9me2). The repressive methyl groups deposited by these HMTs contribute to the maintenance of latency [292–295]. Moreover, EZH2 is suspected to recruit additional repressive proteins such as HDACs and other HMTs [294].

DNA methylation at CpG dinucleotides represses transcription by disrupting the binding of transcription activators to their binding sites or indirectly through the binding methyl-CpG binding proteins (MeCPs). In cell line models of latency, the HIV-1 LTR contains two CpG islands that are hypermethylated (Figure 3) [296]. Methyl-CpG binding domain protein 2 (MDB2) and HDAC-2 bind to the second CpG island on the HIV LTR and are displaced from there when cells are treated with cytosine-methylation inihibitor 5-aza-2′deoxycytidine [296]. In memory CD4+ T-cells from long-term aviremic and viremic patients, an increase in HIV LTR DNA methylation was observed in the aviremic patients [297]. The methylation of the HIV LTR in long-term non-progressors and elite controllers is increased compared to the LTR of aviremic patients on cART [298]. In contrast, this difference was not found in the first CpG island of resting memory CD4+ T-cells from aviremic patients, indicating that the mechanism by which DNA-methylation regulates latency deserves further exploration.

4.17. Viral and host non-coding RNAs regulate viral expression

Non-coding RNAs exert post transcriptional control on gene expression. Small non-coding RNAs (<200 nt) and in particular microRNAs (miRNAs) are well established to have regulatory function. The study of long non-coding RNAs (lncRNA, >200 nt) is an emerging field because of their epigenetic regulatory potential. Both viral and host miRNAs and lncRNAs affect replication of HIV-1 [146,299–301].

RNA interference (RNAi) is a post-transcriptional gene silencing mechanism. miRNAs post-transcriptionally suppress or silence gene expression as part of the RNA-induced silencing complex (RISC) forming a protein–RNA complex. Pri-miRNAs are generated by RNAPII and are subsequently processed by microprocessor into pre-miRNAs in the nucleus. Following export to the cytoplasm, they are cleaved by Dicer and incorporated into RISC. RISC generally binds in the 3′-untranslated region (3′UTR) of a target mRNA. The bound transcript is degraded or transcription is impeded depending on the level of homology, resulting in translational repression. The RNAi affects the infectivity of monocytes and macrophages [302]. Comparisons of productively infected, suppressed, and uninfected patients found difference in miRNA profiles, but it is very unlikely that the observed effects are due to viral activity because the number of infected cells is low in elite controllers or under cART [303–305]. Knockdown of Dicer or Drosha, a component of microprocessor, stimulates HIV-1 replication, indicating that miRNA generally are responsible for suppression of proviral transcription [299,300]. However, phenotypic effects are hard to interpret due to the pleiotropic side effects of microprocessor depletion. RNAi affects infectivity by targeting transcripts of key host factors and viral proteins involved in HIV-1 repression. In resting T-cells, the polycistronic miRNA cluster miR-17/92 is suppressed by HIV, resulting in PCAF upregulation [299]. Additionally, CycT1 is negatively regulated by miR27b [306]. Moreover, during differentiation from monocytes to macrophages, expression of miRNA198 and miR27b decreases relieving suppression of CycT1 [307,308]. In infected cells Tat, and possibly Vpr, inhibit RNAi [309–311]. In resting, but not activated, CD4+ T-cells a cluster of five miRNAs (miR-28, miR-125b, miR-150, miR-223, and miR-382) were found to be upregulated. They all target viral mRNAs for degradation; therefore, these miRNAs are contributing to latency maintenance [312]. However, further studies are required as results thus far are inconsistent [313–319].

The viral protein Nef is targeted by miR29a which interferes with HIV replication [300,320]. TRIM32 activates HIV-1 expression through the NF-kB pathway and is downregulated by miRNA-155 [321]. Tat-induced upregulation of miR34a and miR217 inhibits SIRT1 expression, which in turn results in high abundance of NF-kB, enhancing proviral transcription [322,323]. miRNA-182 has a positive effect on LTR activation by Tat [324]. miR-1236 restricts viral replication by repressing Vpr (HIV-1)-binding protein expression, VprBP [325].

HIV-1-derived miRNAs (vmiRNAs) were predicted *in silico* [326]. Applying deep sequencing technologies vmiRNAs were observed in cell line model systems of latency [327,328]. The TAR-derived miRNA-TAR5p and miR-TAR3p are asymmetrically processed and both repress LTR activity [329]. The *Nef*-derived miR-N367 inhibits viral promotor activity [330]. Nevertheless, relevance of vmiRNAs is debatable as no vmiRNAs were detected in PBMCs or macrophages of infected patients [331].

lncRNAs can modulate gene expression through different proposed mechanisms: (1) affecting mRNAs through sequence recognition, (2) recruiting proteins to DNA, (3) blocking host factors by assuming a secondary structure, (4) functioning as a scaffold for protein complexes. An anti-sense lncRNA of HIV-1 inhibits viral replication[146]. The non-coding repressor of NFAT (NRON) inhibits LTR activity in a NFAT-dependent manner [301].

4.18. Stochastic gene expression

The current model of HIV latency proposes that resting memory CD4+ T-cells are deprived of host factors that are necessary for viral expression. An alternative model proposes that expression is highly stochastic. Due to fluctuations in chromatin state and availability of the transcription factors, the latent and productive state co-exist [332]. In support, clonal lines (containing the same integration) showed binominal distributions of viral expression [333]. Transcriptional bursts of 2–10 mRNA transcripts were estimated to be the source of HIV-1 gene expression [334]. Tat-controlled positive feedback extends the expression reactivation [335]. The sensitivity to reactivation is also stochastic, as cells derived from patients remained latent during a first round of activation and were reactivatable in the next round of activation [83]. Moreover, molecules that increase gene expression fluctuations synergistically enhance HIV-1 reactivation [336].

5. HIV cure

Mechanistic insight into the complex nature of latent HIV-1 infection provides a rationale for eradication strategies. Therefore, identification of molecules that inhibit activity of repressors or potentiate HIV-1 activators alongside with immune system boosting are important objectives in eradication strategies.

5.1. Shocking the virus: screening for Latency Reversal Agents (LRAs)

The initial step of LRA discovery is screening drug libraries with cell-line-based models. Positive hits are evaluated further using primary-cell-based models as they better recapitulate the nature of latent reservoirs. If effective and not toxic, putative LRAs should undergo reactivation studies using primary cells derived from HIV-1-positive individuals that are on cART as well as toxicology studies in animal models, in case of novel molecules. It is advantageous to include molecules that are already approved drugs in such putative LRAs libraries, employing them into clinical practice would be time and resources effective. Moreover, in order to easily diffuse through cell membranes, ideal LRAs are small molecules, with molecular weight below 900 daltons, although clinical practice shows that most effective compounds do not exceed 500 daltons [337,338].

The first attempts to reactivate proviral DNA failed, due to the use of agents (e.g., IL-2 or a monoclonal antibody against CD3 receptor) which resulted in global T-cell activation. Indeed, viral p24 and plasma HIV-1 RNA levels increased, but the toxicity of such treatment left this approach useless [339–341]. Therefore, there is a need for more specific agents, which are able to reactivate proviral transcription without T-cell activation.

5.2. HDAC inhibitors (HDACis)

Histone deacetylase inhibitors (HDACis) are a very promising class of LRAs which include valporic acid (VPA), Vorinostat (SAHA), Romidepsin, Panobinostat, Givinostat, Droxinostat, or Entinostat. Some (Vorinostat (SAHA), Romidepsin, Panobinostat) are undergoing clinical trials [94,342–344].

The focus on HDACis is due to their ability to loosen up the compact chromatin structure at the latent proviral promoter. Inhibition of HDACs results in an increase of histone acetylation level by HATs. HDACs 1, 2, and 3 are of particular interest as they considerably contribute to HIV-1 repression [287]. Fortunately, HDACis are already used in clinical therapies, e.g., VPA is used in epilepsy and bipolar disorders, Vorinostat and Romidepsin are used to treat cutaneous T-cell lymphoma (CTCL) while Panabinostat is used in patients with multiple myeloma. In a very promising study by Archin et al., a single treatment with Vorinostat resulted in an increase in proviral RNA [345]. Unfortunately, the follow-up study with additional, multiple-dose rounds of treatment showed that increase on HIV-1 transcription is neither sustained nor elevated [346]. It is possible that other mechanisms maintaining latency compensate histone acetylation, in order to restrain proviral transcription. Alternatively such low concentrations of Vorinostat result in activation of pTEF-b instead of HDAC inhibition [347]. Since HDACs are involved in general regulation of gene expression; they have pleiotropic effects causing toxicities. Therefore, their use must be strictly controlled and monitored in order to provide maximal safety [348]. Nevertheless, HDACis are still under much interest. Especially, finding more specific HDAC inhibitors is very appealing, as current drugs are inhibiting a wide range of different HDACs, contributing to high toxicity [349].

5.3. BET inhibitors (BETi's)

Since BET proteins repress the HIV-1 promoter, it is worth to use their inhibitors in latency reversal strategies. Treatment with BET protein inhibitor JQ1 reactivates HIV-1 transcription in Tat-independent fashion [247]. Furthermore, BET inhibitor activity was positively tested in more relevant primary model system of latency [249]. Unfortunately, JQ-1 is not clinically available, due to its short half-life.

5.4. HMT inhibitors (HMTis)

Several histone methyltransferases (HMTs) such as EZH2, SUV39H1, and G9a interact with 5′ LTR contributing to maintenance of latency by deposition of repressive methyl groups on nucleosomal proteins [292–295]. Moreover, EZH2 recruits additional repressive proteins such as HDACs and other HMTs [294]. Several inhibitors of these proteins were tested in cell lines or primary cells from HIV-1 positive patients. Among which, Chaetocin (SUV39H1 inhibitor) and BIX-01294 (G9a inhibitor) were most potent [292,350]. However, high toxicity, due to pleiotropic effects, makes them unsuitable for clinical practice. Therefore, identification of novel compounds that are able to inhibit the activity of HMTs is needed.

5.5. DNMT inhibitors (DNMTis)

Inhibition of DNA methyltransferases (DNMTs) with 5-aza-2′ deoxycytidine (aza-CdR or Decitabine) leads to modest reactivation of latent HIV-1. This activity can be further enhanced with PKC agonists [351]. However, 5′ LTR methylation in patients material remains controversial [352]. Thus, further investigation of provirus methylation *in vivo* is needed.

5.6. Toll-like receptors (TLRs) stimulation

TLRs recently gained more attention, as theirs agonists are strong reactivators of HIV-1 [353–357]. The main role of these receptors is to activate an immune response against bacterial or viral infections [358]. Stimulating TLRs (as adjuvants in immunization) as well as opportunistic bacterial infections elevate plasma HIV-RNA and improve immune function [359–363].

Vaccine adjuvant – CPG 7909 (TLR 9 agonist) is able to decrease plasma HIV-1 RNA via activation of HIV-specific CD8+ T-cells in peripheral blood [359]. More recently, in SIV-positive rhesus monkeys undergoing cART were treated with GS-9620, a TLR7 agonist, reversible CD8 cytotoxic T-cells activation alongside with modest CD4 T-cell activation were observed. Moreover, elevated plasma viremia was observed as well as decrease in HIV-1 DNA in blood, colon, and lymph nodes. Interestingly, viral load returned back to undetectable levels when GS-9620 was no longer administrated. More strikingly, when cART was stopped, GS-9620-treated monkeys had 0.5 log lower viral set-point than untreated, infected animals. Additionally, in cells isolated from HIV-positive individuals transcription of HIV-1 was observed. However, some variability between samples was noticed. Clinical trials with the use of this compound are planned [364,365].

5.7. Super elongation complex stimulation

Treatment of cell lines and cells isolated from aviremic patients on cART with hexamethylene bisacetamide (HMBA), an anticancer drug that transiently activates PI3K/Akt pathway, results in phosphorylation of HEXIM1. P-TEFb is subsequently released and interacts with RNAP II, resulting in latency reversal [366–368]. Moreover, HMBA provides CDK9 recruitment to the viral promoter by interaction with SP1, which enhances transcription from proviral DNA. Furthermore, Klichko et al. showed that treatment with HMBA resulted in a decrease of CD4 receptor expression without affecting transcription of CCR5 and CXCR4 co-receptors [369]. Moreover, HMBA does not trigger activation of T-cells. Studies on P-TEFb's role in HIV-1 latency indicate that this heterocomplex might be an interesting target for inclusion in "shock and kill" therapies.

5.8. PKC pathway activation

Another interesting approach is the use of molecules that are able to selectively activate the protein kinase C (PKC) pathway. PKC pathway agonists trigger nuclear localization of NF-kB, NFAT, and AP-1 transcription factors. Therefore, PKC agonists are one of the most potent activators of HIV-1 transcription. Currently, two PKC agonists are being scrutinized clinically: prostratin and bryostatin, due to their safety and specificity toward HIV-1 reactivation. The latter is a clinically available drug [370]. Moreover, these two compounds prevent *de novo* infections, as they downregulate viral receptor and co-receptors CD4, CCR5 and CXCR4 in PBMCs [371]. A rather controversial molecule that reactivates HIV-1 transcription via NF-κB pathway is arsenic trioxide (As_2O_3). In the Jurkat model system of latency, As_2O_3 activates NF-κB leading to HIV-1 replication. Moreover, it synergizes with prostratin, tumor necrosis factor alpha (TNFα), and VPA [372]. Interestingly, arsenic is already used in clinical practice to treat acute promyelocytic leukemia (APL). Therefore, it would be interesting to test this compound in more relevant models of HIV-1 latency such as primary cells infected *ex vivo* and in cells derived from aviremic patients.

The use of PKC agonists raises concerns about their safety in a clinical setting. The protein kinase enzyme family consists of several isoenzymes that play important roles in signal transduction cascades [373]. As activation of latent HIV-1 is mediated via PKCα and PKCθ, the identification of more specific agonists of PKCα and PKCθ is needed. Alternatively, lowering the concentration of a specific agonists might decrease toxicity and contribute to latency reversal [374].

5.9. JNK/MAPK pathway activation

Studies employing mutagenesis of binding sites for activator protein-1 (AP-1) within the proviral genome showed that the AP-1 transcription factor is a crucial activator of proviral transcription, as proviruses with altered AP-1 binding sites were less prone to reactivation even if treated with a strong activator such as phorbol 12-myristate 13-acetate – PMA [191]. Furthermore, the latent pool of cells infected by virus with deletion in AP-1 sites was bigger, implicating that AP-1 is necessary for provirus transcription [192]. Heterodimeric protein AP-1 is formed upon phosphorylation of c-Jun N-terminal kinase (JNK) in JNK/MAPK pathway [193]. It is well established that activation of TLR signaling induces nuclear localization of NF-kB and AP-1 mediated via JNK pathway [194,196,376,377].

Virtual screening followed by validation of positive hits in cell line model systems for HIV-1 latency discovered 8-methoxy-6-methylquinolin-4-ol (MMQO) as a specific activator of the JNK-AP-1 pathway, which is able to reactivate HIV-1 from its latent state. Interestingly, MMQO inhibits IL-2 and TNFa expression, contributing to maintenance of resting state of CD4+ T-cells [378]. The recently synthetized panel of inhibitors of farnesyl transferase (FTase) are able to moderately reactivate HIV-1 transcription via JNK pathway. Interestingly, strong synergy with other LRAs, such as Vorinostat or TNF-a, was observed for these molecules in latency reversal [379,380].

5.10. Canonical Wnt signaling pathway activation

Recently, our group showed that treatment with Wnt3A/Rsp (natural stimulators of Wnt pathway) and lithium (inhibitor of Wnt repressor protein GSK3) leads to latency reversal in latent cell lines and enhances the latency reversal potential of HDAC inhibitors in CD4+ T primary cells obtained from patient volunteers when co-treated [381]. This observation shows a functional role for three LEF1 binding sites in the 5′ LTR contains, which are downstream targets of the classical Wnt pathway [381,382]. It would be very interesting to find more potent and selective inducers of Wnt pathway, as lithium exhibits many pleiotropic, toxic effects [383,384].

5.11. Chromatin loosening

It was discovered by our group that a main player in the establishment and maintenance of latency is the BAF complex (SWI/SNF-A), which belongs to ATP-dependent chromatin remodelers' family. Interestingly, Dykhuizen et al. [378] screened a library of compounds that would be able to mimic BRG-1 knock out. In their study, they found 20 compounds that were transcriptionally mimicking BAF complex disruption. We showed that several of those molecules were able to decrease the frequency of latency establishment and reactivate HIV-1 in cell line and primary cells models of latency [386, in press]. Moreover, they synergize with other LRAs – SAHA and prostratin. Two most potent inhibitors – caffeic acid phenethyl ester (CAPE) and pyrimethamine (PYR) did not activate T-cells derived from healthy donors and cells obtained from aviremic patients. Moreover, PYR is a registered drug used in malaria treatment. Therefore, these inhibitors are promising molecules to include in eradication strategies.

5.12. Multifunctional LRAs

In vitro treatment with cocaine leads to increase in HIV- replication in PBMCs as well as increased viral load in mouse models of HIV infection [387–389]. Interestingly, in *ex vivo* infected primary CD4+ cocaine treatment resulted in downregulation of miR125-b expression, which led to enhanced replication of HIV-1 [314]. In primary human macrophages and myeloid cell systems of latency, cocaine increased replication of HIV-1. Cocaine treatment activates NF-κB and leads to phosphorylation of mitogen- and stress-activated kinase 1 (MSK1). Furthermore, pMSK1 phosphorylates RELA (p65), a subunit of NF-κB promoting the interaction of NF-κB with p300 and recruitment of P-TEFb to the proviral 5′ LTR [390]. Moreover, treatment with cocaine results in histone H3 phosphorylation, thus increasing accessibility of HIV-1 promoter for transcription factors [390]. Therefore, cocaine not only reverses latency via NF-κB pathway but also causes epigenetic changes on 5′ LTR as well as blocks repressive miRNA.

Oral bacteria secrete short-chain fatty acids (SCFAs) including butyric acid, propionic acid, isovaleric acid, and isobutyric acid that are capable of HIV-1 and herpesviruses latency reversal [384,385]. Some of these molecules are known HDACis (e.g. Butyric acid) [393]. Moreover, SCFAs not only promotes histone acetylation, but also inhibit repressive histone formation and DNA methylation. Furthermore, they activate P-TEFb resulting in increased elongation of transcription from 5′ LTR. [345,385,386].

5.13. Immune clearance of reactivated cells – "Kill"

The majority of chronic patients are facing immune exhaustion, characterized by low cytokine secretion, smaller proliferative capacity, and low cytopathic potential of CD8+ T-cells [394,395]. Therefore, the first line of action would be reviving normal immune activity. Indeed, inhibition of programmed cell death protein 1 (PD-1) leads to restoration of immune functions in mouse models of HIV-1 infection [396]. However, these results were obtained in viremic animals. Nevertheless, an IgG4 antibody targeting PD-1 receptor is undergoing clinical trials to assess safety, immunotherapeutic activity, and the ability of treatment to reduce pool of latently infected cells [397].

In so-called "elite controllers", CD8+ T-cells effectively restrain infection without intervention of cART, by killing CD4+ T-cells that are actively producing HIV-1 particles [398,399]. The immune system can be boosted by specific amplification of HIV-1-specific CD8+ T-cells. These observations again aroused the idea of developing a vaccine. Indeed, rhesus monkeys vaccinated with CMV vectors resulted in broad cellular immune response to SIV [400–402]. However, safety issues related to the use of such vectors remain to be elucidated. Another platform being investigated to increase immune response against HIV-1 are Ad26 vectors, as it was shown that vaccinated rhesus monkeys were protected against infection with SIV as well as viral loads were lowered after vaccination [403,404].

A very interesting group of immunoglobulins to include in eradication strategies are broadly neutralizing monoclonal antibodies (mAbs or bNAbs) isolated from chronically infected patients. New generations of bNAbs exert higher potency and wider range of activity against many HIV-1 subtypes. It was shown that a combination of bNAbs is potent enough to transiently suppress viremia in rhesus monkeys as well as to reduce the amount of HIV-1 DNA in the blood, lymph nodes, and gastrointestinal mucosa [403,405,406].

6. Future perspectives and challenges

A reservoir of latent HIV is the main obstacle in finding a functional and sterilizing cure. Several challenges need to be addressed in order to overcome this obstacle. Defining the latent reservoir is impeded by the rare occurrence of a latent infection in a high background of defective proviral integration. Although HIV prefers integration in or near transcriptionally active genes which leaves ample room for variation in chromatin environment and available host transcription factors. This puts considerable demands on LRAs. LRAs should be effective, yet specific, without being toxic. As LRAs act via pathways involved in distinct cellular processes, pleiotropic effects are to be expected. Furthermore, recent studies on material obtained from HIV-1-positive suppressed patients revealed that currently available LRAs are not strong enough to reactivate the whole pool of latent proviruses, even after multiple rounds of stimulation. One of the concerns arising from "shock and kill" therapy is whether putative LRAs are strong enough to drive virus production to a level at which the immune system will be able to recognize and destroy HIV-1-producing cells. Indeed, trials aiming at testing HDAC inhibitors are inconsistent in showing depletion of latently infected cells while showing increased proviral transcription [407–412]. A complementary strategy would be to use multiple LRAs in combination to broadly and potentially synergistically reactivate the diversely integrated latent proviruses. Synergism between LRAs was already identified, e.g., Vorinostat and Prostratin [84]. Therefore, the quest for identification and characterization of novel compounds which are able to reactivate HIV-1 transcription as well as identifying combinations of drugs that can synergize to reverse latency is needed. Currently, no cell model is able to recapitulate the complexities of latency *in vivo*. A better system that more closely resembles the *in vivo* situation would greatly aid the understanding of molecular mechanisms underlying latency and the screening of new LRA. Moreover, as HIV-1 persists in a silent state, it contributes to a low level of inflammation, which over time leads to immune exhaustion. Furthermore, depletion of cells harboring latent provirus requires antigen-specific CTLs stimulation [399]. Most likely successful eradication therapies will be based on the combination of LRAs coupled with boosting HIV-1-specific immune response. A "shock and kill" approach in combination with immune therapies provides hope for reversing HIV-1 infection.

Author details

Michael D. Röling[#], Mateusz Stoszko[#], Tokameh Mahmoudi[*]

*Address all correspondence to: t.mahmoudi@erasmusmc.nl

Department of Biochemistry, Erasmus Medical Centre, Rottrerdam, The Netherlands

[#]These authors contributed equally to this work.

References

[1] Carpenter CCJ, Fischl MA, Hammer SM, Hirsch MS, Jacobsen DM, Katzenstein DA, et al. Antiretroviral Therapy for HIV Infection in 1998. JAMA. American Medical Association; 1998;280:78.

[2] Dinoso JB, Kim SY, Wiegand AM, Palmer SE, Gange SJ, Cranmer L, et al. Treatment intensification does not reduce residual HIV-1 viremia in patients on highly active antiretroviral therapy. Proc. Natl. Acad. Sci. U. S. A. 2009;106:9403–8.

[3] Davey RT, Bhat N, Yoder C, Chun TW, Metcalf JA, Dewar R, et al. HIV-1 and T cell dynamics after interruption of highly active antiretroviral therapy (HAART) in patients with a history of sustained viral suppression. Proc. Natl. Acad. Sci. U. S. A. 1999;96(26):15109-14.

[4] (WHO) WHO. WHO | Data and statistics [Internet]. World Health Organization; 2014 [cited 2015 Jul 29]. Available from: http://www.who.int/hiv/data/en/

[5] Pau AK, George JM. Antiretroviral Therapy. Infect. Dis. Clin. North Am. Elsevier Inc; 2014;28:371–402.

[6] Siliciano JD, Kajdas J, Finzi D, Quinn TC, Chadwick K, Margolick JB, et al. Long-term follow-up studies confirm the stability of the latent reservoir for HIV-1 in resting CD4+ T cells. Nat. Med. 2003;9:727–8.

[7] Centers for Disease Control and Prevention - CDC. CDC - HIV Cost-effectiveness - Ongoing Research - Prevention Research - HIV/AIDS [Internet]. 2015 [cited 2015 Jul 29]. Available from: http://www.cdc.gov/hiv/prevention/ongoing/costeffectiveness/

[8] Deeks SG. HIV infection, inflammation, immunosenescence, and aging. Annu. Rev. Med. 2011;62:141–55.

[9] Meyerhans A, Vartanian JP, Hultgren C, Plikat U, Karlsson A, Wang L, et al. Restriction and enhancement of human immunodeficiency virus type 1 replication by modulation of intracellular deoxynucleoside triphosphate pools. J. Virol. 1994;68:535–40.

[10] Zhou Y, Zhang H, Siliciano JD, Siliciano RF. Kinetics of human immunodeficiency virus type 1 decay following entry into resting CD4+ T cells. J. Virol. 2005;79:2199–210.

[11] Bukrinsky MI, Stanwick TL, Dempsey MP, Stevenson M. Quiescent T lymphocytes as an inducible virus reservoir in HIV-1 infection. Science. 1991;254:423–7.

[12] Zack JA, Arrigo SJ, Weitsman SR, Go AS, Haislip A, Chen IS. HIV-1 entry into quiescent primary lymphocytes: molecular analysis reveals a labile, latent viral structure. Cell. 1990;61:213–22.

[13] Ganesh L, Burstein E, Guha-Niyogi A, Louder MK, Mascola JR, Klomp LWJ, et al. The gene product Murr1 restricts HIV-1 replication in resting CD4+ lymphocytes. Nature. 2003;426:853–7.

[14] Pan X, Baldauf H-M, Keppler OT, Fackler OT. Restrictions to HIV-1 replication in resting CD4+ T lymphocytes. Cell Res. Shanghai Institutes for Biological Sciences, Chinese Academy of Sciences; 2013;23:876–85.

[15] Donahue D a, Wainberg M a. Cellular and molecular mechanisms involved in the establishment of HIV-1 latency. Retrovirology. Retrovirology; 2013;10:11.

[16] Bleul CC, Wu L, Hoxie JA, Springer TA, Mackay CR. The HIV coreceptors CXCR4 and CCR5 are differentially expressed and regulated on human T lymphocytes. Proc. Natl. Acad. Sci. U. S. A. 1997;94:1925–30.

[17] Stevenson M, Stanwick TL, Dempsey MP, Lamonica CA. HIV-1 replication is controlled at the level of T cell activation and proviral integration. EMBO J. 1990;9:1551–60.

[18] Wang W, Guo J, Yu D, Vorster PJ, Chen W, Wu Y. A dichotomy in cortical actin and chemotactic actin activity between human memory and naive T cells contributes to their differential susceptibility to HIV-1 infection. J. Biol. Chem. 2012;287:35455–69.

[19] Spear M, Guo J, Wu Y. The trinity of the cortical actin in the initiation of HIV-1 infection. Retrovirology. 2012;9:45.

[20] Siliciano RF, Greene WC. HIV latency. Cold Spring Harb. Perspect. Med. 2011;1:a007096.

[21] Ho DD, Neumann AU, Perelson AS, Chen W, Leonard JM, Markowitz M. Rapid turnover of plasma virions and CD4 lymphocytes in HIV-1 infection. Nature. 1995;373:123–6.

[22] Wei X, Ghosh SK, Taylor ME, Johnson VA, Emini EA, Deutsch P, et al. Viral dynamics in human immunodeficiency virus type 1 infection. Nature. 1995;373:117–22.

[23] Chavez L, Calvanese V, Verdin E. HIV Latency Is Established Directly and Early in Both Resting and Activated Primary CD4 T Cells. PLoS Pathog. 2015;11:e1004955.

[24] Eriksson S, Graf EH, Dahl V, Strain MC, Yukl SA, Lysenko ES, et al. Comparative analysis of measures of viral reservoirs in HIV-1 eradication studies. PLoS Pathog. Public Library of Science; 2013;9:e1003174.

[25] Chun T, Carruth L, Finzi D, Shen X, DiGiuseppe J, Taylor H, et al. Quantification of latent tissue reservoirs and total body viral load in HIV-1 infection. Lett. to Nat. 1997;246:170–170.

[26] Finzi D, Blankson J, Siliciano JD, Margolick JB, Chadwick K, Pierson T, et al. Latent infection of CD4+ T cells provides a mechanism for lifelong persistence of HIV-1, even in patients on effective combination therapy. Nat. Med. 1999;5:512–7.

[27] Strain MC, Günthard HF, Havlir D V, Ignacio CC, Smith DM, Leigh-Brown AJ, et al. Heterogeneous clearance rates of long-lived lymphocytes infected with HIV: intrinsic stability predicts lifelong persistence. Proc. Natl. Acad. Sci. U. S. A. 2003;100:4819–24.

[28] Chomont N, El-Far M, Ancuta P, Trautmann L, Procopio F a, Yassine-Diab B, et al. HIV reservoir size and persistence are driven by T cell survival and homeostatic proliferation. Nat. Med. 2009;15:893–900.

[29] Wightman F, Solomon A, Khoury G, Green JA, Gray L, Gorry PR, et al. Both CD31(+) and CD31⁻ naive CD4(+) T cells are persistent HIV type 1-infected reservoirs in individuals receiving antiretroviral therapy. J. Infect. Dis. 2010;202:1738–48.

[30] Costiniuk CT, Jenabian M-A. The lungs as anatomical reservoirs of HIV infection. Rev. Med. Virol. 2014;24:35–54.

[31] Salemi M, Lamers SL, Yu S, de Oliveira T, Fitch WM, McGrath MS. Phylodynamic analysis of human immunodeficiency virus type 1 in distinct brain compartments provides a model for the neuropathogenesis of AIDS. J. Virol. 2005;79:11343–52.

[32] garashi T, Brown CR, Endo Y, Buckler-White A, Plishka R, Bischofberger N, et al. Macrophage are the principal reservoir and sustain high virus loads in rhesus macaques after the depletion of CD4+ T cells by a highly pathogenic simian immunodeficiency virus/HIV type 1 chimera (SHIV): Implications for HIV-1 infections of humans. Proc. Natl. Acad. Sci. U. S. A. 2001;98:658–63.

[33] Gartner S, Markovits P, Markovitz DM, Kaplan MH, Gallo RC, Popovic M. The role of mononuclear phagocytes in HTLV-III/LAV infection. Science. 1986;233:215–9.

[34] Van Lint C, Bouchat S, Marcello A. HIV-1 transcription and latency: an update. Retrovirology. Retrovirology; 2013;10:67.

[35] Eisele E, Siliciano RF. Redefining the viral reservoirs that prevent HIV-1 eradication. Immunity. Elsevier Inc.; 2012;37:377–88.

[36] Tyagi M, Bukrinsky M. Human immunodeficiency virus (HIV) latency: the major hurdle in HIV eradication. Mol. Med. 2012;18:1096–108.

[37] Schnell G, Price RW, Swanstrom R, Spudich S. Compartmentalization and clonal amplification of HIV-1 variants in the cerebrospinal fluid during primary infection. J. Virol. 2010;84:2395–407.

[38] Churchill MJ, Gorry PR, Cowley D, Lal L, Sonza S, Purcell DFJ, et al. Use of laser capture microdissection to detect integrated HIV-1 DNA in macrophages and astrocytes from autopsy brain tissues. J. Neurovirol. 2006;12:146–52.

[39] Wiley CA, Schrier RD, Nelson JA, Lampert PW, Oldstone MB. Cellular localization of human immunodeficiency virus infection within the brains of acquired immune deficiency syndrome patients. Proc. Natl. Acad. Sci. U. S. A. 1986;83:7089–93.

[40] Yukl SA, Gianella S, Sinclair E, Epling L, Li Q, Duan L, et al. Differences in HIV burden and immune activation within the gut of HIV-positive patients receiving suppressive antiretroviral therapy. J. Infect. Dis. 2010;202:1553–61.

[41] Chun T-W, Nickle DC, Justement JS, Meyers JH, Roby G, Hallahan CW, et al. Persistence of HIV in gut-associated lymphoid tissue despite long-term antiretroviral therapy. J. Infect. Dis. 2008;197:714–20.

[42] Lerner P, Guadalupe M, Donovan R, Hung J, Flamm J, Prindiville T, et al. The gut mucosal viral reservoir in HIV-infected patients is not the major source of rebound plasma viremia following interruption of highly active antiretroviral therapy. J. Virol. 2011;85:4772–82.

[43] Yilmaz A, Verhofstede C, D'Avolio A, Watson V, Hagberg L, Fuchs D, et al. Treatment intensification has no effect on the HIV-1 central nervous system infection in patients on suppressive antiretroviral therapy. J. Acquir. Immune Defic. Syndr. 2010;55:590–6.

[44] Symons J, Vandekerckhove L, Hütter G, Wensing AMJ, Van Ham PM, Deeks SG, et al. Dependence on the CCR5 coreceptor for viral replication explains the lack of rebound of CXCR4-predicted HIV variants in the Berlin patient. Clin. Infect. Dis. 2014;59:596–600.

[45] Hütter G, Nowak D, Mossner M, Ganepola S, Müssig A, Allers K, et al. Long-term control of HIV by CCR5 Delta32/Delta32 stem-cell transplantation. N. Engl. J. Med. 2009;360:692–8.

[46] Deng H, Liu R, Ellmeier W, Choe S, Unutmaz D, Burkhart M, et al. Identification of a major co-receptor for primary isolates of HIV-1. Nature. 1996;381:661–6.

[47] Dragic T, Litwin V, Allaway GP, Martin SR, Huang Y, Nagashima KA, et al. HIV-1 entry into CD4+ cells is mediated by the chemokine receptor CC-CKR-5. Nature. 1996;381:667–73.

[48] Libert F, Cochaux P, Beckman G, Samson M, Aksenova M, Cao A, et al. The deltaccr5 mutation conferring protection against HIV-1 in Caucasian populations has a single and recent origin in Northeastern Europe. Hum. Mol. Genet. 1998;7:399–406.

[49] Yukl SA, Boritz E, Busch M, Bentsen C, Chun T-W, Douek D, et al. Challenges in detecting HIV persistence during potentially curative interventions: a study of the Berlin patient. PLoS Pathog. Public Library of Science; 2013;9:e1003347.

[50] Martinson JJ, Chapman NH, Rees DC, Liu YT, Clegg JB. Global distribution of the CCR5 gene 32-basepair deletion. Nat. Genet. 1997;16:100–3.

[51] Sabeti PC, Walsh E, Schaffner SF, Varilly P, Fry B, Hutcheson HB, et al. The case for selection at CCR5-Delta32. PLoS Biol. Public Library of Science; 2005;3:e378.

[52] Yukl SA, Boritz E, Busch M, Bentsen C, Chun T-W, Douek D, et al. Challenges in detecting HIV persistence during potentially curative interventions: a study of the Berlin patient. PLoS Pathog. Public Library of Science; 2013;9:e1003347.

[53] Henrich TJ, Hu Z, Li JZ, Sciaranghella G, Busch MP, Keating SM, et al. Long-term reduction in peripheral blood HIV type 1 reservoirs following reduced-intensity conditioning allogeneic stem cell transplantation. J. Infect. Dis. 2013;207:1694–702.

[54] Passaes CP, Sáez-Cirión A. HIV cure research: advances and prospects. Virology. 2014;454-455:340–52.

[55] Persaud D, Gay H, Ziemniak C, Chen YH, Piatak M, Chun T-W, et al. Absence of detectable HIV-1 viremia after treatment cessation in an infant. N. Engl. J. Med. 2013;369:1828–35.

[56] Huang J, Burke PS, Cung TDH, Pereyra F, Toth I, Walker BD, et al. Leukocyte immunoglobulin-like receptors maintain unique antigen-presenting properties of circulating myeloid dendritic cells in HIV-1-infected elite controllers. J. Virol. 2010;84:9463–71.

[57] Lewin SR, Rouzioux C. HIV cure and eradication: how will we get from the laboratory to effective clinical trials? AIDS. 2011;25:885–97.

[58] Autran B, Descours B, Avettand-Fenoel V, Rouzioux C. Elite controllers as a model of functional cure. Curr. Opin. HIV AIDS. 2011;6:181–7.

[59] Okulicz JF, Lambotte O. Epidemiology and clinical characteristics of elite controllers. Curr. Opin. HIV AIDS. 2011;6:163–8.

[60] Blankson JN. Control of HIV-1 replication in elite suppressors. Discov. Med. 2010;9:261–6.

[61] Shacklett BL. Understanding the 'lucky few': the conundrum of HIV-exposed, seronegative individuals. Curr. HIV/AIDS Rep. 2006;3:26–31.

[62] Sáez-Cirión A, Bacchus C, Hocqueloux L, Avettand-Fenoel V, Girault I, Lecuroux C, et al. Post-treatment HIV-1 controllers with a long-term virological remission after the interruption of early initiated antiretroviral therapy ANRS VISCONTI Study. PLoS Pathog. Public Library of Science; 2013;9:e1003211.

[63] Frange P, Faye A, Avettand-Fenoel V, Bellaton E, Deschamps D, Angin M, et al. HIV-1 virological remission for more than 11 years after interruption of early initiated antiretroviral therapy in a perinatally-infected child. 8th Int. AIDS Soc. Conf. HIV Pathog. Treat. Prev. (IAS 2015) Vancouver. 2015. p. MOAA0105LB.

[64] Ru R, Yao Y, Yu S, Yin B, Xu W, Zhao S, et al. Targeted genome engineering in human induced pluripotent stem cells by penetrating TALENs. Cell Regeneration; 2013;2(1):5.

[65] Mandal PK, Ferreira LMR, Collins R, Meissner TB, Boutwell CL, Friesen M, et al. Efficient Ablation of Genes in Human Hematopoietic Stem and Effector Cells using CRISPR/Cas9. Cell Stem Cell. Elsevier Inc.; 2014;15:643–52.

[66] Tebas P, Stein D, Tang WW, Frank I, Wang SQ, Lee G, et al. Gene Editing of CCR5 in Autologous CD4 T Cells of Persons Infected with HIV. N. Engl. J. Med. 2014;370:901–10.

[67] Allers K, Schneider T. CCR5Δ32 mutation and HIV infection: basis for curative HIV therapy. Curr. Opin. Virol. 2015;14:24–9.

[68] Vrins CLJ, Out R, van Santbrink P, van der Zee A, Mahmoudi T, Groenendijk M, et al. Znf202 affects high density lipoprotein cholesterol levels and promotes hepatosteatosis in hyperlipidemic mice. PLoS One. 2013;8:e57492.

[69] Huelsmann PM, Hofmann AD, Knoepfel SA, Popp J, Rauch P, Di Giallonardo F, et al. A suicide gene approach using the human pro-apoptotic protein tBid inhibits HIV-1 replication. BMC Biotechnol. 2011;11:4.

[70] Hamer DH. Can HIV be Cured? Mechanisms of HIV persistence and strategies to combat it. Curr. HIV Res. 2004;2:99–111.

[71] Deeks SG, Autran B, Berkhout B, Benkirane M, Cairns S, Chomont N, et al. Towards an HIV cure: a global scientific strategy. Nat. Rev. Immunol. Nature Publishing Group; 2012;12:607–14.

[72] Barouch DH, Deeks SG. immunologic strategies for HIV-1 remission and eradication. Science (80-.). 2014;345:169–74.

[73] Archin NM, Margolis DM. Emerging strategies to deplete the HIV reservoir. Curr. Opin. Infect. Dis. 2014;27:29–35.

[74] Folks TM, Clouse KA, Justement J, Rabson A, Duh E, Kehrl JH, et al. Tumor necrosis factor alpha induces expression of human immunodeficiency virus in a chronically infected T-cell clone. Proc. Natl. Acad. Sci. U. S. A. 1989;86:2365–8.

[75] Folks TM, Justement J, Kinter a, Dinarello C a, Fauci a S. Cytokine-induced expression of HIV-1 in a chronically infected promonocyte cell line. Science. 1987;238:800–2.

[76] Emiliani S, Van Lint C, Fischle W, Paras P, Ott M, Brady J, et al. A point mutation in the HIV-1 Tat responsive element is associated with postintegration latency. Proc. Natl. Acad. Sci. U. S. A. 1996;93:6377–81.

[77] Emiliani S, Fischle W, Ott M, Van Lint C, Amella CA, Verdin E. Mutations in the tat Gene Are Responsible for Human Immunodeficiency Virus Type 1 Postintegration Latency in the U1 Cell Line. J. Virol. 1998;72:1666–70.

[78] Jordan A, Bisgrove D, Verdin E. HIV reproducibly establishes a latent infection after acute infection of T cells in vitro. EMBO. 2003;22:1868–77.

[79] Folks TM, Justement J, Kinter A, Dinarello CA, Fauci AS. Cytokine-induced expression of HIV-1 in a chronically infected promonocyte cell line. Science. 1987;238:800–2.

[80] Weiss A, Wiskocil RL, Stobo JD. The role of T3 surface molecules in the activation of human T cells: a two-stimulus requirement for IL 2 production reflects events occurring at a pre-translational level. J. Immunol. 1984;133:123–8.

[81] Schneider U, Schwenk HU, Bornkamm G. Characterization of EBV-genome negative 'null' and 'T' cell lines derived from children with acute lymphoblastic leukemia and leukemic transformed non-Hodgkin lymphoma. Int. J. Cancer. 1977;19:621–6.

[82] Schröder ARW, Shinn P, Chen H, Berry C, Ecker JR, Bushman F. HIV-1 integration in the human genome favors active genes and local hotspots. Cell. 2002;110:521–9.

[83] Ho Y-C, Shan L, Hosmane NN, Wang J, Laskey SB, Rosenbloom DIS, et al. Replication-competent noninduced proviruses in the latent reservoir increase barrier to HIV-1 cure. Cell; 2013;155:540–51.

[84] Spina C a, Anderson J, Archin NM, Bosque A, Chan J, Famiglietti M, et al. An in-depth comparison of latent HIV-1 reactivation in multiple cell model systems and resting CD4+ T cells from aviremic patients. PLoS Pathog. 2013;9:e1003834.

[85] Sahu GK, Lee K, Ji J, Braciale V, Baron S, Cloyd MW. A novel in vitro system to generate and study latently HIV-infected long-lived normal CD4+ T-lymphocytes. Virology. 2006;355:127–37.

[86] Bosque A, Planelles V. Induction of HIV-1 latency and reactivation in primary memory CD4+ T cells. Blood. 2009;113:58–65.

[87] Yang H, Xing S, Shan L, Connell KO, Dinoso J, Shen A, et al. Small-molecule screening using a human primary cell model of HIV latency identifies compounds that reverse latency without cellular activation. 2009;119(11):3473-86..

[88] Marini A, Harper JM, Romerio F. An in vitro system to model the establishment and reactivation of HIV-1 latency. J. Immunol. 2008;181:7713–20.

[89] Chun TW, Finzi D, Margolick J, Chadwick K, Schwartz D, Siliciano RF. In vivo fate of HIV-1-infected T cells: quantitative analysis of the transition to stable latency. Nat. Med. 1995;1:1284–90.

[90] Pierson T, McArthur J, Siliciano RF. Reservoirs for HIV-1: mechanisms for viral persistence in the presence of antiviral immune responses and antiretroviral therapy. Annu. Rev. Immunol. 2000;18:665–708.

[91] Finzi D, Hermankova M, Pierson T, Carruth LM, Buck C, Chaisson RE, et al. Identification of a reservoir for HIV-1 in patients on highly active antiretroviral therapy. Science. 1997;278:1295–300.

[92] Swiggard WJ, Baytop C, Yu JJ, Li C, Schretzenmair R, Doherty UO, et al. Human Immunodeficiency Virus Type 1 Can Establish Latent Infection in Resting CD4 + T Cells in the Absence of Activating Stimuli. J..... 2005;79:14179–88.

[93] De Crignis E, Mahmoudi T. HIV eradication: combinatorial approaches to activate latent viruses. Viruses. 2014;6:4581–608.

[94] Archin NM, Sung JM, Garrido C, Soriano-Sarabia N, Margolis DM. Eradicating HIV-1 infection: seeking to clear a persistent pathogen. Nat. Rev. Microbiol. Nature Publishing Group; 2014;12:750–64.

[95] Denton PW, Olesen R, Choudhary SK, Archin NM, Wahl a., Swanson MD, et al. Generation of HIV Latency in Humanized BLT Mice. J. Virol. 2012;86:630–4.

[96] Melkus MW, Estes JD, Padgett-Thomas A, Gatlin J, Denton PW, Othieno F a, et al. Humanized mice mount specific adaptive and innate immune responses to EBV and TSST-1. Nat. Med. 2006;12:1316–22.

[97] Denton PW, Estes JD, Sun Z, Othieno F a., Wei BL, Wege AK, et al. Antiretroviral pre-exposure prophylaxis prevents vaginal transmission of HIV-1 in humanized BLT mice. PLoS Med. 2008;5:0079–89.

[98] North TW, Higgins J, Deere JD, Hayes TL, Villalobos A, Adamson L, et al. Viral sanctuaries during highly active antiretroviral therapy in a nonhuman primate model for AIDS. J. Virol. 2010;84:2913–22.

[99] Van Rompay KK a. Evaluation of antiretrovirals in animal models of HIV infection. Antiviral Res. 2010;85:159–75.

[100] Hatziioannou T, Ambrose Z, Chung NPY, Piatak M, Yuan F, Trubey CM, et al. A macaque model of HIV-1 infection. Proc. Natl. Acad. Sci. U. S. A. 2009;106:4425–9.

[101] Krebs FC, Hogan TH, Quiterio S, Gartner S, Wigdahl B. Lentiviral LTR-directed Expression, Sequence Variation, and Disease Pathogenesis Reviews. In: CL K, B F, B H, B K, F M, PA M, et al., editors. HIV Seq. Compend. 2001. Los Alamos: Theoretical Biology and Biophysics Group, Los Alamos National Laboratory: Los Alamos, NM; 2001. p. 1–42.

[102] Bruner KM, Hosmane NN, Siliciano RF. Towards an HIV-1 cure: measuring the latent reservoir. Trends Microbiol. Elsevier Ltd; 2015;23:192–203.

[103] Hindson BJ, Ness KD, Masquelier D a., Belgrader P, Heredia NJ, Makarewicz AJ, et al. High-throughput droplet digital PCR system for absolute quantitation of DNA copy number. Anal. Chem. 2011;83:8604–10.

[104] Procopio FA, Fromentin R, Kulpa DA, Brehm JH, Bebin A-G, Strain MC, et al. A Novel Assay to Measure the Magnitude of the Inducible Viral Reservoir in HIV-infected Individuals. EBioMedicine. Elsevier; 2015;

[105] Descours B, Cribier A, Chable-Bessia C, Ayinde D, Rice G, Crow Y, et al. SAMHD1 restricts HIV-1 reverse transcription in quiescent CD4+ T-cells. Retrovirology. Retrovirology; 2012;9:87.

[106] Goldstone DC, Ennis-Adeniran V, Hedden JJ, Groom HCT, Rice GI, Christodoulou E, et al. HIV-1 restriction factor SAMHD1 is a deoxynucleoside triphosphate triphosphohydrolase. Nature. Nature Publishing Group; 2011;480:379–82.

[107] Kim B, Nguyen L a., Daddacha W, Hollenbaugh J a. Tight interplay among SAMHD1 protein level, cellular dNTP levels, and HIV-1 proviral DNA synthesis kinetics in human primary monocyte-derived macrophages. J. Biol. Chem. 2012;287:21570–4.

[108] Lahouassa H, Daddacha W, Hofmann H, Ayinde D, Logue EC, Dragin L, et al. SAMHD1 restricts the replication of human immunodeficiency virus type 1 by depleting the intracellular pool of deoxynucleoside triphosphates. Nat. Immunol. 2012;13:621–621.

[109] Ryoo J, Choi J, Oh C, Kim S, Seo M, Diaz-griffero F, et al. The ribonuclease activity of SAMHD1 is required for HIV-1 restriction. Nat. Med. 2014;20:936–41.

[110] Choi J, Ryoo J, Oh C, Hwang S, Ahn K. SAMHD1 specifically restricts retroviruses through its RNase activity. Retrovirology. BioMed Central; 2015;12:1–12.

[111] Hofmann H, Logue EC, Bloch N, Daddacha W, Polsky SB, Schultz ML, et al. The Vpx lentiviral accessory protein targets SAMHD1 for degradation in the nucleus. J. Virol. 2012;86:12552–60.

[112] Sheehy AM, Gaddis NC, Choi JD, Malim MH. Isolation of a human gene that inhibits HIV-1 infection and is suppressed by the viral Vif protein. Nature. 2002;418:646–50.

[113] Schrijvers R, De Rijck J, Demeulemeester J, Adachi N, Vets S, Ronen K, et al. LEDGF/p75-independent HIV-1 replication demonstrates a role for HRP-2 and remains sensitive to inhibition by LEDGINs. PLoS Pathog. 2012;8.

[114] Ciuffi A, Llano M, Poeschla E, Hoffmann C, Leipzig J, Shinn P, et al. A role for LEDGF/p75 in targeting HIV DNA integration. Nat. Med. 2005;11:1287–9.

[115] Shun MC, Raghavendra NK, Vandegraaff N, Daigle JE, Hughes S, Kellam P, et al. LEDGF/p75 functions downstream from preintegration complex formation to effect gene-specific HIV-1 integration. Genes Dev. 2007;21:1767–78.

[116] Engelman A, Cherepanov P. The lentiviral integrase binding protein LEDGF/p75 and HIV-1 replication. PLoS Pathog. 2008;4.

[117] Wang H, Jurado KA, Wu X, Shun M-C, Li X, Ferris AL, et al. HRP2 determines the efficiency and specificity of HIV-1 integration in LEDGF/p75 knockout cells but does not contribute to the antiviral activity of a potent LEDGF/p75-binding site integrase inhibitor. Nucleic Acids Res. 2012;40:11518–30.

[118] Lesbats P, Botbol Y, Chevereau G, Vaillant C, Calmels C, Arneodo A, et al. Functional coupling between HIV-1 integrase and the SWI/SNF chromatin remodeling complex for efficient in vitro integration into stable nucleosomes. PLoS Pathog. 2011;7:e1001280.

[119] Maroun M, Delelis O, Coadou G, Bader T, Ségéral E, Mbemba G, et al. Inhibition of early steps of HIV-1 replication by SNF5/Ini1. J. Biol. Chem. 2006;281:22736–43.

[120] Turelli P, Doucas V, Craig E, Mangeat B, Klages N, Evans R, et al. Cytoplasmic recruitment of INI1 and PML on incoming HIV preintegration complexes: Interference with early steps of viral replication. Mol. Cell. 2001;7:1245–54.

[121] Ocwieja KE, Brady TL, Ronen K, Huegel A, Roth SL, Schaller T, et al. HIV integration targeting: A pathway involving transportin-3 and the nuclear pore protein RanBP2. PLoS Pathog. 2011;7:19–21.

[122] Pierson TC, Kieffer TL, Ruff CT, Buck C, Gange SJ, Siliciano RF. Intrinsic Stability of Episomal Circles Formed during Human Immunodeficiency Virus Type 1 Replication. J. Virol. 2002;76:4138–44.

[123] Pierson TC, Zhou Y, Kieffer TL, Christian T, Buck C, Siliciano RF, et al. Molecular Characterization of Preintegration Latency in Human Immunodeficiency Virus Type 1 Infection. J. Virol. 2002;76:8518–31.

[124] Zamborlini A, Lehmann-Che J, Clave E, Giron M-L, Tobaly-Tapiero J, Roingeard P, et al. Centrosomal pre-integration latency of HIV-1 in quiescent cells. Retrovirology. 2007;4:63.

[125] Trinité B, Ohlson EC, Voznesensky I, Rana SP, Chan CN, Mahajan S, et al. An HIV-1 replication pathway utilizing reverse transcription products that fail to integrate. J. Virol. 2013;87:12701–20.

[126] Han Y, Lassen K, Monie D, Ahmad R, Shimoji S, Liu X, et al. Resting CD4 + T Cells from Human Immunodeficiency Virus Type 1 (HIV-1) -Infected Individuals Carry Integrated HIV-1 Genomes within Actively Transcribed Host Genes. J. Virol. 2004;78:6122.

[127] Liu H, Dow EC, Arora R, Kimata JT, Bull LM, Arduino RC, et al. Integration of human immunodeficiency virus type 1 in untreated infection occurs preferentially within genes. J. Virol. 2006;80:7765–8.

[128] Lewinski MK, Bisgrove D, Shinn P, Chen H, Hoffmann C, Hannenhalli S, et al. Genome-Wide Analysis of Chromosomal Features Repressing Human Immunodeficiency Virus Transcription. J Virol. 2005;79:6610–9.

[129] Marini B, Kertesz-farkas A, Ali H, Lucic B, Lisek K, Manganaro L, et al. Nuclear architecture dictates HIV-1 integration site selection. Nature. 2015;521(7551):227-31

[130] Wang GP, Ciuffi A, Leipzig J, Berry CC, Bushman FD. HIV integration site selection: analysis by massively parallel pyrosequencing reveals association with epigenetic modifications. Genome Res. 2007;17:1186–94.

[131] Brady T, Agosto LM, Malani N, Berry CC, O'Doherty U, Bushman F. HIV integration site distributions in resting and activated CD4+ T cells infected in culture. AIDS. 2009;23:1461–71.

[132] Albanese A, Arosio D, Terreni M, Cereseto A. HIV-1 pre-integration complexes selectively target decondensed chromatin in the nuclear periphery. PLoS One. 2008; 3(6): e2413.

[133] Dieudonné M, Maiuri P, Biancotto C, Knezevich A, Kula A, Lusic M, et al. Transcriptional competence of the integrated HIV-1 provirus at the nuclear periphery. EMBO J. 2009;28:2231–43.

[134] Cohn LB, Silva IT, Oliveira TY, Rosales RA, Parrish EH, Learn GH, et al. HIV-1 Integration Landscape during Latent and Active Infection. Cell. Elsevier Inc.; 2015;160:420–32.

[135] Lusic M, Marini B, Ali H, Lucic B, Luzzati R, Giacca M. Proximity to PML nuclear bodies regulates HIV-1 latency in CD4+ T cells. Cell Host Microbe. Elsevier Inc.; 2013;13:665–77.

[136] Gallastegui E, Millán-Zambrano G, Terme J-M, Chávez S, Jordan A. Chromatin reassembly factors are involved in transcriptional interference promoting HIV latency. J. Virol. 2011;85:3187–202.

[137] Lenasi T, Contreras X, Peterlin BM. Transcriptional interference antagonizes proviral gene expression to promote HIV latency. Cell Host Microbe. 2008;4:123–33.

[138] Han Y, Lin YB, An W, Xu J, Yang H-C, O'Connell K, et al. Orientation-dependent regulation of integrated HIV-1 expression by host gene transcriptional readthrough. Cell Host Microbe. 2008;4:134–46.

[139] Shan L, Yang H-C, Rabi SA, Bravo HC, Shroff NS, Irizarry R a, et al. Influence of host gene transcription level and orientation on HIV-1 latency in a primary-cell model. J. Virol. 2011;85:5384–93.

[140] De Marco A, Biancotto C, Knezevich A, Maiuri P, Vardabasso C, Marcello A. Intragenic transcriptional cis-activation of the human immunodeficiency virus 1 does not result in allele-specific inhibition of the endogenous gene. Retrovirology. 2008;5:98.

[141] Klaver B, Berkhout B. Comparison of 5′ and 3' long terminal repeat promoter function in human immunodeficiency virus. J. Virol. 1994;68:3830–40.

[142] Cullen BR, Lomedico PT, Ju G. Transcriptional interference in avian retroviruses—implications for the promoter insertion model of leukaemogenesis. Nature. 1984;307:241–5.

[143] Michael NL, Vahey MT, d'Arcy L, Ehrenberg PK, Mosca JD, Rappaport J, et al. Negative-strand RNA transcripts are produced in human immunodeficiency virus type 1-

infected cells and patients by a novel promoter downregulated by Tat. J. Virol. 1994;68:979–87.

[144] Landry S, Halin M, Lefort S, Audet B, Vaquero C, Mesnard J-M, et al. Detection, characterization and regulation of antisense transcripts in HIV-1. Retrovirology. 2007;4:71.

[145] Ludwig LB, Ambrus JL, Krawczyk K a, Sharma S, Brooks S, Hsiao C-B, et al. Human Immunodeficiency Virus-Type 1 LTR DNA contains an intrinsic gene producing antisense RNA and protein products. Retrovirology. 2006;3:80.

[146] Kobayashi-Ishihara M, Yamagishi M, Hara T, Matsuda Y, Takahashi R, Miyake A, et al. HIV-1-encoded antisense RNA suppresses viral replication for a prolonged period. Retrovirology. 2012;9:38.

[147] Saayman S, Ackley A, Turner A-MW, Famiglietti M, Bosque A, Clemson M, et al. An HIV-encoded antisense long noncoding RNA epigenetically regulates viral transcription. Mol. Ther. 2014;22:1164–75.

[148] Karn J, Stoltzfus CM. Regulation of HIV-1 Gene Expression. Cold Spring Harb. Perspect. Med. 2012;1–17.

[149] Peeters a, Lambert PF, Deacon NJ. A fourth Sp1 site in the human immunodeficiency virus type 1 long terminal repeat is essential for negative-sense transcription. J. Virol. 1996;70:6665–72.

[150] Bentley K, Deacon N, Sonza S, Zeichner S, Churchill M. Mutational analysis of the HIV-1 LTR as a promoter of negative sense transcription. Arch. Virol. 2004;149:2277–94.

[151] Gaynor Richard. Cellular transcription factors involved in the regulation of HIV-1 gene expression. Aids. 1992. p. 347–63.

[152] Rosen C a, Sodroski JG, Haseltine W a. Location of cis-acting regulatory sequences in the human T-cell leukemia virus type I long terminal repeat. Proc. Natl. Acad. Sci. U. S. A. 1985;82:6502–6.

[153] Siekevitz M, Josephs SF, Dukovich M, Peffer N, Wong-Staal F, Greene WC. Activation of the HIV-1 LTR by T cell mitogens and the trans-activator protein of HTLV-I. Science. 1987;238:1575–8.

[154] Pereira LA, Bentley K, Peeters A, Churchill MJ, Deacon NJ. SURVEY AND SUMMARY A compilation of cellular transcription factor interactions with the HIV-1 LTR promoter. 2000;28:663–8.

[155] Kinoshita S, Su L, Amano M, Timmerman L a, Kaneshima H, Nolan GP. The T cell activation factor NF-ATc positively regulates HIV-1 replication and gene expression in T cells. Immunity. 1997;6:235–44.

[156] Selliah N, Zhang M, DeSimone D, Kim H, Brunner M, Ittenbach RF, et al. The??c-cytokine regulated transcription factor, STAT5, increases HIV-1 production in primary CD4 T cells. Virology. 2006;344:283–91.

[157] Nabel G, Baltimore D. An inducible transcription factor activates expression of human immunodeficiency virus in T cells. Nature. 1987;326:711–3.

[158] Gerritsen ME, Williams a J, Neish a S, Moore S, Shi Y, Collins T. CREB-binding protein/p300 are transcriptional coactivators of p65. Proc. Natl. Acad. Sci. U. S. A. 1997;94:2927–32.

[159] Tesmer VM, Rajadhyaksha a, Babin J, Bina M. NF-IL6-mediated transcriptional activation of the long terminal repeat of the human immunodeficiency virus type 1. Proc. Natl. Acad. Sci. 1993;90:7298–302.

[160] Henderson a J, Zou X, Calame KL. C/EBP proteins activate transcription from the human immunodeficiency virus type 1 long terminal repeat in macrophages/monocytes. J. Virol. 1995;69:5337–44.

[161] Yang X, Chen Y, Gabuzda D. ERK MAP kinase links cytokine signals to activation of latent HIV-1 infection by stimulating a cooperative interaction of AP-1 and NF-??B. J. Biol. Chem. 1999;274:27981–8.

[162] Krebs FC, Mehrens D, Pomeroy S, Goodenow MM, Wigdahl B. Human immunodeficiency virus type 1 long terminal repeat quasispecies differ in basal transcription and nuclear factor recruitment in human glial cells and lymphocytes. J. Biomed. Sci. 1998;5:31–44.

[163] Coiras M, López-Huertas MR, Rullas J, Mittelbrunn M, Alcamí J. Basal shuttle of NF-kappaB/I kappaB alpha in resting T lymphocytes regulates HIV-1 LTR dependent expression. Retrovirology. 2007;4:56.

[164] Colin L, Van Lint C. Molecular control of HIV-1 postintegration latency: implications for the development of new therapeutic strategies. Retrovirology. 2009;6:111.

[165] Cron RQ, Bartz SR, Clausell A, Bort SJ, Klebanoff SJ, Lewis DB. NFAT1 enhances HIV-1 gene expression in primary human CD4 T cells. Clin. Immunol. 2000;94:179–91.

[166] McKernan LN, Momjian D, Kulkosky J. Protein Kinase C: One Pathway towards the Eradication of Latent HIV-1 Reservoirs. Adv. Virol. 2012;2012:805347.

[167] Mahmoudi T. The BAF complex and HIV latency. Transcription. 2012;3:171–6.

[168] West MJ, Lowe AD, Karn J. Activation of Human Immunodeficiency Virus Transcription in T Cells Revisited: NF- κ B p65 Stimulates Transcriptional Elongation Activation of Human Immunodeficiency Virus Transcription in T Cells Revisited: NF-, B p65 Stimulates Transcriptional Elonga. J. Virol. 2001;75:8524–37.

[169] Li X, Josef J, Marasco W a. Hiv-1 Tat can substantially enhance the capacity of NIK to induce IkappaB degradation. Biochem. Biophys. Res. Commun. 2001;286:587–94.

[170] Pazin MJ, Sheridan PL, Cannon K, Cao Z, Keck JG, Kadonaga JT, et al. NF-κB-mediated chromatin reconfiguration and transcriptional activation of the HIV-1 enhancer in vitro. Genes Dev. 1996;10:37–49.

[171] Steger DJ, Workman JL. Stable co-occupancy of transcription factors and histones at the HIV-1 enhancer. EMBO J. 1997;16:2463–72.

[172] Rothgiesser KM, Erener S, Waibel S, Lüscher B, Hottiger MO. SIRT2 regulates NF-κB dependent gene expression through deacetylation of p65 Lys310. J. Cell Sci. 2010;123:4251–8.

[173] Kwon H-S, Ott M. The ups and downs of SIRT1. Trends Biochem. Sci. 2008;33:517–25.

[174] Zhang JL, Sharma PL, Crumpacker CS. Enhancement of the basal-level activity of HIV-1 long terminal repeat by HIV-1 nucleocapsid protein. Virology. 2000;268:251–63.

[175] Kim YK, Bourgeois CF, Pearson R, Tyagi M, West MJ, Wong J, et al. Recruitment of TFIIH to the HIV LTR is a rate-limiting step in the emergence of HIV from latency. EMBO J. 2006;25:3596–604.

[176] Larochelle S, Amat R, Glover-Cutter K, Sansó M, Zhang C, Allen JJ, et al. Cyclin-dependent kinase control of the initiation-to-elongation switch of RNA polymerase II. Nat. Struct. Mol. Biol. 2012;19:1108–15.

[177] Takahashi Y, Tanaka Y, Yamashita A. OX40 Stimulation by gp34/OX40 ligand enhances prodcuttive human immunodeficiency virus type1 infection. J. Virol. 2001;75:674806757.

[178] Kundu M, Srinivasan a, Pomerantz RJ, Khalili K. Evidence that a cell cycle regulator, E2F1, down-regulates transcriptional activity of the human immunodeficiency virus type 1 promoter. J. Virol. 1995;69:6940–6.

[179] Majello B, De Luca P, Hagen G, Suske G, Lania L. Different members of the Sp1 multigene family exert opposite transcriptional regulation of the long terminal repeat of HIV-1. Nucleic Acids Res. 1994;22:4914–21.

[180] Millhouse S, Krebs FC, Yao J, McAllister JJ, Conner J, Ross H, et al. Sp1 and related factors fail to interact with the NF-kappaB-proximal G/C box in the LTR of a replication competent, brain-derived strain of HIV-1 (YU-2). J. Neurovirol. 1998;4:312–23.

[181] Garcia-Rodriguez C, Rao A. Nuclear Factor of Activated T Cells (NFAT)-dependent Transactivation Regulated by the Coactivators p300/CREB-binding Protein (CBP). J. Exp. Med. 1998;187:2031–6.

[182] Wang FX, Xu Y, Sullivan J, Souder E, Argyris EG, Acheampong E a., et al. IL-7 is a potent and proviral strain-specific inducer of latent HIV-1 cellular reservoirs of infected individuals on virally suppressive HAART. J. Clin. Invest. 2005;115:128–37.

[183] Shuai K, Liu B. Regulation of JAK-STAT signalling in the immune system. Nat. Rev. Immunol. 2003;3:900–11.

[184] Bovolenta C, Camorali L, Lorini a L, Ghezzi S, Vicenzi E, Lazzarin a, et al. Constitutive activation of STATs upon in vivo human immunodeficiency virus infection. Blood. 1999;94:4202–9.

[185] Crotti A, Lusic M, Lupo R, Lievens PMJ, Liboi E, Della Chiara G, et al. Naturally occurring C-terminally truncated STAT5 is a negative regulator of HIV-1 expression. Blood. 2007;109:5380–9.

[186] Della Chiara G, Crotti A, Liboi E, Giacca M, Poli G, Lusic M. Negative regulation of HIV-1 transcription by a heterodimeric NF-??B1/p50 and C-terminally truncated STAT5 complex. J. Mol. Biol. Elsevier Ltd; 2011;410:933–43.

[187] Henderson AJ, Connor RI, Calame KL. C/EBP activators are required for HIV-1 replication and proviral induction in monocytic cell lines. Immunity. 1996;5:91–101.

[188] Henderson a J, Calame KL. CCAAT/enhancer binding protein (C/EBP) sites are required for HIV-1 replication in primary macrophages but not CD4(+) T cells. Proc. Natl. Acad. Sci. U. S. A. 1997;94:8714–9.

[189] Lee ES, Zhou H, Al LEEET, Irol J V. Endothelial Cells Enhance Human Immunodeficiency Virus Type 1 Replication in Macrophages through a C / EBP-Dependent Mechanism. Society. 2001;75:9703–12.

[190] Combates J, Kwon P, Rzepka W, Cohen D. Involvement of the Transcription Factor NF-1L6 in Phorbol Ester Induction of P-glycoprotein in U937 Cells. Cell. 1997;8:213–9.

[191] Colin L, Vandenhoudt N, de Walque S, Van Driessche B, Bergamaschi A, Martinelli V, et al. The AP-1 binding sites located in the pol gene intragenic regulatory region of HIV-1 are important for viral replication. PLoS One. Public Library of Science; 2011;6:e19084.

[192] Duverger A, Wolschendorf F, Zhang M, Wagner F, Hatcher B, Jones J, et al. An AP-1 binding site in the enhancer/core element of the HIV-1 promoter controls the ability of HIV-1 to establish latent infection. J. Virol. 2013;87:2264–77.

[193] Hess J, Angel P, Schorpp-Kistner M. AP-1 subunits: quarrel and harmony among siblings. J. Cell Sci. 2004;117:5965–73.

[194] Challacombe SJ, Naglik JR. The effects of HIV infection on oral mucosal immunity. Adv. Dent. Res. 2006;19:29–35.

[195] Long J, Wang Y, Wang W, Chang BHJ, Danesh FR. Identification of microRNA-93 as a novel regulator of vascular endothelial growth factor in hyperglycemic conditions. J. Biol. Chem. 2010;285:23457–65.

[196] Novis CL, Archin NM, Buzon MJ, Verdin E, Round JL, Lichterfeld M, et al. Reactivation of latent HIV-1 in central memory $CD4^+$ T cells through TLR-1/2 stimulation. Retrovirology. 2013;10:119.

[197] Pearson R, Kim YK, Hokello J, Lassen K, Friedman J, Tyagi M, et al. Epigenetic silencing of human immunodeficiency virus (HIV) transcription by formation of restrictive chromatin structures at the viral long terminal repeat drives the progressive entry of HIV into latency. J. Virol. 2008;82:12291–303.

[198] Kim YK, Mbonye U, Hokello J, Karn J. T-cell receptor signaling enhances transcriptional elongation from latent HIV proviruses by activating P-TEFb through an ERK-dependent pathway. J. Mol. Biol. 2011;410:896–916.

[199] Herrmann CH, Rice a P. Lentivirus Tat proteins specifically associate with a cellular protein kinase, TAK, that hyperphosphorylates the carboxyl-terminal domain of the large subunit of RNA polymerase II: candidate for a Tat cofactor. J. Virol. 1995;69:1612–20.

[200] Wei P, Garber ME, Fang SM, Fischer WH, Jones K a. A novel CDK9-associated C-type cyclin interacts directly with HIV-1 Tat and mediates its high-affinity, loop-specific binding to TAR RNA. Cell. 1998;92:451–62.

[201] Bieniasz PD, Grdina T a, Bogerd HP, Cullen BR. Recruitment of a protein complex containing Tat and cyclin T1 to TAR governs the species specificity of HIV-1 Tat. EMBO J. 1998;17:7056–65.

[202] Fujinaga K, Cujec TP, Peng J, Garriga J, Price DH, Graña X, et al. The ability of positive transcription elongation factor B to transactivate human immunodeficiency virus transcription depends on a functional kinase domain, cyclin T1, and Tat. J. Virol. 1998;72:7154–9.

[203] Garber ME, Wei P, KewalRamani VN, Mayall TP, Herrmann CH, Rice AP, et al. The interaction between HIV-1 Tat and human cyclin T1 requires zinc and a critical cysteine residue that is not conserved in the murine CycT1 protein. Genes Dev. 1998;12:3512–27.

[204] Felzien LK, Woffendin C, Hottiger MO, Subbramanian R a, Cohen E a, Nabel GJ. HIV transcriptional activation by the accessory protein, VPR, is mediated by the p300 co-activator. Proc. Natl. Acad. Sci. U. S. A. 1998;95:5281–6.

[205] Wang L, Mukherjee S, Jia F, Narayan O, Zhao LJ. Interaction of virion protein Vpr of human immunodeficiency virus type 1 with cellular transcription factor Sp1 and trans-activation of viral long terminal repeat. J. Biol. Chem. 1995;270:25564–9.

[206] Agostini I, Navarro JM, Rey F, Bouhamdan M, Spire B, Vigne R, et al. The human immunodeficiency virus type 1 Vpr transactivator: cooperation with promoter-bound activator domains and binding to TFIIB. J. Mol. Biol. 1996;261:599–606.

[207] He G, Margolis DM. Counterregulation of chromatin deacetylation and histone deacetylase occupancy at the integrated promoter of human immunodeficiency virus type 1 (HIV-1) by the HIV-1 repressor YY1 and HIV-1 activator Tat. Mol. Cell. Biol. 2002;22:2965–73.

[208] Tyagi M, Karn J. CBF-1 promotes transcriptional silencing during the establishment of HIV-1 latency. EMBO J. 2007;26:4985–95.

[209] Tyagi M, Pearson RJ, Karn J. Establishment of HIV latency in primary CD4+ cells is due to epigenetic transcriptional silencing and P-TEFb restriction. J. Virol. 2010;84:6425–37.

[210] Jiang G, Espeseth A, Hazuda DJ, Margolis DM. c-Myc and Sp1 contribute to proviral latency by recruiting histone deacetylase 1 to the human immunodeficiency virus type 1 promoter. J. Virol. 2007;81:10914–23.

[211] Wen Y, Shatkin AJ. Transcription elongation factor hSPT5 stimulates mRNA capping Transcription elongation factor hSPT5 stimulates mRNA capping. Genes Dev. 1999; 13(14): 1774–1779.

[212] Cheng B, Price DH. Analysis of factor interactions with RNA polymerase II elongation complexes using a new electrophoretic mobility shift assay. Nucleic Acids Res. 2008;36:1–10.

[213] Missra A, Gilmour DS. Interactions between DSIF (DRB sensitivity inducing factor), NELF (negative elongation factor), and the Drosophila RNA polymerase II transcription elongation complex. Proc. Natl. Acad. Sci. U. S. A. 2010;107:11301–6.

[214] Yamaguchi Y, Inukai N, Narita T, Wada T, Handa H. Evidence that Negative Elongation Factor Represses Transcription Elongation through Binding to a DRB Sensitivity-Inducing Factor / RNA Polymerase II Complex and RNA. Mol. Cell. Biol. 2002;22:2918–27.

[215] Renner DB, Yamaguchi Y, Wada T, Handa H, Price DH. A Highly Purified RNA Polymerase II Elongation Control System. J. Biol. Chem. 2001;276:42601–9.

[216] Zhang Z, Klatt A, Gilmour DS, Henderson AJ. Negative elongation factor NELF represses human immunodeficiency virus transcription by pausing the RNA polymerase II complex. J. Biol. Chem. 2007;282:16981–8.

[217] Natarajan M, Schiralli Lester GM, Lee C, Missra A, Wasserman G a., Steffen M, et al. Negative elongation factor (NELF) coordinates RNA polymerase II pausing, premature termination, and chromatin remodeling to regulate HIV transcription. J. Biol. Chem. 2013;288:25995–6003.

[218] Jadlowsky JK, Wong JY, Graham AC, Dobrowolski C, Devor RL, Adams MD, et al. Negative Elongation Factor Is Required for the Maintenance of Proviral Latency but Does Not Induce Promoter-Proximal Pausing of RNA Polymerase II on the HIV Long Terminal Repeat. Mol. Cell. Biol. 2014;34:1911–28.

[219] Wagschal A, Rousset E, Basavarajaiah P, Contreras X, Harwig A, Laurent-Chabalier S, et al. Microprocessor, Setx, Xrn2, and Rrp6 co-operate to induce premature termination of transcription by RNAPII. Cell. 2012;150:1147–57.

[220] Kao SY, Calman a F, Luciw P a, Peterlin BM. Anti-termination of transcription within the long terminal repeat of HIV-1 by tat gene product. Nature. 1987;330:489–93.

[221] Laspia MF, Rice a P, Mathews MB. HIV-1 Tat protein increases transcriptional initiation and stabilizes elongation. Cell. 1989;59:283–92.

[222] Dingwall C, Ernberg I, Gait MJ, Green SM, Heaphy S, Karn J, et al. HIV-1 tat protein stimulates transcription by binding to a U-rich bulge in the stem of the TAR RNA structure. EMBO J. 1990;9:4145–53.

[223] Tahirov TH, Babayeva ND, Varzavand K, Cooper JJ, Sedore SC, Price DH. Crystal structure of HIV-1 Tat complexed with human P-TEFb. Nature. 2010;465:747–51.

[224] Fujinaga K, Irwin D, Huang Y, Taube R, Kurosu T, Peterlin BM. Dynamics of human immunodeficiency virus transcription: P-TEFb phosphorylates RD and dissociates negative effectors from the transactivation response element. Mol. Cell. Biol. 2004;24:787–95.

[225] Komarnitsky P, Cho EJ, Buratowski S. Different phosphorylated forms of RNA polymerase II and associated mRNA processing factors during transcription. Genes Dev. 2000;14:2452–60.

[226] Kim YK, Bourgeois CF, Isel C, Churcher MJ, Karn J. Phosphorylation of the RNA polymerase II carboxyl-terminal domain by CDK9 is directly responsible for human immunodeficiency virus type 1 Tat-activated transcriptional elongation. Mol. Cell. Biol. 2002;22:4622–37.

[227] Czudnochowski N, Bösken C a., Geyer M. Serine-7 but not serine-5 phosphorylation primes RNA polymerase II CTD for P-TEFb recognition. Nat. Commun. 2012;3:842.

[228] Ahn SH, Kim M, Buratowski S. Phosphorylation of serine 2 within the RNA polymerase II C-terminal domain couples transcription and 3J end. Process. Mol. Cell. 2004;13:67–76.

[229] Lenasi T, Peterlin BM, Barboric M. Cap-binding protein complex links pre-mRNA capping to transcription elongation and alternative splicing through positive transcription elongation factor b (P-TEFb). J. Biol. Chem. 2011;286:22758–68.

[230] Brиs V, Gomes N, Pickle L, Jones K a. A human splicing factor, SKIP, associates with P-TEFb and enhances transcription elongation by HIV-1 Tat. Genes Dev. 2005;19:1211–26.

[231] Bourgeois CF, Kim YK, Churcher MJ, West MJ, Karn J. Spt5 cooperates with human immunodeficiency virus type 1 Tat by preventing premature RNA release at terminator sequences. Mol. Cell. Biol. 2002;22:1079–93.

[232] Yamada T, Yamaguchi Y, Inukai N, Okamoto S, Mura T, Handa H. P-TEFb-mediated phosphorylation of hSpt5 C-terminal repeats is critical for processive transcription elongation. Mol. Cell. 2006;21:227–37.

[233] Keen NJ, Churcher MJ, Karn J. Transfer of Tat and release of TAR RNA during the activation of the human immunodeficiency virus type-1 transcription elongation complex. EMBO J. 1997;16:5260–72.

[234] Sobhian B, Laguette N, Yatim A, Nakamura M, Levy Y, Kiernan R, et al. HIV-1 Tat Assembles a Multifunctional Transcription Elongation Complex and Stably Associates with the 7SK snRNP. Mol. Cell. Elsevier Ltd; 2010;38:439–51.

[235] Nguyen VT, Kiss T, Michels a a, Bensaude O. 7SK small nuclear RNA binds to and inhibits the activity of CDK9/cyclin T complexes. Nature. 2001;414:322–5.

[236] Yang Z, Zhu Q, Luo K, Zhou Q. The 7SK small nuclear RNA inhibits the CDK9/cyclin T1 kinase to control transcription. Nature. 2001;414:317–22.

[237] Yik JHN, Chen R, Nishimura R, Jennings JL, Link AJ, Zhou Q. Inhibition of P-TEFb (CDK9/cyclin T) kinase and RNA polymerase II transcription by the coordinated actions of HEXIM1 and 7SK snRNA. Mol. Cell. 2003;12:971–82.

[238] Li Q, Price JP, Byers SA, Cheng D, Peng J, Price DH. Analysis of the large inactive P-TEFb complex indicates that it contains one 7SK molecule, a dimer of HEXIM1 or HEXIM2, and two P-TEFb molecules containing Cdk9 phosphorylated at threonine 186. J. Biol. Chem. 2005;280:28819–26.

[239] Peterlin BM, Brogie JE, Price DH. 7SK snRNA: A noncoding RNA that plays a major role in regulating eukaryotic transcription. Wiley Interdiscip. Rev. RNA. 2012;3:92–103.

[240] Jeronimo C, Forget D, Bouchard A, Li Q, Chua G, Poitras C, et al. Systematic Analysis of the Protein Interaction Network for the Human Transcription Machinery Reveals the Identity of the 7SK Capping Enzyme. Mol. Cell. 2007;27:262–74.

[241] Krueger BJ, Varzavand K, Cooper JJ, Price DH. The mechanism of release of P-TEFb and HEXIM1 from the 7SK snRNP by viral and cellular activators includes a conformational change in 7SK. PLoS One. 2010;5.

[242] Markert A, Grimm M, Martinez J, Wiesner J, Meyerhans A, Meyuhas O, et al. The La-related protein LARP7 is a component of the 7SK ribonucleoprotein and affects transcription of cellular and viral polymerase II genes. EMBO Rep. 2008;9:569–75.

[243] Schröder S, Cho S, Zeng L, Zhang Q, Kaehlcke K, Mak L, et al. Two-pronged binding with bromodomain-containing protein 4 liberates positive transcription elongation factor b from inactive ribonucleoprotein complexes. J. Biol. Chem. 2012;287:1090–9.

[244] Bisgrove D a, Mahmoudi T, Henklein P, Verdin E. Conserved P-TEFb-interacting domain of BRD4 inhibits HIV transcription. Proc. Natl. Acad. Sci. U. S. A. 2007;104:13690–5.

[245] Jang MK, Mochizuki K, Zhou M, Jeong H-S, Brady JN, Ozato K. The bromodomain protein Brd4 is a positive regulatory component of P-TEFb and stimulates RNA polymerase II-dependent transcription. Mol. Cell. 2005;19:523–34.

[246] Yang Z, Yik JHN, Chen R, He N, Jang MK, Ozato K, et al. Recruitment of P-TEFb for stimulation of transcriptional elongation by the bromodomain protein Brd4. Mol. Cell. 2005;19:535–45.

[247] Zhu J, Gaiha GD, John SP, Pertel T, Chin CR, Gao G, et al. Reactivation of latent HIV-1 by inhibition of BRD4. Cell Rep. 2012;2:807–16.

[248] Wu S-Y, Chiang C-M. The double bromodomain-containing chromatin adaptor Brd4 and transcriptional regulation. J. Biol. Chem. 2007;282:13141–5.

[249] Boehm D, Calvanese V, Dar RD, Xing S, Schroeder S, Martins L, et al. BET bromodomain-targeting compounds reactivate HIV from latency via a Tat-independent mechanism. Cell Cycle. 2013;12:452–62.

[250] Denis G V, McComb ME, Faller D V, Sinha A, Romesser PB, Costello CE. Identification of transcription complexes that contain the double bromodomain protein Brd2 and chromatin remodeling machines. J. Proteome Res. 2006;5:502–11.

[251] Cherrier T, Le Douce V, Eilebrecht S, Riclet R, Marban C, Dequiedt F, et al. CTIP2 is a negative regulator of P-TEFb. Proc. Natl. Acad. Sci. U. S. A. 2013;110:12655–60.

[252] Mbonye UR, Wang B, Gokulrangan G, Chance MR, Karn J. Phosphorylation of HEXIM1 at Tyr271 and Tyr274 Promotes Release of P-TEFb from the 7SK snRNP Complex and Enhances Proviral HIV Gene Expression. Proteomics. 2015;15:2078–86.

[253] Ji X, Zhou Y, Pandit S, Huang J, Li H, Lin CY, et al. SR proteins collaborate with 7SK and promoter-associated nascent RNA to release paused polymerase. Cell. 2013;153:855–68.

[254] Suñé C, Goldstrohm a C, Peng J, Price DH, Garcia-Blanco M a. An in vitro transcription system that recapitulates equine infectious anemia virus tat-mediated inhibition of human immunodeficiency virus type 1 Tat activity demonstrates a role for posi-

tive transcription elongation factor b and associated proteins in th. Virology. 2000;271:356 66.

[255] Lu H, Li Z, Xue Y, Schulze-Gahmen U, Johnson JR, Krogan NJ, et al. AFF1 is a ubiquitous P-TEFb partner to enable Tat extraction of P-TEFb from 7SK snRNP and formation of SECs for HIV transactivation. Proc. Natl. Acad. Sci.. 2014;111 :E15–24.

[256] He N, Liu M, Hsu J, Xue Y, Chou S, Burlingame A, et al. HIV-1 Tat and host AFF4 recruit two transcription elongation factors into a bifunctional complex for coordinated activation of HIV-1 transcription. Mol. Cell. 2010;38:428–38.

[257] Mueller D, García-Cuéllar MP, Bach C, Buhl S, Maethner E, Slany RK. Misguided transcriptional elongation causes mixed lineage leukemia. PLoS Biol. 2009;7.

[258] Lin C, Smith ER, Takahashi H, Lai K, Martin- S, Florens L, et al. AFF4, a component of the ELL/p-TEFb elongation complex and a shared subunit of MLL chimeras can link transcription elongation to leukemia. Mol. Cell. 2010;37:429–37.

[259] Yokoyama A, Lin M, Naresh A, Kitabayashi I, Cleary ML. A Higher-Order Complex Containing AF4 and ENL Family Proteins with P-TEFb Facilitates Oncogenic and Physiologic MLL-Dependent Transcription. Cancer Cell. 2010;17:198–212.

[260] Smith E, Lin C, Shilatifard A. The super elongation complex (SEC) and MLL in development and disease. Genes Dev. 2011;25:661–72.

[261] Chou S, Upton H, Bao K, Schulze-Gahmen U, Samelson AJ, He N, et al. HIV-1 Tat recruits transcription elongation factors dispersed along a flexible AFF4 scaffold. Proc. Natl. Acad. Sci. U. S. A. 2013;110:E123–31.

[262] Liu M, Hsu J, Chan C, Li Z, Zhou Q. The Ubiquitin Ligase Siah1 Controls ELL2 Stability and Formation of Super Elongation Complexes to Modulate Gene Transcription. Mol. Cell. Elsevier Inc.; 2012;46:325–34.

[263] Ammosova T, Berro R, Jerebtsova M, Jackson A, Charles S, Klase Z, et al. Phosphorylation of HIV-1 Tat by CDK2 in HIV-1 transcription. Retrovirology. 2006;3:78.

[264] Kiernan RE, Vanhulle C, Schiltz L, Adam E, Xiao H, Maudoux F, et al. HIV-1 tat transcriptional activity is regulated by acetylation. EMBO J. 1999;18:6106–18.

[265] Brès V, Tagami H, Péloponèse JM, Loret E, Jeang KT, Nakatani Y, et al. Differential acetylation of Tat coordinates its interaction with the co-activators cyclin T1 and PCAF. EMBO J. 2002;21:6811–9.

[266] Huo L, Li D, Sun X, Shi X, Karna P, Yang W, et al. Regulation of Tat acetylation and transactivation activity by the microtubule-associated deacetylase HDAC6. J. Biol. Chem. 2011;286:9280–6.

[267] Ott M, Schnölzer M, Garnica J, Fischle W, Emiliani S, Rackwitz HR, et al. Acetylation of the HIV-1 tat protein by p300 is important for its transcriptional activity. Curr. Biol. 1999;9:1489–92.

[268] Col E, Caron C, Seigneurin-Berny D, Gracia J, Favier A, Khochbin S. The Histone Acetyltransferase, hGCN5, Interacts with and Acetylates the HIV Transactivator, Tat. J. Biol. Chem. 2001;276:28179–84.

[269] Dorr A, Kiermer V, Pedal A, Rackwitz HR, Henklein P, Schubert U, et al. Transcriptional synergy between Tat and PCAF is dependent on the binding of acetylated Tat to the PCAF bromodomain. EMBO J. 2002;21:2715–23.

[270] Kaehlcke K, Dorr A, Hetzer-Egger C, Kiermer V, Henklein P, Schnoelzer M, et al. Acetylation of Tat defines a CyclinT1-independent step in HIV transactivation. Mol. Cell. 2003;12:167–76.

[271] Mahmoudi T, Parra M, Vries RGJ, Kauder SE, Verrijzer CP, Ott M, et al. The SWI/SNF chromatin-remodeling complex is a cofactor for Tat transactivation of the HIV promoter. J. Biol. Chem. 2006;281:19960–8.

[272] Tréand C, du Chéné I, Brès V, Kiernan R, Benarous R, Benkirane M, et al. Requirement for SWI/SNF chromatin-remodeling complex in Tat-mediated activation of the HIV-1 promoter. EMBO J. 2006;25:1690–9.

[273] Agbottah E, Deng L, Dannenberg LO, Pumfery A, Kashanchi F. Effect of SWI/SNF chromatin remodeling complex on HIV-1 Tat activated transcription. Retrovirology. 2006;3:48.

[274] Pagans S, Pedal A, North BJ, Kaehlcke K, Marshall BL, Dorr A, et al. SIRT1 regulates HIV transcription via Tat deacetylation. PLoS Biol. 2005;3:0210–20.

[275] Pagans S, Kauder SE, Kaehlcke K, Sakane N, Schroeder S, Dormeyer W, et al. The Cellular lysine methyltransferase Set7/9-KMT7 binds HIV-1 TAR RNA, monomethylates the viral transactivator Tat, and enhances HIV transcription. Cell Host Microbe. 2010;7:234–44.

[276] Sakane N, Kwon HS, Pagans S, Kaehlcke K, Mizusawa Y, Kamada M, et al. Activation of hiv transcription by the viral tat protein requires a demethylation step mediated by lysine-specific demethylase 1 (LSD1/KDM1). PLoS Pathog. 2011;7:1–12.

[277] Brès V, Kiernan RE, Linares LK, Chable-Bessia C, Plechakova O, Tréand C, et al. A non-proteolytic role for ubiquitin in Tat-mediated transactivation of the HIV-1 promoter. Nat. Cell Biol. 2003;5:754–61.

[278] Verdin E. DNase I-hypersensitive sites are associated with both long terminal repeats and with the intragenic enhancer of integrated human immunodeficiency virus type 1. J. Virol. 1991;65:6790–9.

[279] Verdin E, Paras P, Van Lint C. Chromatin disruption in the promoter of human immunodeficiency virus type 1 during transcriptional activation. EMBO J. 1993;12:3249–59.

[280] Van Lint C, Emiliani S, Ott M, Verdin E. Transcriptional activation and chromatin remodeling of the HIV-1 promoter in response to histone acetylation. EMBO J. 1996;15:1112–20.

[281] Rafati H, Parra M, Hakre S, Moshkin Y, Verdin E, Mahmoudi T. Repressive LTR nucleosome positioning by the BAF complex is required for HIV latency. PLoS Biol. 2011;9:e1001206.

[282] Cismasiu VB, Paskaleva E, Suman Daya S, Canki M, Duus K, Avram D. BCL11B is a general transcriptional repressor of the HIV-1 long terminal repeat in T lymphocytes through recruitment of the NuRD complex. Virology. 2008;380:173–81.

[283] Xue Y, Wong J, Moreno GT, Young MK, Côté J, Wang W. NURD, a novel complex with both ATP-dependent chromatin-remodeling and histone deacetylase activities. Mol. Cell. 1998;2:851–61.

[284] Zhang Y, Li Y. The Expanding Mi-2/NuRD Complexes: A Schematic Glance. Proteomics Insights. Libertas Academica; 2011;2010:79.

[285] Perkins ND, Felzien LK, Betts JC, Leung K, Beach DH, Nabel GJ. Regulation of NF-kappaB by cyclin-dependent kinases associated with the p300 coactivator. Science. 1997;275:523–7.

[286] Williams SA, Chen L-F, Kwon H, Ruiz-Jarabo CM, Verdin E, Greene WC. NF-kappaB p50 promotes HIV latency through HDAC recruitment and repression of transcriptional initiation. EMBO J. 2006;25:139–49.

[287] Keedy KS, Archin NM, Gates AT, Espeseth A, Hazuda DJ, Margolis DM. A limited group of class I histone deacetylases acts to repress human immunodeficiency virus type 1 expression. J. Virol. 2009;83:4749–56.

[288] Huber K, Doyon G, Plaks J, Fyne E, Mellors JW, Sluis-Cremer N. Inhibitors of histone deacetylases: Correlation between isoform specificity and reactivation of HIV type 1 (HIV-1) from latently infected cells. J. Biol. Chem. 2011;286:22211–8.

[289] Ying H, Zhang Y, Zhou X, Qu X, Wang P, Liu S, et al. Selective Histonedeacetylase Inhibitor M344 Intervenes in HIV-1 Latency through Increasing Histone Acetylation and Activation of NF-kappaB. PLoS One. 2012;7.

[290] Marban C, Suzanne S, Dequiedt F, de Walque S, Redel L, Van Lint C, et al. Recruitment of chromatin-modifying enzymes by CTIP2 promotes HIV-1 transcriptional silencing. EMBO J. 2007;26:412–23.

[291] Marban C, Redel L, Suzanne S, Van Lint C, Lecestre D, Chasserot-Golaz S, et al. COUP-TF interacting protein 2 represses the initial phase of HIV-1 gene transcription in human microglial cells. Nucleic Acids Res. 2005;33:2318–31.

[292] Bouchat S, Gatot J-S, Kabeya K, Cardona C, Colin L, Herbein G, et al. Histone methyltransferase inhibitors induce HIV-1 recovery in resting CD4(+) T cells from HIV-1-infected HAART-treated patients. AIDS. 2012;26:1473–82.

[293] Du Chéné I, Basyuk E, Lin Y-L, Triboulet R, Knezevich A, Chable-Bessia C, et al. Suv39H1 and HP1gamma are responsible for chromatin-mediated HIV-1 transcriptional silencing and post-integration latency. EMBO J. 2007;26:424–35.

[294] Friedman J, Cho W-K, Chu CK, Keedy KS, Archin NM, Margolis DM, et al. Epigenetic silencing of HIV-1 by the histone H3 lysine 27 methyltransferase enhancer of Zeste 2. J. Virol. 2011;85:9078–89.

[295] Imai K, Togami H, Okamoto T. Involvement of histone H3 lysine 9 (H3K9) methyltransferase G9a in the maintenance of HIV-1 latency and its reactivation by BIX01294. J. Biol. Chem. 2010;285:16538–45.

[296] Kauder SE, Bosque A, Lindqvist A, Planelles V, Verdin E. Epigenetic regulation of HIV-1 latency by cytosine methylation. PLoS Pathog. 2009;5:e1000495.

[297] Blazkova J, Trejbalova K, Gondois-Rey F, Halfon P, Philibert P, Guiguen A, et al. CpG methylation controls reactivation of HIV from latency. PLoS Pathog. 2009;5.

[298] Palacios JA, Pérez-Piñar T, Toro C, Sanz-Minguela B, Moreno V, Valencia E, et al. Long-term nonprogressor and elite controller patients who control viremia have a higher percentage of methylation in their HIV-1 proviral promoters than aviremic patients receiving highly active antiretroviral therapy. J. Virol. 2012;86:13081–4.

[299] Triboulet R, Mari B, Lin Y, Chable-bessia C, Bennasser Y, Lebrigand K, et al. Suppression of MicroRNA-Silencing Pathway by HIV-1 During Virus Replication. Science (80-.). 2007;1579–82.

[300] Nathans R, Chu C-Y, Serquina AK, Lu C-C, Cao H, Rana TM. Cellular microRNA and P bodies modulate host-HIV-1 interactions. Mol. Cell. Elsevier Ltd; 2009;34:696–709.

[301] Imam H, Shahr Bano A, Patel P, Holla P, Jameel S. The lncRNA NRON modulates HIV-1 replication in a NFAT-dependent manner and is differentially regulated by early and late viral proteins. Sci. Rep. 2015;5:8639.

[302] Wang X, Ye L, Hou W, Zhou Y, Wang Y-J, Metzger DS, et al. Cellular microRNA expression correlates with susceptibility of monocytes/macrophages to HIV-1 infection. Blood. 2009;113:671–4.

[303] Houzet L, Yeung ML, de Lame V, Desai D, Smith SM, Jeang K-T. MicroRNA profile changes in human immunodeficiency virus type 1 (HIV-1) seropositive individuals. Retrovirology. 2008;5:118.

[304] Witwer KW, Watson AK, Blankson JN, Clements JE. Relationships of PBMC microRNA expression, plasma viral load, and CD4+ T-cell count in HIV-1-infected elite suppressors and viremic patients. Retrovirology. 2012;9:5.

[305] Bignami F, Pilotti E, Bertoncelli L, Ronzi P, Gulli M, Marmiroli N, et al. Stable changes in CD4 + T lymphocyte miRNA expression after exposure to HIV-1 Stable changes in CD4 T lymphocyte miRNA expression after exposure to HIV-1. Blood. 2013;119:6259–67.

[306] Chiang K, Sung T-L, Rice a. P. Regulation of Cyclin T1 and HIV-1 Replication by MicroRNAs in Resting CD4+ T Lymphocytes. J. Virol. 2012;86:3244–52.

[307] Sung TL, Rice AP. miR-198 inhibits HIV-1 gene expression and replication in monocytes and its mechanism of action appears to involve repression of cyclin T1. PLoS Pathog. 2009;5.

[308] Chiang K, Rice AP. MicroRNA-mediated restriction of HIV-1 in resting CD4+ T cells and monocytes. Viruses. 2012;4:1390–409.

[309] Qian S, Zhong X, Yu L, Ding B, de Haan P, Boris-Lawrie K. HIV-1 Tat RNA silencing suppressor activity is conserved across kingdoms and counteracts translational repression of HIV-1. Proc. Natl. Acad. Sci. U. S. A. 2009;106:605–10.

[310] Hayes AM, Qian S, Yu L, Boris-Lawrie K. Tat RNA silencing suppressor activity contributes to perturbation of lymphocyte miRNA by HIV-1. Retrovirology. BioMed Central Ltd; 2011;8:36.

[311] Coley W, Van Duyne R, Carpio L, Guendel I, Kehn-Hall K, Chevalier S, et al. Absence of DICER in monocytes and its regulation by HIV-1. J. Biol. Chem. 2010;285:31930–43.

[312] Huang J, Wang F, Argyris E, Chen K, Liang Z, Tian H, et al. Cellular microRNAs contribute to HIV-1 latency in resting primary CD4+ T lymphocytes. Nat. Med. 2007;13:1241–7.

[313] Jiménez VC, Booiman T, de Taeye SW, van Dort K a., Rits M a. N, Hamann J, et al. Differential expression of HIV-1 interfering factors in monocyte-derived macrophages stimulated with polarizing cytokines or interferons. Sci. Rep. 2012;2:1–7.

[314] Mantri CK, Pandhare Dash J, Mantri JV, Dash CC V. Cocaine enhances HIV-1 replication in CD4+ T cells by down-regulating MiR-125b. PLoS One. Public Library of Science; 2012;7:e51387.

[315] Wang X, Ye L, Zhou Y, Liu MQ, Zhou DJ, Ho WZ. Inhibition of anti-HIV microRNA expression: A mechanism for opioid-mediated enhancement of HIV infection of monocytes. Am. J. Pathol. 2011;178:41–7.

[316] Swaminathan S, Murray DD, Kelleher AD. Mirnas and HIV: Unforeseen Determinants Of Host-Pathogen Interaction. Immunol. Rev. 2013;254:265–80.

[317] Sun G, Li H, Wu X, Covarrubias M, Scherer L, Meinking K, et al. Interplay between HIV-1 infection and host microRNAs. Nucleic Acids Res. 2012;40:2181–96.

[318] Betel D, Wilson M, Gabow A, Marks DS, Sander C. The microRNA.org resource: Targets and expression. Nucleic Acids Res. 2008;36:149–53.

[319] Landgraf P, Rusu M, Sheridan R, Sewer A, Iovino N, Aravin A, et al. A Mammalian microRNA Expression Atlas Based on Small RNA Library Sequencing. Cell. 2009;129:1401–14.

[320] Ahluwalia JK, Khan SZ, Soni K, Rawat P, Gupta A, Hariharan M, et al. Human cellular microRNA hsa-miR-29a interferes with viral nef protein expression and HIV-1 replication. Retrovirology. 2008;5:117.

[321] Ruelas DS, Chan JK, Oh E, Heidersbach AJ, Hebbeler AM, Chavez L, et al. MicroRNA-155 Reinforces HIV Latency. J. Biol. Chem. 2015;290:jbc.M115.641837.

[322] Zhang HS, Chen XY, Wu TC, Sang WW, Ruan Z. MiR-34a is involved in Tat-induced HIV-1 long terminal repeat (LTR) transactivation through the SIRT1/NF??B pathway. FEBS Lett. Federation of European Biochemical Societies; 2012;586:4203–7.

[323] Zhang H-S, Wu T-C, Sang W-W, Ruan Z. MiR-217 is involved in Tat-induced HIV-1 long terminal repeat (LTR) transactivation by down-regulation of SIRT1. Biochim. Biophys. Acta. 2012;1823:1017–23.

[324] Chen XY, Zhang HS, Wu TC, Sang WW, Ruan Z. Down-regulation of NAMPT expression by miR-182 is involved in Tat-induced HIV-1 long terminal repeat (LTR) transactivation. Int. J. Biochem. Cell Biol. Elsevier B.V.; 2013;45:292–8.

[325] Ma L, Shen CJ, Cohen É a., Xiong SD, Wang JH. MiRNA-1236 inhibits HIV-1 infection of monocytes by repressing translation of cellular factor VprBP. PLoS One. 2014;9:1–7.

[326] Bennasser Y, Le S-Y, Yeung ML, Jeang K-T. HIV-1 encoded candidate micro-RNAs and their cellular targets. Retrovirology. 2004;1:43.

[327] Yeung ML, Houzet L, Yedavalli VSRK, Jeang K-T. A genome-wide short hairpin RNA screening of jurkat T-cells for human proteins contributing to productive HIV-1 replication. J. Biol. Chem. 2009;284:19463–73.

[328] Schopman NCT, Willemsen M, Liu YP, Bradley T, Van Kampen A, Baas F, et al. Deep sequencing of virus-infected cells reveals HIV-encoded small RNAs. Nucleic Acids Res. 2012;40:414–27.

[329] Ouellet DL, Plante I, Landry P, Barat C, Janelle M-E, Flamand L, et al. Identification of functional microRNAs released through asymmetrical processing of HIV-1 TAR element. Nucleic Acids Res. 2008;36:2353–65.

[330] Omoto S, Fujii YR. Regulation of human immunodeficiency virus 1 transcription by nef microRNA. J. Gen. Virol. 2005;86:751–5.

[331] Whisnant AW, Bogerd HP, Flores O, Ho P, Powers JG, Sharova N, et al. In-depth analysis of the interaction of HIV-1 with cellular microRNA biogenesis and effector mechanisms. MBio. 2013;4:e000193.

[332] Raj A, van Oudenaarden A. Nature, Nurture, or Chance: Stochastic Gene Expression and Its Consequences. Cell. 2008;135:216–26.

[333] Weinberger LS, Burnett JC, Toettcher JE, Arkin AP, Schaffer D V. Stochastic gene expression in a lentiviral positive-feedback loop: HIV-1 Tat fluctuations drive phenotypic diversity. Cell. 2005;122:169–82.

[334] Singh A, Razooky B, Cox CD, Simpson ML, Weinberger LS. Transcriptional bursting from the HIV-1 promoter is a significant source of stochastic noise in HIV-1 gene expression. Biophys. J. Biophysical Society; 2010;98:L32–4.

[335] Weinberger AD, Weinberger LS. Stochastic fate selection in HIV-infected patients. Cell. Elsevier; 2013;155:497–9.

[336] Dar RD, Hosmane NN, Michelle RA, Siliciano RF, Weinberger LS. Screening for noise in gene expression identifies drug synergies. Science (80-.). 2014;344:1392–6.

[337] Lipinski CA. Lead- and drug-like compounds: the rule-of-five revolution. Drug Discov. Today. Technol. 2004;1:337–41.

[338] Leeson PD, Springthorpe B. The influence of drug-like concepts on decision-making in medicinal chemistry. Nat. Rev. Drug Discov. 2007;6:881–90.

[339] Chun TW, Engel D, Mizell SB, Ehler LA, Fauci AS. Induction of HIV-1 replication in latently infected CD4+ T cells using a combination of cytokines. J. Exp. Med. 1998;188:83–91.

[340] Prins JM, Jurriaans S, van Praag RM, Blaak H, van Rij R, Schellekens PT, et al. Immuno-activation with anti-CD3 and recombinant human IL-2 in HIV-1-infected patients on potent antiretroviral therapy. AIDS. 1999;13:2405–10.

[341] Brooks DG, Hamer DH, Arlen PA, Gao L, Bristol G, Kitchen CMR, et al. Molecular characterization, reactivation, and depletion of latent HIV. Immunity. 2003;19:413–23.

[342] Rasmussen TA, Schmeltz Søgaard O, Brinkmann C, Wightman F, Lewin SR, Melchjorsen J, et al. Comparison of HDAC inhibitors in clinical development: effect on HIV production in latently infected cells and T-cell activation. Hum. Vaccin. Immunother. 2013;9:993–1001.

[343] Wightman F, Lu HK, Solomon AE, Saleh S, Harman AN, Cunningham AL, et al. Entinostat is a histone deacetylase inhibitor selective for class 1 histone deacetylases and activates HIV production from latently infected primary T cells. AIDS. 2013;27:2853–62.

[344] Wei DG, Chiang V, Fyne E, Balakrishnan M, Barnes T, Graupe M, et al. Histone deacetylase inhibitor romidepsin induces HIV expression in CD4 T cells from patients

on suppressive antiretroviral therapy at concentrations achieved by clinical dosing. PLoS Pathog. Public Library of Science; 2014;10:e1004071.

[345] Archin NM, Liberty AL, Kashuba AD, Choudhary SK, Kuruc JD, Crooks AM, et al. Administration of vorinostat disrupts HIV-1 latency in patients on antiretroviral therapy. Nature. 2012;487:482–5.

[346] Archin NM, Bateson R, Tripathy MK, Crooks AM, Yang K-H, Dahl NP, et al. HIV-1 expression within resting CD4+ T cells after multiple doses of vorinostat. J. Infect. Dis. 2014;210:728–35.

[347] Bartholomeeusen K, Xiang Y, Fujinaga K, Peterlin BM. Bromodomain and extra-terminal (BET) bromodomain inhibition activate transcription via transient release of positive transcription elongation factor b (P-TEFb) from 7SK small nuclear ribonucleoprotein. J. Biol. Chem. 2012;287:36609–16.

[348] Falkenberg KJ, Johnstone RW. Histone deacetylases and their inhibitors in cancer, neurological diseases and immune disorders. Nat. Rev. Drug Discov. Nature Publishing Group, a division of Macmillan Publishers Limited. All Rights Reserved.; 2014;13:673–91.

[349] Xing S, Siliciano RF. Targeting HIV latency: pharmacologic strategies toward eradication. Drug Discov. Today. Elsevier Ltd; 2013;18:541–51.

[350] Bernhard W, Barreto K, Saunders A, Dahabieh MS, Johnson P, Sadowski I. The Suv39H1 methyltransferase inhibitor chaetocin causes induction of integrated HIV-1 without producing a T cell response. FEBS Lett. 2011;585:3549–54.

[351] Fernandez G, Zeichner SL. Cell line-dependent variability in HIV activation employing DNMT inhibitors. Virol. J. 2010;7:266.

[352] Blazkova J, Murray D, Justement JS, Funk EK, Nelson AK, Moir S, et al. Paucity of HIV DNA methylation in latently infected, resting CD4+ T cells from infected individuals receiving antiretroviral therapy. J. Virol. 2012;86:5390–2.

[353] Thibault S, Imbeault M, Tardif MR, Tremblay MJ. TLR5 stimulation is sufficient to trigger reactivation of latent HIV-1 provirus in T lymphoid cells and activate virus gene expression in central memory CD4+ T cells. Virology. 2009;389:20–5.

[354] Chang JJ, Altfeld M. Immune activation and the role of TLRs and TLR agonists in the pathogenesis of HIV-1 infection in the humanized mouse model. J. Infect. Dis. 2013;208 Suppl :S145–9.

[355] De Jong MAWP, de Witte L, Oudhoff MJ, Gringhuis SI, Gallay P, Geijtenbeek TBH. TNF-alpha and TLR agonists increase susceptibility to HIV-1 transmission by human Langerhans cells ex vivo. J. Clin. Invest. American Society for Clinical Investigation; 2008;118:3440–52.

[356] Moody MA, Santra S, Vandergrift NA, Sutherland LL, Gurley TC, Drinker MS, et al. Toll-like receptor 7/8 (TLR7/8) and TLR9 agonists cooperate to enhance HIV-1 envelope antibody responses in rhesus macaques. J. Virol. 2014;88:3329–39.

[357] Sanders CM, Cruse JM, Lewis RE. Toll-like receptors, cytokines and HIV-1. Exp. Mol. Pathol. 2008;84:31–6.

[358] De Nardo D. Toll-like receptors: Activation, signalling and transcriptional modulation. Cytokine. 2015;74:181–9.

[359] Winckelmann AA, Munk-Petersen L V, Rasmussen TA, Melchjorsen J, Hjelholt TJ, Montefiori D, et al. Administration of a Toll-like receptor 9 agonist decreases the proviral reservoir in virologically suppressed HIV-infected patients. PLoS One. Public Library of Science; 2013;8:e62074.

[360] Offersen R, Melchjorsen J, Paludan SR, Østergaard L, Tolstrup M, Søgaard OS. TLR9-adjuvanted pneumococcal conjugate vaccine induces antibody-independent memory responses in HIV-infected adults. Hum. Vaccin. Immunother. 2012;8:1042–7.

[361] Scheller C, Ullrich A, Lamla S, Dittmer U, Rethwilm A, Koutsilieri E. Dual activity of phosphorothioate CpG oligodeoxynucleotides on HIV: reactivation of latent provirus and inhibition of productive infection in human T cells. Ann. N. Y. Acad. Sci. 2006;1091:540–7.

[362] Scheller C, Ullrich A, McPherson K, Hefele B, Knöferle J, Lamla S, et al. CpG oligodeoxynucleotides activate HIV replication in latently infected human T cells. J. Biol. Chem. 2004;279:21897–902.

[363] Søgaard OS, Lohse N, Harboe ZB, Offersen R, Bukh AR, Davis HL, et al. Improving the immunogenicity of pneumococcal conjugate vaccine in HIV-infected adults with a toll-like receptor 9 agonist adjuvant: a randomized, controlled trial. Clin. Infect. Dis. 2010;51:42–50.

[364] Sloan DD, Irrinki A, Tsai A, Kaur J, Lalezari J, Murry J, et al. TLR7 Agonist GS-9620 Activates HIV-1 in PBMCs From HIV-Infected Patients on cART. Conf. Retroviruses Opportunistic Infect. 2015, Bost. Massachusetts. 2015. p. P – F7, 417.

[365] Whitney JB, Lim S-Y, Osuna CE, Sanisetty S, Barnes TL, Hraber PT, et al. Treatment With a TLR7 Agonist Induces Transient Viremia in SIV-Infected ART-Suppressed Monkeys. Conf. Retroviruses Opportunistic Infect. 2015, Bost. Massachusetts. 2015. p. O – 9, 108.

[366] Antoni BA, Rabson AB, Kinter A, Bodkin M, Poli G. NF-kappa B-dependent and -independent pathways of HIV activation in a chronically infected T cell line. Virology. 1994;202:684–94.

[367] Contreras X, Barboric M, Lenasi T, Peterlin BM. HMBA releases P-TEFb from HEXIM1 and 7SK snRNA via PI3K/Akt and activates HIV transcription. PLoS Pathog. 2007;3:1459–69.

[368] Choudhary SK, Archin NM, Margolis DM. Hexamethylbisacetamide and disruption of human immunodeficiency virus type 1 latency in CD4(+) T cells. J. Infect. Dis. 2008;197:1162–70.

[369] Klichko V, Archin N, Kaur R, Lehrman G, Margolis D. Hexamethylbisacetamide remodels the human immunodeficiency virus type 1 (HIV-1) promoter and induces Tat-independent HIV-1 expression but blunts cell activation. J. Virol. 2006;80:4570–9.

[370] Pérez M, de Vinuesa AG, Sanchez-Duffhues G, Marquez N, Bellido ML, Muñoz-Fernandez MA, et al. Bryostatin-1 synergizes with histone deacetylase inhibitors to reactivate HIV-1 from latency. Curr. HIV Res. 2010;8:418–29.

[371] Biancotto A, Grivel J-C, Gondois-Rey F, Bettendroffer L, Vigne R, Brown S, et al. Dual role of prostratin in inhibition of infection and reactivation of human immunodeficiency virus from latency in primary blood lymphocytes and lymphoid tissue. J. Virol. 2004;78:10507–15.

[372] Wang P, Qu X, Wang X, Liu L, Zhu X, Zeng H, et al. As2O3 synergistically reactivate latent HIV-1 by induction of NF-κB. Antiviral Res. 2013. p. 688–97.

[373] Mochly-Rosen D, Khaner H, Lopez J. Identification of intracellular receptor proteins for activated protein kinase C. Proc. Natl. Acad. Sci. 1991;88:3997–4000.

[374] Trushin SA, Bren GD, Asin S, Pennington KN, Paya C V, Badley AD. Human immunodeficiency virus reactivation by phorbol esters or T-cell receptor ligation requires both PKCalpha and PKCtheta. J. Virol. 2005;79:9821–30.

[375] Colin L, Vandenhoudt N, de Walque S, Van Driessche B, Bergamaschi A, Martinelli V, et al. The AP-1 binding sites located in the pol gene intragenic regulatory region of HIV-1 are important for viral replication. PLoS One. Public Library of Science; 2011;6:e19084.

[376] Hirsch I, Caux C, Hasan U, Bendriss-Vermare N, Olive D. Impaired Toll-like receptor 7 and 9 signaling: from chronic viral infections to cancer. Trends Immunol. 2010;31:391–7.

[377] Chang JJ, Altfeld M. Immune activation and the role of TLRs and TLR agonists in the pathogenesis of HIV-1 infection in the humanized mouse model. J. Infect. Dis. 2013;208 Suppl :S145–9.

[378] Gallastegui E, Marshall B, Vidal D, Sanchez-Duffhues G, Collado JA, Alvarez-Fernández C, et al. Combination of biological screening in a cellular model of viral latency and virtual screening identifies novel compounds that reactivate HIV-1. J. Virol. 2012;86:3795–808.

[379] Das B, Dobrowolski C, Mao H, Powell D, Miller M, Hazuda D, et al. Farnesyl transferase: A new target for eradication of latent HIV-1 provirus in jurkat T-cells. Proc. 6th Int. Work. HIV Persistence Dur. Ther. Miami, FL, USA, 3–6 December 2013. 2013.

[380] Hazuda D, Barnard R, Wolkenberg S, Powell D, Karn J, Das B, et al. HIV latency drug discovery: Optimizing drugs to induce latent HIV expression. Proc. 6th Int. Work. HIV Persistence Dur. Ther. Miami, FL, USA, 3–6 December 2013. 2013;

[381] Rafati H, LeMasters E, Lennert VDD, El-Sayyed M, Boucher C, Vries R, et al. Activation of the Wnt pathway by natural ligands or small molecule inhibitors activates latent HIV. Proc. 7th IAS Conf. HIV Pathog. Treat. Prev. (IAS), Kuala Lumpur, Malaysia, 30 June–3 July 2013.

[382] Sheridan PL, Sheline CT, Cannon K, Voz ML, Pazin MJ, Kadonaga JT, et al. Activation of the HIV-1 enhancer by the LEF-1 HMG protein on nucleosome-assembled DNA in vitro. Genes Dev. 1995;9:2090–104.

[383] McKnight RF, Adida M, Budge K, Stockton S, Goodwin GM, Geddes JR. Lithium toxicity profile: a systematic review and meta-analysis. Lancet. 2012;379:721–8.

[384] Oruch R, Elderbi MA, Khattab HA, Pryme IF, Lund A. Lithium: a review of pharmacology, clinical uses, and toxicity. Eur. J. Pharmacol. 2014;740:464–73.

[385] Dykhuizen EC, Carmody LC, Tolliday N, Crabtree GR, Palmer M a J. Screening for inhibitors of an essential chromatin remodeler in mouse embryonic stem cells by monitoring transcriptional regulation. J. Biomol. Screen. 2012;17:1221–30.

[386] Stoszko; M, Crignis; E De, Khalid; MM, Lungu; C, Palstra; R-J, Dykhuizen; EC, et al. Small molecule inhibitors of BAF; a new family of compounds in HIV latency reversal Article. EBioMedicine. 2015, submitted.

[387] Roth MD, Tashkin DP, Choi R, Jamieson BD, Zack JA, Baldwin GC. Cocaine Enhances Human Immunodeficiency Virus Replication in a Model of Severe Combined Immunodeficient Mice Implanted with Human Peripheral Blood Leukocytes. J. Infect. Dis. 2002;185:701–5.

[388] Bagasra O, Pomerantz RJ. Human immunodeficiency virus type 1 replication in peripheral blood mononuclear cells in the presence of cocaine. J. Infect. Dis. 1993;168:1157–64.

[389] Peterson PK, Gekker G, Chao CC, Schut R, Molitor TW, Balfour HH. Cocaine potentiates HIV-1 replication in human peripheral blood mononuclear cell cocultures. Involvement of transforming growth factor-beta. J. Immunol. 1991;146:81–4.

[390] Sahu G, Farley K, El-Hage N, Aiamkitsumrit B, Fassnacht R, Kashanchi F, et al. Cocaine promotes both initiation and elongation phase of HIV-1 transcription by activating NF-κB and MSK1 and inducing selective epigenetic modifications at HIV-1 LTR. Virology. 2015;483:185–202.

[391] Imai K, Yamada K, Tamura M, Ochiai K, Okamoto T. Reactivation of latent HIV-1 by a wide variety of butyric acid-producing bacteria. Cell. Mol. Life Sci. 2012;69:2583–92.

[392] Ye F, Karn J. Bacterial Short Chain Fatty Acids Push All The Buttons Needed To Reactivate Latent Viruses. Stem cell epigenetics. 2015;2.

[393] Shirakawa K, Chavez L, Hakre S, Calvanese V, Verdin E. Reactivation of latent HIV by histone deacetylase inhibitors. Trends Microbiol. Elsevier Ltd; 2013;21:277–85.

[394] Wherry EJ, Blattman JN, Murali-Krishna K, van der Most R, Ahmed R. Viral persistence alters CD8 T-cell immunodominance and tissue distribution and results in distinct stages of functional impairment. J. Virol. 2003;77:4911–27.

[395] Khaitan A, Unutmaz D. Revisiting immune exhaustion during HIV infection. Curr. HIV/AIDS Rep. 2011;8:4–11.

[396] Palmer BE, Neff CP, Lecureux J, Ehler A, Dsouza M, Remling-Mulder L, et al. In vivo blockade of the PD-1 receptor suppresses HIV-1 viral loads and improves CD4+ T cell levels in humanized mice. J. Immunol. 2013;190:211–9.

[397] (NIAID) NI of A and ID. Safety and Immune Response of BMS-936559 in HIV-Infected People Taking Combination Antiretroviral Therapy. 2015.

[398] Migueles SA, Osborne CM, Royce C, Compton AA, Joshi RP, Weeks KA, et al. Lytic granule loading of CD8+ T cells is required for HIV-infected cell elimination associated with immune control. Immunity. 2008;29:1009–21.

[399] Shan L, Deng K, Shroff NS, Durand CM, Rabi SA, Yang H-C, et al. Stimulation of HIV-1-specific cytolytic T lymphocytes facilitates elimination of latent viral reservoir after virus reactivation. Immunity. 2012;36:491–501.

[400] Hansen SG, Ford JC, Lewis MS, Ventura AB, Hughes CM, Coyne-Johnson L, et al. Profound early control of highly pathogenic SIV by an effector memory T-cell vaccine. Nature. 2011;473:523–7.

[401] Hansen SG, Piatak M, Ventura AB, Hughes CM, Gilbride RM, Ford JC, et al. Immune clearance of highly pathogenic SIV infection. Nature. 2013;502:100–4.

[402] Hansen SG, Sacha JB, Hughes CM, Ford JC, Burwitz BJ, Scholz I, et al. Cytomegalovirus vectors violate CD8+ T cell epitope recognition paradigms. Science. 2013;340:1237874.

[403] Barouch DH, Whitney JB, Moldt B, Klein F, Oliveira TY, Liu J, et al. Therapeutic efficacy of potent neutralizing HIV-1-specific monoclonal antibodies in SHIV-infected rhesus monkeys. Nature.; 2013;503:224–8.

[404] Barouch DH, Stephenson KE, Borducchi EN, Smith K, Stanley K, McNally AG, et al. Protective efficacy of a global HIV-1 mosaic vaccine against heterologous SHIV challenges in rhesus monkeys. Cell. 2013;155:531–9.

[405] Klein F, Halper-Stromberg A, Horwitz JA, Gruell H, Scheid JF, Bournazos S, et al. HIV therapy by a combination of broadly neutralizing antibodies in humanized mice. Nature. 2012;492:118–22.

[406] Shingai M, Nishimura Y, Klein F, Mouquet H, Donau OK, Plishka R, et al. Antibody-mediated immunotherapy of macaques chronically infected with SHIV suppresses viraemia. Nature. 2013;503:277–80.

[407] Lehrman G, Hogue IB, Palmer S, Jennings C, Spina C a, Wiegand A, et al. Depletion of latent HIV-1 infection in vivo: a proof-of-concept study. Lancet. 2005;366:549–55.

[408] Steel A, Clark S, Teo I, Shaunak S, Nelson M, Gazzard B, et al. No change to HIV-1 latency with valproate therapy. AIDS. 2006;20:1681–2.

[409] Siliciano JD, Lai J, Callender M, Pitt E, Zhang H, Margolick JB, et al. Stability of the latent reservoir for HIV-1 in patients receiving valproic acid. J. Infect. Dis. 2007;195:833–6.

[410] Archin NM, Eron JJ, Palmer S, Hartmann-Duff A, Martinson JA, Wiegand A, et al. Valproic acid without intensified antiviral therapy has limited impact on persistent HIV infection of resting CD4+ T cells. AIDS. 2008;22:1131–5.

[411] Archin NM, Cheema M, Parker D, Wiegand A, Bosch RJ, Coffin JM, et al. Antiretroviral intensification and valproic acid lack sustained effect on residual HIV-1 viremia or resting CD4+ cell infection. PLoS One. 2010;5:e9390.

[412] Sagot-Lerolle N, Lamine A, Chaix M-L, Boufassa F, Aboulker J-P, Costagliola D, et al. Prolonged valproic acid treatment does not reduce the size of latent HIV reservoir. AIDS. 2008;22:1125–9.

7

Difficulties and Coping Strategies Experienced by Employed People with HIV in Japan: A Qualitative Study Comparing High and Low Sense of Coherence Groups

Tomoko Omiya, Yoshihiko Yamazaki,
Megumi Shimada, Kazuko Ikeda,
Seiko Ishiuchi-Ishitani and Katsumi Ohira

Abstract

People with HIV experience anxiety about discrimination in the workplace and disclosing their disease. Effective coping ability toward HIV-related challenges may be associated with a person's sense of coherence (SOC). This study describes the range of difficulties HIV-positive individuals experience and their coping strategies, especially in the workplace. The experiences of those with high and low SOC are compared. Data were collected in Japan from 2007 to 2009 using a qualitative approach. Semistructured interviews were conducted with 40 participants with HIV with work experience. Interviews focused on individual's perspectives, including self-perceptions of physical and mental functioning, work conditions, and perceived changes in their circumstances. Participants were divided into high and low SOC groups based on SOC-13 scores. A number of categories and subcategories of experiences were extracted, including "acute feeling of the severe social positioning of HIV," with some categories specific to those with low SOC. Those with high SOC appeared to have a unique perspective that supported more successful coping, for example, "Awareness of death is linked to valuing living in the present," "Do not be discouraged by uncertainties and difficulties," and so on. It suggests that development of coping skills may help people with HIV.

Keywords: coping strategies, qualitative study, salutogenesis, sense of coherence, Japan

1. Introduction

Acquired immunodeficiency syndrome (AIDS) is characterized by infection with human immunodeficiency virus (HIV) and serious, systemic dysfunction of immunity. Although its global incidence rate is declining, the rate of HIV infection is increasing in Japan, reaching approximately 16,000 cases in 2014 [1]. In the last decade, new treatments for HIV infection and AIDS have improved health and life expectancy for many people who are HIV-positive. In the recent era of highly active antiretroviral therapy, the estimated median survival for a young person diagnosed with HIV infection is >35 years [2]. Most people with HIV are in a stable and manageable condition [3], with this group accounting for the majority of people infected with HIV in Japan, particularly males aged 20–40 years. For this group, infection was diagnosed at a time critical for career development [1].

The importance of employment has been emphasized in many studies on chronic diseases [4]. Employment helps people to function as adults and find self-worth, therefore playing an important role in maintaining human dignity [5]. Mental health is reported to be better in people with HIV who are employed than in those who are unemployed [6]. However, in the workplace, people with HIV suffer from anxiety about discrimination and layoff [7]. Disclosing the name of their disease may also be highly problematic for them [8, 9].

In many life situations, people with HIV experience various stressors [10]; for example, HIV is perceived as a more stigmatized disease than cancer [11]. People with HIV are also faced with problems unique to HIV, which further affect their vulnerability and makes psychological adjustment more difficult [12]. People with HIV are, therefore, forced to cope with highly stressful situations, brought about by stigma and their own anxiety about experiencing stigma.

Sense of coherence (SOC), a concept proposed by the health sociologist Antonovsky, was conceptualized and standardized as the ability to cope successfully [13]. SOC focuses on salutary factors (i.e., health factors) described as "salutogenesis" [14]. Rather than focusing on pathogenesis, or a conventional medical line of questioning regarding the causes of disease, salutogenesis aims to shed light on what creates health.

Antonovsky created the salutogenic model, which illustrates relationships among stressors, coping (tension coping and coping resources), and SOC. The salutogenic model comprises two theoretical models. First, in the face of stressors and the resulting strain, SOC copes by mobilizing generalized resistance resources. The success or failure of coping depends on the richness of coping resources and the strength of SOC. The second theoretical model explains that SOC is formed by good life experiences and strengthened by successful experiences of coping with tension. The quality of these good life experiences is formed by "generalized resistance resources" (GRRs) [13]. GRRs can be identified as resources bound to an individual's capacities and include material and nonmaterial qualities ranging from individual level factors to those of the person's culture and/or society [15]. That is, GRRs are the physical, biological, artifactual-material, cognitive, emotional, valuative-attitudinal, interpersonal-relational, and macro-sociocultural characteristics of an individual or a group that are effective in avoiding or combating a wide variety of stressors [14].

The salutogenic model indicates that success or failure of stress coping depends on the level of SOC. Higher SOC brings more successful coping, which results in further strengthening SOC. Therefore, a positive spiral relationship has been suggested between SOC and successful coping experiences. In other words, high SOC helps stress coping, which promotes redefinition and reconstruction of the experience, creating a virtuous cycle [14, 15].

Describing coping experiences of people with high SOC is to describe successful coping with stressors. It is also important to describe how flexibly and successfully those with high SOC are able to cope. This may lead to useful suggestions for supporting people with HIV. In addition, comparing different coping styles of people with HIV who have high or low SOC, and examining their unique experiences and living environments may provide clues to their different perspectives and coping behaviors. Particular difficulties experienced by a person with HIV may also be related to low SOC or a decline in SOC.

There is a lack of information on the appropriate types of workplace support for people with HIV in the workforce. The present study aimed to describe the difficulties and coping strategies experienced by people with HIV in the workplace and compare the experiences of those with high and low SOC using the 13-item SOC scale [16]. It is anticipated that the results may provide clues to appropriate types of workplace support for people with HIV.

2. Method

2.1. Study design

Antonovsky stated that qualitative studies are useful to better understand the function of SOC, including its strength and flexibility [13]. The present study wanted to examine participants' experiences from their perspectives and analyze their work life from a new standpoint based on the salutogenic model. A qualitative approach was considered appropriate for these goals.

2.2. Participant recruitment

First, medical facilities with specialized HIV outpatient clinics in Tokyo were asked to invite patients to participate in the study; 15 patients were recruited in total. Inclusion criteria were patients in their twenties to early fifties whose symptoms had been stabilized and who had work experience. Participants were recruited by nurses when visiting the facilities for treatment. Participants chose where the interviews took place, with most taking place at the medical facilities. NPO corporations and social welfare corporations were also contacted and asked to assist with recruitment of participants, and a further 25 participants were recruited. This second round of recruitment increased the diversity of the sampling routes as access to participants living in different areas (Kansai and Kyushu) was made possible. Three pilot interviews and the first 15 interviews for the present study were conducted by two interviewers. The interviewers were the first author and a researcher with a medical degree (Seiko Ishiuchi-Ishitani, fifth author) who was familiar with the interview questions and had worked as a special consultant for a social welfare corporation offering assistance to people with HIV. These interviews were conducted by two interviewers because the purpose of the present study was to collect explorative data, and it was considered beneficial to observe participants from multiple angles. It was also thought that the presence of an interviewer who was affiliated with a social welfare corporation assisting people with HIV may give participants a sense of security and facilitate development of rapport. The 25 interviews in the latter half of the study were conducted by the first author only. The question items were more narrowly focused and based on the earlier data, and as participants introduced by the medical facilities were cooperative, no problems arising from one interviewer were anticipated. During the analysis of participant interviews, it became clear that the results would need to be further evaluated depending on infection route (homosexual contact, heterosexual contact, and tainted blood products), sex, type of employment (regular or irregular), and progression to AIDS. Therefore, it was decided that throughout the study, interviews would cover people with diverse characteristics. As the majority of patients infected through homosexual contact were men, female patients and patients infected by tainted blood products were considered to have different experiences. Therefore, these patients were invited to participate at slightly higher rates than the actual infection rate. We stopped recruiting participants after the number of interviews reached 40, as this was deemed to have reached saturation. Participant details are shown in **Table 1**.

2.3. Data collection

During recruitment and on the day of the interview, participants were assured of privacy through verbal explanations and in written documentation. Before their interview began, participants signed a consent form that included permission to record the interview. The interviews took place in situations where privacy was secured, such as conference rooms and training rooms at a library. The interview duration ranged from 40 to 135 min, with a mean duration of 75 min. Interviews were conducted from September 2007 to September 2009. The interview questions covered: participants' perspectives of their physical and mental functioning since HIV infection was identified, working conditions and the type of job at the time, reactions of people around them, disclosure of infection, relationship with a partner, what HIV means to them, whether their views about HIV and feelings about life and work had changed, what kinds of change occurred, and how they evaluated these changes. The interview was particularly focused on participants' ways of thinking, asking "Why did you behave that way? (or not behave that way)"; "What does the experience mean to you?"; and "Why did you think that way?"

2.4. SOC scale

We used the 13-item, 5-point version of the SOC scale, because the interviews were expected to take a long time and to allow comparison with survey data from a nationwide representative sample [16]. The reliability validity of SOC-13 Japanese edition was determined in a randomly selected nationwide sample of 1800 men and women aged over 20 years. The SOC mean for the sample was 44.06 ± 8.83 [16].

2.5. Ethical considerations

The first author has significant experience working as an occupational health nurse, as well as in supporting people who have a disease that is difficult to disclose to others; this breadth

	n	%
Demographics		
Gender		
Male	35	87.5
Female	5	12.5
Age group		
<30	5	12.5
30 ≤ 39	17	42.5
40 ≤ 49	15	37.5
50 ≤ 59	3	7.5
Education		
University, graduate school	18	45.0
Junior/high school and other	13	32.5
No answer	9	22.5
HIV-associated indicators		
The length of time since HIV diagnose		
<1 year	0	0.0
1–4 years	15	37.5
5–10 years	12	30.0
11 years and above	13	32.5
Route of HIV infection		
Tainted blood products and blood transfusion	5	12.5
Sexual contact	34	85.0
Unknown	1	2.5
CD4 cell counts		
200 ≤ 500/μl	19	47.5
500/μl≤	21	52.5
Sexuality		
Heterosexual	10	25.0
Homosexual	24	60.0
Bisexual	6	15.0

Table 1. Demographic characteristics of participants (n = 40).

of experience enhanced understanding of the difficulties in interpersonal relationships in the workplace. After consulting with the facilities several times, careful consideration was given to the protection of privacy, participants' physical condition at the time of the interview, and arrangement of a comfortable interview place for participants. The purpose of the study, methods, protection of privacy, and disclosure of the results were explained to participants orally and in writing. Participants were informed that they would be able to participate with a fictitious name, to ask any questions during the interview, would not have to answer if they did not want to, and would be able to stop participating at any point. Participants recruited through medical facilities were informed that the interviewer was not associated with the facilities and that their treatment would not be affected in any way, even if they withdrew from participation. The recordings, verbatim transcripts, and analysis notes were stored in a locked room, and the data were stored with real names and other personal information converted into codes. These materials could only be accessed with a password.

The present study was approved by the Medical Research Ethics Committee of Tokyo University, Graduate School (Approval No. 2403), and the Ethics Committee of the National Center for Global Health and Medicine (Approval No. 675).

2.6. Analysis

2.6.1. Interview data

The method of Lofland [17] was used to analyze interview data. First, a transcript of the interview was read repeatedly to grasp the whole picture of the interview. The information was then coded, categorized, and analyzed, with reference to the results of intergroup comparisons between participants with high and low SOC. To ensure the validity of the results, discussions and member checking were conducted with coresearchers [18].

2.6.2. Measuring SOC

SOC was measured after the interview. With the permission of participants, responses were collected while the interview was still being recording, and the majority of their responses were confirmed. According to Söderhamn is collect! [19], an official cut-off point is not prescribed for SOC, and the cut-off point differed in quantitative studies comparing high and low SOC [20, 21]. In qualitative research, the SOC score analysis cannot be conducted by performing group division. However, there is an exception in a study conducted in Croatia [22] that used the SOC-29 (7-point scale), which is the most commonly used version globally. In our study, we used the SOC-13 (5-point scale), as we intended to divide participants based on Japanese mean score. No previous research is available about group division of the SOC-13. Therefore, this was discussed among the present researchers while referring to a Japanese average score. Participants' average SOC-13 score was 43.0 ± 7.9. Given that the scale ranged from 13 to 60, this score was slightly higher than the nationwide sample average (the average score was 41.15 for those in their thirties and 42.16 for those in their forties) [16]. Based on the average score, median score, scores from previous studies, and the nationwide sample scores, participants scoring over 42 (n = 22) were categorized as the high SOC group, with those scoring 39 or less (n = 12) defined as the low SOC group. The remaining six participants scored 40–42 and were categorized as the middle SOC group.

3.1. Difficulties faced by participants

In the present paper, [ ] indicates a category, << >> a sub-category, and < > a code. Relevant quotations from the interviews have been included to illustrate key themes. Details in parentheses after the quotations indicate the participant's ID number, sex, and SOC score (range 13–65).

Difficulties experienced by participants were divided into three domains: physical, social, and personal. Physical domain categories were [Awareness of death] and [Low possibility of maintaining one's physical condition]. Social (employment, interpersonal) domain categories were [Inability to maintain or weakening of coherence with respect to work], [Being made aware of the lack of understanding and knowledge about HIV in society], [Cut off from society because of the name of the illness], and [Keeping love and marriage at a distance]. The personal domain was represented by the categories [Feelings of guilt and self-reproach] and [Having complicated feelings about being infected]. No distinctive difficulties were observed in the high SOC group.

3.1.1. Difficulties specific to patients with low SOC

Four distinctive subcategories found in the low SOC group were the following: <<Being at work becomes difficult after infection is determined>>; <<Leaving one's job due to the fear of HIV becoming known>>; <<Being seized by the idea that working hard has no meaning>>; and <<Just getting by is enough for my life>> (**Table 2**).

> *I don't find any meaning in working so hard. To be honest, I just think it's enough to do whatever is in front of me. That's the only prospect I have at the moment. (#31, male, score: 33)*

Some participants in the low SOC group experienced [Being made to realize the lack of understanding and knowledge about HIV in society].

> *During a job interview, people ask how I got the disease. My answer is "because I had sex without using a condom." They probably don't understand much about immunodeficiency, even people who want to hire people to whom the Disabled People Employment Promotion Act applies.(#9, male, score: 34)*

In the category [Cut off from society because of the name of the illness], participants in the low SOC group reported experiencing severe stigma, including: <<Being told that my handicap isn't normal>> and <<Being told that you don't get that disease if you live a normal life>>. Participants reported that stigma by people they were close to and had a good relationship with in the workplace or where they received treatment was most hurtful. This stigma was particularly felt when a participant was hired under the Disabled People Employment Promotion Act, and for some, this became a major reason to give up working.

> *(As a worker covered by the Disabled People Employment Promotion Act) when I was having my individual counseling, the first thing they said was "we didn't want to hire you from the start." Loud and clear. Looking back now, the president of the company must have told them to hire me. They perhaps couldn't say no and hired me unwillingly. They even told me, "We wanted to employ a normal disabled person, so to speak." (#43, male, score: 28)*

Domain	Categories	Subcategories **Difficulties peculiar to patients with low SOC**
Physical	[Awareness of death] [Low possibility of maintaining one's physical condition]	
Social (employment, interpersonal)	[Inability to maintain/weakening of coherence with respect to work]	<<Being at work becomes difficult after infection is determined>> <<Leaving one's job due to the fear of HIV becoming known>> <<Being seized by the idea that working hard is no meaning>> <<Just getting by is enough for my life>>
	[Being made to realize the lack of understanding and knowledge about HIV in society] low SOC only	<<Being asked that why you were infected>> <<Being asked the meaning of immune dysfunction>>
	[Cut off from society by virtue of the disease's name]	<< Being told that my handicap isn't normal>> <<Being told that you don't get that disease if you live a normal life>>
	[Keeping love and marriage at a distance]	<<Arguments about who gave who the infection with partner>> <<A poor relationship with a lover or a partner>>
Personal	[Feelings of guilt and self-reproach] [Having complicated feelings about being infected]	<<Victims who had been infected by someone else>> <<Anger towards the person who passed on the infection>>

Table 2. Difficulties experienced by participants

Besides difficulties at work, participants experienced anguish on an interpersonal level about disclosure of their infection to significant others and about lovers and marriage. Particularly in the low SOC group, participants felt there were <<Arguments about who gave who the infection>> which led to <<A poor relationship with a lover or a partner>>, and as a result they (sexually infected homosexual males) experienced [Keeping love and marriage at a distance].

> *The person I was going out with had shingles twice in a row. Then I thought I could also have it (HIV) and so I checked. He probably gave it to me, but he didn't tell me anything. In the end, I lost my trust in him and we broke up. (#31, male, score: 33)*

Participants expressed [Feelings of guilt and self-reproach] for having become infected; particularly, participants in the low SOC group felt very strongly that they could not understand and accept why they had been infected. As a result, they perceived themselves as <<Victims who had been infected by someone else>>. This feeling of being a victim was linked to <<Anger towards the person who passed on the infection>> who they felt was to blame.

I trusted the pitcher (the person who inserts his penis) and didn't wear a rubber. That's how I got it, and the guilty party, so to speak, was my partner and he is responsible. I can't forgive him for that. (#43, male, score: 28)

3.2. Characteristic coping experiences in the high SOC group

Coping experiences characteristic of the high SOC group are presented in **Table 3**.

These experiences were classified by encounter environment and way of coping. In terms of the environment, employment and personal relationships were extracted as categories in the social domain. Coping may also be classified as being cognitive or behavioral.

3.2.1. Social domain

In the category [A workplace environment enabling maintenance of coherence with respect to work], working conditions were important, such as access to a paid vacation and a fully equipped welfare system. Other important conditions were no shift work, preservation of privacy, minimal overwork, minimal other physical burdens, and stable work. In addition, <<A workplace climate appreciating diversity>> was important for men who have sex with men. This enabled them to continue doing the same job in the same way as before infection.

In our corporate climate, people don't get involved with each other unless it concerns business. There are quite a few people who take sick leave in my company because of bad physical and mental condition. When they are back in the office, everyone behaves normally as though nothing special has happened. (#39, male, score: 50)

The category [Opportunity to have a workplace where one is needed and where colleagues trust each other] reflected the importance of personal relationships in the workplace. One participant who became infected through sexual contact with another man commented on informing his superior of his need for leave of absence due to the infection.

Since I was infected with HIV, my condition was bad and I decided to tell my superior. When I was about to tell him how I was infected, he said, "Take a rest" and "How you got the disease doesn't matter to me at all. You are still you and I understand very well how hard you have been working." (#4, male, score: 49)

In this way, <<Having the confidence that even though infected, one is still trusted as a member of society>> provided substantial moral support.

The category [Had opportunity to know someone who understands about the infection] indicated understanding of HIV infection by significant others, such as parents and siblings, friends, lovers, and partners. Many participants commented on how, at difficult times, such as the onset of AIDS and when they lost their jobs, they had been helped by others who <<Offered comfort during times of physical and mental stress>>. Among their significant others, it was important that there were <<Friends who remained as close as they had been before hearing of the infection>> and <<Support from the company's occupational health doctor>> in the workplace. However, only participants who were hired because of a disability or who had hemophilia told their company's occupational health doctor about their disease. Even if the company's occupational health doctor said they were thorough about

Domain	Categories	Subcategories	Coping caracteristics
Social (employment, personal relationships)	[A workplace environment enabling maintenance of coherence with respect to work]	<<A workplace climate appreciating diversity>>	Coping whth the environment they encounter
	[Opportunity to have a workplace where one is needed and where colleagues trust each other]	<<Having the confidence that even though infected, one is still trusted as a member of society>>	
	[Had opportunity to know someone who understands about the infection]	<<Offered confort during times of physical and mental stress>> <<Friends who remained as close as they had been before hearing of the infection>> <<Support from the company's occupational health doctor>> <<No change in love and affection from spouse, lover or partner after informing them of the infection>>	
	[The infection provided an opportunity to build/rebuild important bonds]	<<ebuilding relationships with significant others as a result of infection>> <<Infection led to meeting irreplaceable people>>	
	[No perception of direct stigma]	<<The attitude was the same as that towards other disabilities>>	
	[Treat the infection and related events neutrally]	<<Being infected is unlucky but not a disaster>> <<Apart from the infection, I'm happy so it's OK>> <<Everyone faces their own difficulties and anxieties>> <<Is the problem really caused by HIV?>>	Cognitive coping
	[Awareness of death is linked to valuing living in the present]	<<Think about what kind of work I really want to do and how to live>>	
	[Judging and assessing events from a long-term point of view]	<<Particular events in the past resulted in me being in this position now>>	
	[Create boundary lines for important things, do a reality check, and then actively change them]	<<Reaching a compromise between the content and conditions of work and one's physical condition and or environment>> <<Changing one's work goals and aim in life>>	

Domain	Categories	Subcategories	Coping caracteristics
	["Anyway, give it a try" behavior]	<<Disclosed the infection to a partner or lover in an attempt to have them accept it>> <<Disclosure of the infection at the company to gain the support of superiors and colleagues at the workplace>> <<Disclosure of the infection to friends to confirm the way of socializing in the future>> <<Ask for help myself>>	Behavioral coping
	[Do not be discouraged by uncertainties and difficulties]		Cognitive coping
	[Being infected cannot be helped and I am prepared for the worst]	<<I accept responsibility for becoming HIV-infected (infection between homosexuals)>> <<I am not going to be at the mercy of anger due to the infection (harmful effects of medicines, heterosexual)>>	
	[Ready to live one's own life]	<<Live while regretting one's behavior that led to infection (homosexual infection)>> <<I will go straight>>	
		<<Be thoroughly prepared for the onset of AIDS and dying before others>>	

Table 3. Coping experiences observed in high SOC participants

protecting privileged information, many participants did not tell anyone in the company about their HIV infection.

> *The drugs I was taking were no longer suitable for me and I really thought of suicide then. It took me about half a year to get settled, and my mother came regularly from my hometown to stay with me because she thought I shouldn't be left alone. She really helped me a lot.(#23, male, score: 49)*

Almost all participants felt they had to tell their spouse, lover, or partner about their infection to prevent them also becoming infected. In this situation, many participants in the high SOC group experienced <<No change in love and affection from spouse, lover, or partner after informing them of the infection>>. Some received considerable support from the presence of significant others who understood about HIV infection and continued to accept them.

> *I have only dated two people since I found out about my disease. I would tell him/her about my condition (HIV) and ask if he/she is still sure. Interviewer: "And if he/she says it's OK, then the relationship could start?" I would feel that I should do my best for them.(#39, male, score: 50)*

The category [The infection provided an opportunity to build/rebuild important bonds] included the subcategory <<Rebuilding relationships with significant others as a result of infection>>. This was reflected by participants who reported that disclosing HIV infection improved their relationships with other people, particularly parents, siblings, and other blood relatives. Participants in the high SOC group experienced love and affection from their parents and siblings, and felt disclosing the infection provided a chance to rebuild relationships.

> *Since our points of view have been always different, my brother and I weren't so close once we had both grown up. However, because he is younger, my brother was very understanding, and said "anybody could be infected." That changed my relationship with him completely. Now we are very close. If I hadn't been infected, things probably wouldn't have turned out this way. (#26, female, score: 53)*

Another subcategory, <<Infection led to meeting irreplaceable people>>, referred to those who felt lucky because they had met people they would never have met if they had not been infected. As well as attaching a more positive meaning to HIV infection, this was a source of energy for some participants to live with HIV and continue living.

> *Then I met this man and realized that he loved me for everything, including my disease. I thought that even if I never go out with another man until I die, that's OK, because this experience was quite enough for me. Looking back now, I wouldn't have met this man who really loved me if I hadn't had my disease. As he said himself, to find each other I had to have been infected. We wouldn't have shared any common ground, otherwise. (#26, female, score: 53)*

The category [No perception of direct stigma] was common for participants in the high SOC group. These participants reported that regardless of the route of infection, when the name of their disease was disclosed when applying for a job open to disabled people, they experienced <<The attitude was the same as that toward other disabilities>>, and even if there was concern for their physical condition, the attitudes of people around them did not change.

> *The top people of the company weren't prejudiced and the company's philosophy was to let more disabled people have jobs and participate in society. So, I thought I preferred to tell them and be employed. At the interview, they asked me, as they do normally, "Is there any difficulty when you work?" and "Do you visit hospital regularly?" and so on. I told them "There are no problems when I work because my condition is stable." (#10, male, score: 46)*

3.2.2. Cognitive and behavioral coping

3.2.2.1. Cognitive coping

The category [Treat the infection and related events neutrally] reflected how participants in the high SOC group tended to view things objectively and look at them calmly from a distance. This was observed in the high SOC group, where even if participants experienced feeling guilty or depressed, they felt that <<Being infected is unlucky but not a disaster>>. When re-evaluating their current lives, they felt <<Apart from the infection, I'm happy, so it's OK>>. When comparing their past with the present, they thought about past hardships with the infection in the context of <<Everyone faces their own difficulties and anxieties>>.

Some participants also reported that when others knew of the infection, they sometimes reacted negatively. Even without experiencing strong stigma, this response made participants feel bitter, sad, or angry. However, those in the high SOC group reflected on the situation later and wondered <<Is the problem really caused by HIV?>>. They perceived hard experiences as not necessarily all being a result of HIV. They thought objectively about their own HIV infection and looked at themselves with a calm, neutral attitude.

> *Well, it wasn't a friend of mine but an acquaintance of my spouse. She knew about my infection and someone told me that she was talking about me behind my back. Apparently, she said that she didn't want to have meals with me, or something. But of course, that isn't all about my disease. I reckon that's something to do with liking or disliking each other. Me being an HIV carrier is the excuse she uses. She probably just hated my personality (laughs). (#26, female, score: 53)*

The category [Awareness of death is linked to valuing living in the present] reflected how participants assumed there was a high possibility of dying prematurely. Those in the high SOC group were observed to live life to the fullest, do what they wanted to do now, and <<Think about what kind of work I really want to do and how to live>>.

> *It's true that I can work harder since I got this disease. Before, when I was healthy, I had so little motivation. After I got ill, I became very grateful to my company. I became ill and they still employ me. They allow me to take leave, too. Then, I remembered that I really wanted to continue working because when I left my hometown, I made a strong resolution. (#37, male, score: 57)*

The category [Judging and assessing events from a long-term point of view] represented those who considered that <<Particular events in the past resulted in me being in this position now>> rather than making fragmentary judgments or assessments. Furthermore, they reported that "what I am experiencing now will be in some way useful in the future." Inevitably, perceiving that the past, present, and future are joined was linked to comments about belief in invisible powers such as "believing in fate" and "believing in God's will."

> *I got this (HIV) and it had an influence on my field of specialization. I had to give up. I was disappointed, but somehow I was able to think positively that something good would turn up and that this infection must be useful for something in the future. Interviewer: "What made you think so?" I've always been like that. I think positively and believe in what I think (laughs). That's all. (#33, male, score: 44)*

The category [Create boundary lines for important things, do a reality check, and then actively change them] described how, for many participants, HIV infection led to letting go of things that were important or giving up long-term dreams. This was particularly true for work. In the high SOC group, there were some who accepted this, coping by <<Reaching a compromise between the content and conditions of work and one's physical condition and/or environment>> and <<Changing one's work goals and aim in life>>. Being aware that decisions lie within oneself was particularly important. Even if the current situation involved unavoidable reconciliation, awareness that one must make the final decision alone, be confident, and make decisions independently was important.

> *(Because of the infection, this person was transferred to a clerical position from working outside the office) I really wanted to continue the job I was doing until I had gained one year of experience. But, thinking about the trouble I might cause other people if I insisted on doing the former job, and the company's offer of allowing me to continue working, in the end I decided by myself that I should do my best in the new position. (#4, male, employed, score: 49)*

3.2.2.2. Behavioral coping

The category ["Anyway, give it a try" behavior] often applied when infection was disclosed to a lover or a partner. Nearly all participants in the low SOC group had given up the idea of having a lover saying, "After all, I can't make love" and "Nobody would understand." In contrast, participants in the high SOC group reported that they carefully planned the timing and <<Disclosed the infection to a partner or a lover in an attempt to have them accept it>>. This resulted in the relationship continuing in some cases and ending in others. Either way, participants accepted the outcome. In addition to affectionate relationships, there was positive behavior shown by <<Disclosure of the infection at the company to gain the support of superiors and colleagues in the workplace>> and <<Disclosure of the infection to friends to confirm the way of socializing in the future>>. Whether or not infection was disclosed, a "give it a try" attitude was characteristic of the general behavior of many participants, for example, <Ask for help myself>.

> *I learned a lot by asking the doctor at the hospital. "...This medicine works this way so the virus reacts this way and is deactivated." I am given explanations like that so I thoroughly understand. (#39, male, score: 50)*

The category [Do not be discouraged by uncertainties and difficulties] reflected the tendency of participants in the high SOC group to meet challenges even if they had initially failed. One participant disclosed his infection to a person he had become fond of, which ended the relationship. He also disclosed the infection to the next person he came to love, feeling a moral obligation to tell the other party because of the infection risk. Despite the fact that a relationship ending is hurtful, the participant maintained his stance about disclosing infection.

> *Being rejected by the person you want to go out with... I remember three times. Interviewer: "Three times? Did you have any fears about being rejected again (if you disclose the infection)?" Well, it would be a lie if I said no. Interviewer: "After being turned down by several people, don't you feel that you don't want to disclose your infection anymore? Because the person before rejected you, do you think the next person must do the same?" I don't think so. In fact, some people didn't reject me. I don't think that everyone is the same. There are many different people living in this world. (#10, male, score: 56)*

Participants held similar attitudes regarding work. In cases where a participant decided their infection should be disclosed at work, their behavior was to disclose the infection. Even if one company did not hire them, they tried talking to another company about the infection.

3.2.3. *High SOC group attitudes as a result of coping*

Experiences in the category [Being infected cannot be helped and I am prepared for the worst] differed between the high and low SOC groups. Participants in the low SOC group experienced becoming infected with HIV as "the result of giving in to the demand of the other party (sexual contact without using a condom)" or "due to betrayal by a person I trusted." In contrast, those in the high SOC group felt that "It was my own fault," <<I accept responsibility for becoming HIV-infected (infection between homosexuals)>>, and <<I am not going to be at the mercy of anger due to the infection (harmful effects of medicines, heterosexual)>>.

> *Probably he did not know he was infected with HIV, that he did not pass on the infection with any feelings of malice, and that passing on the infection was not intentional.(#26, female, score: 53)*

The category [Ready to fully live one's own life] encompassed subcategories that described participants' motivation to <<Live while regretting one's behavior that led to infection (homosexual infection)>>, <<I will go straight>>, and to <<Be thoroughly prepared for the onset of AIDS and dying before others>>. Some participants reported that this mental state was not reached immediately after discovering the infection, and was not easy. At the time the infection was discovered, some participants became depressed and desperate. However, having people around them providing support allowed them to organize things in their minds and behave in ways to help discover how to live their life.

> *What happened has happened and there is nothing I can do about it. I can't hide from reality. So, go back to point zero and think about how I want to live my life, that's what I've done. Speaking from experience, having done my best including trying to be mentally positive, I think in the end it's best to live my life honestly and properly. (#34, male, score: 44)*

4. Discussion

4.1. Difficulties experienced by people with HIV

Previous studies have shown that major barriers for people infected with HIV in remaining motivated about re-employment are anxiety about their health, education and skills, and workplace discrimination [23, 24]. Although the present study largely focused on those who were already working, there are a range of difficulties faced by people with HIV in terms of their physical and social condition and self-concept. The experience of having been [Cut off from society because of the name of the illness] was only found in the low SOC group. This suggests they had experienced direct (enacted) stigma, such as <<Being told that my disability was not normal>> or <<Being told that you do not get that disease if you live a normal life>>. Most participants felt that although stigma from the community was unfair, they could not do anything about it and had to accept it. A previous study [25] found that enacted stigma and vicarious stigma (where a person hears of another's experience) were significantly associated with depression and self-stigma. These experiences are likely to damage a person's SOC and prevent its restoration. This was true for the low SOC group in the present study. A study focused on mental illness by Lundberg et al. is the only research to date that has examined the relationship between SOC and stigma [26]. The present study is the first to examine the relationship between the SOC of people with HIV and their experiences of stigma.

Lundberg et al. [26] found the experience of having been socially rejected was significantly associated with low SOC. This association was stronger ($\beta = -0.357$, $p < 0.001$) than for empowerment ($p < 0.02$) or self-esteem ($p < 0.01$). The results of their research, and those of the present study, confirm the close relationship between SOC and stigma. This is a significant finding; however, the ways in which experiences of stigma impact on SOC have not yet been sufficiently investigated.

The present study found that people with HIV experienced direct stigma in medical settings and in the workplace. In particular, two participants who reported experiencing stigma at work were employed under the Disability Act. This suggests that experiencing stigma in medical facilities and workplaces, where a higher level of understanding is usually expected, may result in an unmanageable and incomprehensible situation that causes confusion and a sense of powerlessness. If people working under the Disability Act experience stigma at work, they have lost a place to feel safe, which may result in despair. Furthermore, unlike vicarious stigma, enacted stigma is inescapable, and may result in beliefs such as HIV infection being the reason for stigma. Therefore, stigma may negatively affect SOC, and this may explain why a person decides not to reveal their illness at work or in other situations.

4.2. Coping by people with HIV

Coping strategies of participants with high SOC in the present study were classified as coping with the environments they encountered and cognitive coping. The findings showed that encounters with favorable environments maintained or improved SOC. However, in those who did not report good encounters with people or favorable environments, their high SOC was attributed to cognitive and behavioral coping. Cognitive coping referred to how encountered environments were perceived. Behavioral coping referred to how they changed their own environment. High SOC is considered to make cognitive and behavioral coping possible.

4.2.1. The surrounding environment

Categories extracted relating to the surrounding environment represented experiences of favorable working conditions and workplace cultures, as well as positive human relationships. Previous theoretical [13] and qualitative studies have indicated that there is a significant relationship between working environment and SOC [27]. SOC reflects one's trust toward one's life and the wider context (surrounding people and environment). In SOC theory, "legitimate others" are those who provide this sense of being trusted, loved, watched, and recognized. Legitimate others bring a sense of security and the feeling that one is not alone. They also give people meaning in life, energy, and courage [13].

4.3. High SOC coping strategies

A coping strategy in participants with high SOC concerned the challenge of how they should behave in a situation they could not control (e.g., strong stigma against HIV, a workplace culture that did not allow diversity, difficult work conditions, unstable physical condition, and relationship breakup). These are situations that participants could not do anything about by themselves. Participants in the high SOC group reported trying their best to cope with these stressors.

According to Antonovsky [13], people with high SOC tend to view the world as consistent. An effective way of holding this perspective is flexibly controlling the boundaries of important areas in life. For example, to avoid distress, they might bring part of their lives to a peripheral area that was not as important to them. Participants with high SOC in the present study tried to actively change the boundaries between what was important to them and reality, including compromising on job content and conditions, depending on their own physical condition and environment, and changing the goals of their work or life. They coped with events that had become incomprehensible and unmanageable by bringing them to areas that were less important to them. Kraaij found that people with HIV who were capable of making goal adjustment in their lives were able to maintain positive mental health [28]. The present study confirmed the importance of flexibly adjusting goals.

The group with high SOC escaped from the chaos of their reality by neutrally perceiving the events relating to their infection and by calmly and objectively observing their reality. Antonovsky [13] stated that people with high SOC are not trapped by their emotions too long; instead, they define the nature and dimension of their problems, deal with them, and explore ways to move from chaos to order. The present study found the high SOC group used behavioral coping strategies, deciding to do something about it, taking action, and not allowing themselves to be defeated by a sense of uncertainty or difficulties. Antonovsky [13] regarded participation in consequences as an important element of meaningfulness. Participation in consequences encompasses factors such as autonomy and participation in decision-making; for example, accepting current challenges, taking responsibility, and making decisions as to what to do or not to do. The accumulation of these experiences nurtures a sense of meaningfulness. In the present study, many participants in the low SOC group had given up on having an intimate relationship. In contrast, those in the high SOC group took action and tried not to be defeated by uncertainty or difficulties. Even if the consequence of their action did not turn out as expected, this group considered their judgment to be meaningful because their will and behavior had been reflected in the consequences.

Participants in the high SOC group who were infected through sexual contact tried to accept their responsibility for the infection. In contrast, those in the low SOC group were not able to overcome their sense of being victimized. Antonovsky [13] suggests that many stressors cause problems of blame where responsibility is attributed to others. Those with low SOC tend to blame other people or factors for their problems. In the present study, some participants with high SOC reported experiencing confusion and depression when they learned about their infection or progression to AIDS, despairing and not caring anymore about what they did. However, they reported being able to find ways to cognitively and emotionally cope with their problems, taking responsibility for their infection, placing the infection within an area of life they could control, and viewing their problems objectively. These participants coped with the difficulties of HIV infection by feeling that they were participating in the consequences.

4.4. Suggestions for practice

Although it is not surprising that only those with low SOC reported experiencing direct stigma, it is a reality that should not be ignored. Direct stigma has a serious, negative impact on people with HIV. In the present study, direct stigma was reported by people who were working under the framework of the Disability Act. Even if an employer or a human resources manager has knowledge about HIV infection, other colleagues may not share the same level of understanding. HIV infection is an invisible disability, and those employed under the Disability Act tend to be regarded by others with suspicion. Some participants in the present study reported that they did not know what to say when asked by fellow workers what disease they had. Educating employers, human resource managers, and other staff about HIV through corporate training is urgently needed.

In addition, from an industrial health perspective, it may be necessary to develop workplace cultures in which people with health conditions can work and receive treatment without distress. A workplace in which workers with HIV can feel comfortable will be a good workplace for all employees. Everyone risks losing their health at some point. Therefore, it is important to improve working conditions so employees can work according to their health conditions and lifestyles. However, it is also important that good relationships are developed with managers and colleagues through regular communication, allowing people with HIV to gain trust, and be seen as a reliable working member of society. The present analysis showed that participants' social skills were an important factor for SOC, and although changes are needed in the workplace, people with HIV also need to make their own efforts to fulfill the role of a worker.

The attitudes of those with high SOC make them more likely to cope successfully. This provides important clues for future interventions and education. Although international studies have accumulated a wide knowledge base about interventions for HIV infection [29, 30], there have been few studies in Japan. It is important to increase coping skills to support people with HIV, including suggesting alternative ways of thinking about their situation. Unconditional support from families and significant others is important.

4.5. Limitations

First, no participants in the high SOC group reported experiencing direct stigma. However, this may not mean that they never experienced direct stigma. They may have had experiences they did not report or did not recognize as stigma. Future studies should examine whether or not participants had real experience of stigma, quantitatively clarify how the impact of stigma was recognized, and examine the association between stigma and SOC.

Second, participants in the present study might have been patients in particularly good physical and mental condition. Participants were selected by the nurses working in the specialized medical facilities, and limited to those considered by the nurses to be in a good enough condition to be interviewed. It may be that recruited participants were those who had good relationships with the nurses and who were considered easy to communicate with. The facilities advised that 5–10 patients declined to participate because they came for treatment during working hours and did not have time for an interview or did not feel well. Some of those who were not asked to participate may not have been physically or mentally well, or may not have had a good relationship with their medical professionals. The present study stopped recruiting participants after 40 interviews, as this was deemed the saturation level. However, it is possible that if those who declined had been included, other categories of experiences might have been extracted. Therefore, the interpretation of the present results requires some caution.

Acknowledgements

This study was supported by JSPS KAKENHI Grant Number 24530731.

Author details

Tomoko Omiya*, Yoshihiko Yamazaki, Megumi Shimada, Kazuko Ikeda,
Seiko Ishiuchi-Ishitani and Katsumi Ohira

*Address all correspondence to: toomiya-tky@umin.ac.jp

Toho University, Tokyo, Japan

References

[1] AIDS surveillance committee of Ministry of Health, Labour and Welfare. 2010 AIDS outbreak trend annual report in Japan. [Internet]. 2011/05/23 [Updated: 2011/05/23]. Available from: http://api-net.jfap.or.jp/status/2014/14nenpo/h26gaiyo.pdf [Accessed: 2012/06/27.]

[2] Lohse, N., Hansen, A. B. E., Pedersen, G., Kronborg, G., Gerstoft, J., Sorensen, H. T. Survival of persons with and without HIV infection in Denmark, 1995–2005. Annals of Internal Medicine. 2007; **146**(2); 87–95.

[3] Mizushima, D., Oka, S. HIV infection in Japan. Clinical Microbiology. 2010; **37**(6):684–689.

[4] McGurk, S. R., Mueser, K. T., DeRosa, T. J., Wolfe, R. Work, recovery, and comorbidity in schizophrenia: a randomized controlled trial of cognitive remediation. Schizophrenia Bulletin. 2009; **35**(2):319–335.

[5] Swindells, S., Mohr, J., Justis, J. C., Berman, S., Squier, C., Wagener, M. M. Quality of life in patients with human immunodeficiency virus infection: impact of social support, coping style and hopelessness. International Journal of STD & AIDS. 1999; **10**(6):383–91.

[6] Omiya, T., Yamazaki, Y., Shimada, M., Ikeda, K., Ishiuchi-Ishitani, S., Ysuno, Y. S. Mental health of patients with human immunodeficiency virus in Japan: a comparative analysis of employed and unemployed patients. AIDS Care. 2014; **26**(11):1370–1378. DOI: 10.1080/09540121.2014.913765

[7] Brooks, R. A., Klosinski, L. E. Assisting persons living with HIV AIDS to return to work: programmatic steps for AIDS service organizations. AIDS Education and Prevention. 1999; **11**(3):212–223.

[8] Hergenrather, K. C., Rhodes, S. D., Clark, G. The employment perspectives study: identifying factors influencing the job-seeking behavior of persons living with HIV/AIDS. AIDS Education and Prevention. 2005; **17**(2):131–142. DOI: 10.1521/aeap.17.3.131.62905

[9] Medley, A. M., Kennedy, C. E., Lunyolo, S., Sweat, M. D. Disclosure outcomes, coping strategies, and life changes among women living with HIV in Uganda. Qualitative Health Research. 2009; **19**(12):1744–1754. DOI: 10.1177/1049732309353417

[10] Cohen, M., Hoffman, R. G., Cromwell, C., Schmeidler, J., Ebrahim, F., Carrera, G. The prevalence of distress in persons with human immunodeficiency virus infection. Psychosomatics. 2002; **43**(1):10–15.

[11] Fesko, S. L. Workplace experiences of individuals who are HIV plus and individuals with cancer. Rehabilitation Counseling Bulletin. 2001; **45**(1):2–11.

[12] Heckman, T. G., Anderson, E. S., Sikkema, K. J., Kochman, A., Kalichman, S. C., Anderson, T. Emotional distress in nonmetropolitan persons living with HIV disease enrolled in a telephone-delivered, coping improvement group intervention. Health Psychology. 2004; **23**(1):94–100. DOI: 10.1037/0278-6133.23.1.94

[13] Antonovsky, A. Unraveling the Mystery of Health: How People Manage Stress and Stay Well. 1st ed. San Francisco, California: Jossey-Bass Publishers; 1987.

[14] Antonovsky, A. Health, Stress, and Coping: New Perspectives on Mental and Physical Well-Being. San Francisco, California: Jossey-Bass Publishers; 1979.

[15] Eriksson, M., Lindstrom, B. Antonovsky's sense of coherence scale and its relation with quality of life: a systematic review. Journal of Epidermal Community Health. 2007; **61**(11):938–944. DOI: 10.1136/jech.2006.056028

[16] Togari, T., Yamazaki, Y. Examination of the reliability and factor validity of 13-item five-point version sense of coherence scale. Journal of Health and Human Ecology. 2005; **71**(4):168–182.

[17] Lofland, J. Analyzing Social Settings: A Guide to Qualitative Observation and Analysis. 4th ed. Belmont, California: Wadsworth; 2006. pages.

[18] Creswell, J W. Qualitative Inquiry and Research Design: Choosing Among Five Traditions. Thousand Oaks, California: Sage Publications; 2007. pages.

[19] Söderhamn, U., Dale B., Söderhamn, O. Narrated lived experiences of self-care and health among rural-living older persons with a strong sense of coherence. Psychology Research and Behavior Management. 2011; **4**:151–158.

[20] Ahola, A. J., Saraheimo, M., Forsblom, C., Hietala, K., Groop, P. H. The cross-sectional associations between sense of coherence and diabetic microvascular complications, glycaemic control, and patients' conceptions of type 1 diabetes. Health and Quality of Life Outcomes. 2010; **8**:142. DOI: 10.1186/1477-7525-8-142.

[21] Urakawa, K., Yokoyama, K., Itoh, H. Sense of coherence is associated with reduced psychological responses to job stressors among Japanese factory workers. BMC Research Notes. 2012; **5**. DOI: 10.1186/1756-0500-5-247

[22] Ebina, R., Yamazaki, Y. Sense of coherence and coping in adolescents directly affected by the 1991–5 war in Croatia. Promotion & Education. 2008; **15**(4):5–10.

[23] Brooks, R. A., Martin, D. J., Ortiz, D. J., Veniegas, R. C. Perceived barriers to employment among persons living with HIV/AIDS. AIDS Care. 2004; **16**(6):756–766. DOI: 10.1080/09540120412331269594

[24] Martin, D. J, Brooks, R. A., Ortiz, D. J., Veniegas, R. C. Perceived employment barriers and their relation to workforce-entry intent among people with HIV/AIDS. Journal of Occupational Health Psychology. 2003; **8**(3):181–194.

[25] Steward, W. T., Herek, G. M., Ramakrishna, J., Bharat, S., Chandy, S., Wrubel, J. HIV-related stigma: adapting a theoretical framework for use in India. Social Science & Medicine. 2008; **67**(8):1225–1235. DOI: 10.1016/j.socscimed.2008.05.032

[26] Lundberg, B., Hansson, L., Wentz, E., Bjorkman, T. Are stigma experiences among persons with mental illness, related to perceptions of self-esteem, empowerment and sense of coherence? Journal of Psychiatric and Mental Health Nursing. 2009; **16**(6):516–522. DOI: 10.1111/j.1365-2850.2009.01418.x

[27] Feldt, T., Kinnunen, U., Mauno, S. A mediational model of sense of coherence in the work context: a one-year follow-up study. Journal of Organizational Behavior. 2000; **21**(4):461–476.

[28] Kraaij, V., Van der Veek, S. M., Garnefski, N., Schroevers, M., Witlox, R., Maes, S. Coping, goal adjustment, and psychological well-being in HIV-infected men who have sex with men. AIDS Patient Care and STDs. 2008; **22**(5):395–402. DOI: 10.1089/apc.2007.0145

[29] Antoni, M. H., Carrico, A. W., Duran, R. E., Spitzer, S., Penedo, F., Ironson, G. Randomized clinical trial of cognitive behavioral stress management on human immunodeficiency virus viral load in gay men treated with highly active antiretroviral therapy. Psychosomatic Medicine. 2006; **68**(1):143–151. DOI: 10.1097/01.psy.0000195749.60049.63

[30] Carrico, A. W., Antoni, M. H., Pereira, D. B., Fletcher, M. A., Klimas, N., Lechner, S. C. Cognitive behavioral stress management effects on mood, social support, and a marker of antiviral immunity are maintained up to 1 year in HIV-infected gay men. International Journal of Behavioral Medicine. 2005; **12**(4):218–216. DOI: 10.1207/s15327558ijbm1204_2

8

Tuberculosis and HIV — Doubling the Fatality

Tatina T. Todorova, Gabriela Tsankova, Neli Lodozova and Tcvetelina Kostadinova

Abstract

Tuberculosis (TB) and HIV/AIDS infection are one of the most ubiquitous and deadliest communicable diseases in the world. They cause millions of deaths each year and are recognized as major threats for public health worldwide. The corresponding pathogens (*Mycobacterium tuberculosis* and HIV) share overlapping epidemiology—they affect low-income countries and place an immense burden on their feeble health care systems. Over the last decades, the natural history of both diseases has changed; in addition to devastating single HIV and TB infections, the coinfection with both pathogens has emerged and has spread in pandemic scale. When present as dual infection in an individual, *Mycobacterium tuberculosis* and HIV potentiate each other and kill in cooperation the host. TB is the leading cause of death in HIV-positive patients and in turn HIV infection is the strongest risk factor for the development of new or reactivation of dormant TB disease. Both pathogens (as single or dual infection) provoke a robust immune response in the infected host but the immune system does not achieve to eliminate the infectious agent(s). The failure of immune defense results in vulnerable immune balance between the micro- and the macroorganism and often ends up in a fatal outcome.

Keywords: Tuberculosis, HIV, immunity, co-infection

1. Introduction

Human immunodeficiency virus (HIV) and tuberculosis (TB) represent, respectively, the first and the second leading cause of death from infectious disease in the world. Both are responsible for approximately 3 million deaths annually [1].

Either HIV or TB, when present as a single infection, irreversibly affects and exhausts the immune system of the infected person. Moreover, if they simultaneously coexist in an individual (coinfection), they act in synergy to deteriorate the defense mechanisms of the host's immunity and to accelerate the fatal scenario.

In this chapter, we will review current knowledge of innate and adaptive immune responses against TB and HIV infections. We will discuss in detail the immunological basis behind the dual threat of TB/HIV coinfection.

2. Epidemiology

2.1. Epidemiology of HIV pandemic

HIV infection is a viral disease that affects host immune system and makes the host strongly susceptible to opportunistic infections. It spreads among human population via sexual contact, sharing needles during drug injection, transfusion of contaminated blood products, or during births from HIV-infected women.

Since the late 20th century, HIV infection has become a global pandemic and a major challenge for public health authorities at the national and international levels. At the end of 2013, 35 million people were living with HIV worldwide [2]. During the same year, approximately 2.1 million people were newly infected with HIV. Sub-Saharan Africa is the most affected region in the world—almost 70% of the prevalent and the new HIV-positive cases are diagnosed there. The socio-economic status of the countries in the core of HIV pandemic determines the low number of infected people currently on adequate antiretroviral therapy (only 36% of overall cases).

2.2. Epidemiology of tuberculosis

Tuberculosis (TB) is an infectious disease caused by bacterial species grouped in *Mycobacterium tuberculosis* complex—MBTC (*M. bovis, M. africanum, M. canetti, M. caprae, M. microti, M. pinnipedii)*. Among these mycobacterial species, the most important and major cause of human tuberculosis is *Mycobacterium tuberculosis*. It is a widespread microorganism that readily colonizes and infects humans. Primary infection represents clinical manifestation in only 10% of infected individuals, while in the remaining 90%, *M. tuberculosis* stays in latent form without showing any obvious clinical signs—latent (dormant) tuberculosis [3].

The World Health Organization (WHO) recognizes TB as "a global public health emergency" and "one of the world's deadliest communicable diseases" [1]. At least one-third of the world population (approx. 2 billion people) is currently infected with latent mycobacteria and has a risk, although low (5–10%), to develop an active disease during the life course [1]. In 2013, 9 million new TB cases occurred worldwide (TB incidence: 126 cases per 100,000 population) and the prevalent cases were 11 million (TB prevalence: 159 cases per 100,000 population). Despite the efforts at the international, national, and regional level and the significant progress in the detection and management of TB infection, still the incidence, prevalence, and mortality rate of TB are unacceptably high.

2.3. Epidemiology of TB/HIV coinfection

People living with HIV have 26–31 times higher risk to develop active TB than the normal population [1]. Both diseases are epidemiologically and biologically connected—TB is the leading cause of death in HIV-positive patients and in turn HIV infection exacerbates the gravity of TB. Due to the global circulation of HIV, the incidence of TB —an infection previously thought to be almost eliminated at least in developed countries—is still high in both developing and high-income countries. HIV disrupts the host immune system through significant depletion of CD4+ lymphocytes, a mechanism that readily facilitates the reactivation of latent TB to an active disease. Therefore, HIV is the strongest risk factor for the development of new or the reactivation of dormant TB disease, including multidrug-resistant TB, an infection resistant to at least two of the first choice drugs for TB treatment, isoniazid and rifampicin. HIV infection predisposes TB-infected patients to antibiotic (rifampicin) resistance through gastrointestinal malabsorption of TB medications [4]. On the other hand, *M. tuberculosis* enhances HIV replication [5] and decreases the CD4+ T cell counts in HIV-positive patients [6].

As one-third of the total world population is currently infected with latent *M. tuberculosis* [1] and almost 1% of the adult population is living with HIV, it is not surprising that 1.1 million (13%) of the 9 million people who developed TB in 2013 were at the same time HIV-positive and 360,000 of the overall 1.5 million TB deaths for 2013 were HIV-positive. Most of them (78%) were living in low-income economies in Sub-Saharan Africa, a region where 50–80% of TB patients have HIV coinfection[1].

WHO recommends regular screening of TB for all people living with HIV at every visit to a health care specialist [7]. WHO also recommends that routine HIV testing should be offered to all patients with presumptive and diagnosed TB, as well as to partners of known HIV-positive TB patients.

In addition to the increase in TB incidence, the worldwide HIV pandemic changed the average age of TB-infected people. In contrast to normal populations where TB is most prevalent among elderly people, in regions with significant number of HIV-positive cases, the most affected age by TB is the reproductive age (20–45 years). This leads to the consecutive increase in the number of TB-infected children [8].

3. Immunology of tuberculosis

3.1. The first date

Primary infection with *M. tuberculosis* occurs after inhalation of aerosolized infectious nuclei containing mycobacterial cells [9]. Any person with active TB can transmit the pathogen through coughing or sneezing, infecting 2–10 healthy individuals. Tubercle bacilli survive in the air for a short time (few hours), but the infective dose is relatively low (only 1–10 living cells). Infectious nuclei bigger than 10 μm gravitate in the nasal conchae and the nasopharynx. Those measuring between 5 and 10 μm enter the lower respiratory tract and mucociliary escalator eliminates them. Only infectious droplets smaller than 5 μm persist in the distal lung alveoli and can cause infection.

In most cases, the non-immune mechanisms do not allow the development of the infectious process. If infection occurs, the immune system in the lungs activates the first-line innate defense and then, several weeks later, an adaptive anti-mycobacterial immune response is activated. The strong immune response against *M. tuberculosis* works in two warring interests —on one hand, it restricts *M. tuberculosis* dissemination outside the initial infection place, and on the other hand, it supports its survival and silent presence for years in healthy individuals. The human immune system succeeds to completely eliminate *M. tuberculosis* in only 10% of infected cases, while in the remaining 90%, it fulfills in different degrees and controls the infection by turning it into the latent state [3].

3.2. Innate immunity

The early stages of TB infection consist of inhalation of tubercle bacilli and initial encounter between the immune system and the pathogen. Alveolar macrophages and sometimes nonprofessional phagocytic cells (alveolar epithelial cells) are the first to recognize *M. tuberculosis* cells [10, 11, 12]. Still, unknown intrinsic virulent features of *M. tuberculosis* strains and individual host immune differences are crucial for the fate of tubercle bacilli in the early days of infection. The most favorable outcome is the definitive destruction of *M. tuberculosis* by non-specific defense mechanisms in the macrophages. In this case, adaptive immunity does not develop and participate in the protection.

If bacteria survive bactericidal macrophage action, they can multiply intracellularly to destroy the infected macrophage and to release attractants for monocyte and dendritic cells accumulation. The attracted monocytes will differentiate into macrophages that in turn can recognize new *M. tuberculosis* cells to increase the population size of infected cells in the lung and sometimes in extra pulmonary locations. All these immune cells readily engulf *M. tuberculosis* cells but are unable to completely destroy them. Thus, the number of *M. tuberculosis* in the place of infection progressively increases.

Macrophages and dendritic cells bind *M. tuberculosis* cells via different receptors: toll-like receptors (TLRs), nucleotide-binding oligomerization domain (NOD-) like receptors (NLRs), mannose receptors (CD207), dendritic cell-specific intercellular adhesion molecule grabbing nonintegrins (DC-SIGN), Dectin-1 receptors, complement receptors, and others [3]. Among TLRs, the most important for pulmonary TB cases are TLR2, TLR4, and TLR9 [10–12]. TLR2 recognizes tubercle polysaccharides and via binding with TLR1 can identify tubercle cell wall 19 and 27 kDa lipoproteins—important *M. tuberculosis* cell surface ligands. Furthermore, bacterial DNA released after bacterial destruction in lisosomes activates TLR9.

The interaction between *M. tuberculosis* and TLRs induces a signal proinflammatory cascade and provokes secretion of cellular signals—TNF-alpha, IL-1, IL-6, IL-12, IL-18, IL-15, IL-23, IFN-gamma, and chemokinases. The infected macrophages also release small molecules—chemokines CCL, CCL3, CCL4, CCL5 (8–10 κDa)—to attract other blood monocytes and neutrophils [13], which after differentiation can directly display bactericidal action towards

M. tuberculosis. Interleukins and chemokines serve both to attract other immune cells (lymphocytes) and to activate them.

3.3. Cell-mediated immunity

A fundamental characteristic of *M. tuberculosis* infection is the considerable delay in the onset of adaptive immunity, achieved by efficient control and management of the innate immunity; the host establishes an effective cell-mediated immune response several weeks (2–8) after the initial infection [3]. Nonetheless, the initiation of cell-mediated adaptive immunity, though delayed, is crucial for efficient control of further TB invasion.

The matured dendritic cells move to the regional lymph nodes where they initiate specific cell immune response by presenting the ingested mycobacterial antigens to the naïve T cells. Dendritic cells are a primary target for *M. tuberculosis* after aerosolic lung infection [14, 15]. They are professional antigen presenting cells (more effective than macrophages) and strong T cell activators. One of the mechanisms used by *M. tuberculosis* to delay the cell-mediated immunity is the efficient postponement of the movement of dendritic cells towards regional lymph nodes. In the lymph nodes, infected dendritic cells produce IL-12 [16] for the activation of NK cells and stimulation of INF-gamma release from T-lymphocytes [17]. Antigen presenting dendritic cells prompts T cells to differentiate and to migrate, under the navigation of secreted adhesion molecules and chemokines, to the initial site of infection.

The concentration of macrophages, T-lymphocytes, dendritic cells, and other immune and lung cells (epithelial, giant multinuclear Langerhans' cells, plasma cells, neutrophils, fibroblasts) in the place of infection is known as granuloma. The process of granuloma formation limits the spread of *M. tuberculosis* to other organs and restricts tissue's damage by separating the infected place [18]. But at the same time, granuloma microenvironment ensures the needed conditions for mycobacterial growth and multiplication.

Both human and animal granulomas contain giant multinuclear Langerhans' cells produced after the fusion of macrophages [18, 19]. In these cells, tubercle bacilli cannot multiply and survive successfully.

Neutrophils are important for early control of acute bacterial infection [20] as they immediately migrate to the place of mycobacterial infection and start bacterial phagocytosis [21]. Infected neutrophils produce IL-8 and TNF for activation of alveolar macrophages and limitation of the infection [22].

Both CD4+ and CD8+[23] contribute to the stimulation of macrophages and lysis of chronically infected macrophages (via INF-gamma action). The principal role in cell-mediated immunity against tuberculosis is played by CD4+ T-lymphocytes. CD4+ express *a*/*b* T cell receptors to recognize mycobacterial antigens on the surface of antigen-presenting cells such as monocytes, macrophages, or dendritic cells [24]. Then, CD4+ lymphocytes efficiently induce apoptosis of macrophages [25] and stimulate the cytotoxic function of CD8+ [26].

CD8+ cells play an important role in IFN-gamma release, cell lysis and bacterial killing [27]. Some CD8+ lymphocytes may also recognize surface antigens presented by Class I MHC molecules—MHC class I-restricted cytotoxic T-lymphocytes (CTL). They are able to eliminate infected macrophages and also to kill intracellular bacteria via production of granulysin (a cytolytic and proinflammatory substance) [28].

Other immune cells—CD1 restricted T cells, γ/δ-T cells, and cytotoxic T-cells—also protect lung tissue against tuberculosis. T cells of type γ/δ are the first line of defense against microbial antigens and the connection between innate and adaptive immune response [29]. They have cytotoxic activity and may present mycobacterial antigens to CD8+ and CD4+ lymphocytes. In response to IL-23 secreted from infected dendritic cells, the γ/δ-T cells start to release IL-17 for accumulation of additional immune cells in the place of infection.

Activated macrophages represent higher phagocytic activity against extracellular mycobacteria. On the base of T-lymphocyte stimulation, two types of macrophages are known: classically activated macrophages (CAM) and alternatively activated macrophages (AAM). During the immune response against tubercle bacilli, activation of macrophages by T-lymphocytes is achieved mainly through release of IFN-gamma and other Th-1 cytokines. The Th-1 cytokines (INF-gamma, TNF-alpha, IL-1beta) induce CAM to kill tubercle bacilli via production of nitric oxide synthetase (iNOS). This enzyme catalyzes synthesis of nitric oxide (NO), a powerful antimicrobial substance. The Th-2 cytokines (IL-4 and IL-13) activate AAM to produce anti-inflammatory cytokines and arginase. They both compete for arginine utilization with iNOS [30]. The increased arginase activity stimulates tissue repair but at the same time restricts bacterial killing [31].

M. tuberculosis (particularly the virulent strains and not the attenuated ones) can survive in phagosomes of macrophages by suppressing the fusion between formed mycobacterial phagosome and lysosomes [32]. Other mechanisms to overcome bactericidal activity of macrophages include the prevention of phagosomal acidification and guidance of infected cells towards necrosis. Necrosis is a form of cellular death characterized by plasma and mitochondrial membrane disruption. In this way, tubercle bacilli leave infected macrophages and spread to other cells. Moreover, *M. tuberculosis* may inhibit the programmed cell death or apoptosis, a cellular death that protects further bacterial spread by preserving the cellular integrity of infected macrophage. Apoptotic macrophages transmit mycobacterial antigens to dendritic cells and induce more efficient T cell response.

3.4. Humoral immunity

In addition to cell-mediated immunity, humoral immune response plays a major role in TB infection control. The formed antibodies cannot transfer immunity but have an opsoning role and facilitate the phagocytosis by the macrophages and the cytotoxic function of T-lymphocytes [33]. Besides their antibody synthetic function [34], B-lymphocytes can present mycobacterial antigens to T cells [35]. They stimulate proliferation and differentiation of T-lymphocytes by the production of different cytokines. Specific effector B1-cells secrete Th1-cytokines—IFN-gamma and IL-12—while B2-cells secrete IL-4, typical for Th2-cells. Furthermore, activated B cells can produce IL-6 for T cell stimulation and IL-10 for inhibition of dendritic cells and macrophages.

3.5. Latent tuberculosis

The late stage of TB infection represents a prolonged (in many cases lifelong) suppression of mycobacterial cells as a result of the dynamic balance between the pathogen and the host immunity. *M. tuberculosis* persists within the granulomas and escapes total disruption by the immune system. In latent TB, the host and tubercle bacilli coexist in "perfect" synergy; the granuloma represents a place for bacterial survival and place for host attack [36]. Usually, the host immune system succeeds to manage the infectious process, but in extreme conditions (starving, diabetes, alcohol abuse, corticosteroid treatment, and especially supplementary HIV infection) the disease can progress. This progression is linked to granuloma disruption and further dissemination of *M. tuberculosis*. The late tuberculosis occurs in the presence of sensitized T-lymphocytes and already existing specific defense mechanisms. This determines rapid limitation of the process with strong caseous necrosis, cavern formation, and fibrosis.

4. Immunology of HIV

4.1. Entry through the mucosal barrier

The principal route of HIV entry into the human body is through the mucosal epithelial surfaces (mainly genital or rectal). The virus prefers to infect immune cells expressing CD4+ receptors on their surface—CD4+ helper T cells, macrophages, and dendritic cells—all present in activated state in the mucosal lymphoid tissues.

HIV crosses the intact epithelial layers via interaction with dendritic cells and/or CD4+ helper T cells. The CD4+ receptor of these cells recognizes the viral envelope glycoprotein 120 (gp120) and causes its conformational change. This makes possible the binding with one of the auxiliary co-receptors: CCR5 or CXCR4. The second binding allows viral glycoprotein 41 (gp41) to integrate within the cell membrane and viral genome to access the host cytoplasm.

After entry into the cell, viral RNA—under the action of reverse transcriptase and integrase—turns into double-strand DNA and integrates into the host DNA. The integrated copy of HIV nucleic acid (named provirus) can stay in latent form for years and can become active at any time to complete the viral life cycle and produce new virions.

The principal target for HIV is the activated CD4+ T-lymphocyte expressing CCR5 or CXCR4 co-receptor. The high number of CD4+ T cells (especially memory CD4+CCR5+ T-lymphocytes) in the mucosa is ideal for HIV replication [37]. In contrast, mucosal dendritic cells do not express CD4+ or CCR5 receptors [38] but they do express other receptors that successfully recognize HIV envelope proteins—dendritic cell-specific intercellular adhesion molecule grabbing nonintegrins (DC-SIGN) and langerin [39].

4.2. HIV expansion

Early after the entry of HIV, the primary infected T-lymphocytes attract and activate other immune cells to expand the initial place of infection. The infected local site starts to grow until the detachment of the infected cells. Thus, the virus disseminates from the mucosal surfaces to the regional lymph nodes (usually in 10 days after the infection) and then throughout the body. The virus can be detected in all lymphoid organs but the highest number of viral particles concentrates in the mucosal lymphoid tissues (such as gastro-intestinal associated lymphoid tissue). Dendritic cells in lymph nodes and mucosal lymphoid tissues present the HIV antigens to naïve B cells and T cells, prompting them to differentiate and activate. In these first stages, the viral load is significant and CD4+ T cells count starts to decline rapidly.

In many cases, the early events of viral expansion (acute stage) are not clinically manifested. In some people, influenza-like or mononucleosis-like symptoms may occur several weeks after the exposure to infection but they are not specific and often misdiagnosed.

4.3. T cell-mediated immune response during HIV latency

Several months after the initial infection, a precise balance between the virus and the immune response (both cell-mediated and humoral) is established. Host immune system (especially CD8+ lymphocytes) succeeds to control viral replication at some degree but the elimination of target CD4+ population continues. This represents the chronic (latent) phase in HIV infection, clinically manifested with decreased viral load and appearance of specific anti-HIV antibodies in the blood of infected individuals.

Although the major characteristic of HIV infection is the depletion of CD4+ T cells, other lymphocyte types are also affected. HIV notably influences naïve T cells (both CD4 T naïve cells and CD8 T naïve cells) during the asymptomatic phase of the infection [40]. Any T cell-mediated immune response requires new naïve T cells and their depletion results in progressively compromised immunity. The reduction in naïve T cell counts is probably due to decreased thymic output and increased T cell turnover in HIV-positive patients [41]. Furthermore, during HIV asymptomatic phase, the overall CD8+ count remains the same as before infection but significant alteration in the ratio memory/naïve CD8+ cells occurs, the normal predominance of naïve CD8+ is replaced by the domination of memory cells (in many patients, the compartment of CD8+ memory cells represents more than 80% of all CD8+ circulating cells) [40].

The cellular immune response mediated by CD8+ cytotoxic T-lymphocytes (CTLs) plays a crucial role in HIV infection [42]. The precursor CTLs recognize viral antigens expressed on the surface of presenting cells. They become active with the help of IL-2, IFN-gamma, and TNF-alpha (produced from CD4+ T cells) and can directly eliminate infected CD4+ lymphocytes via secretion of perforin (a cytolytic protein) and granzymes (serine proteases). The increased ability to secrete perforin is specific for CD8+ T cells from small group HIV-positive individuals who maintain HIV replication in undetectable levels (elite controllers) [43] and who do not progress immunologically towards AIDS in the absence of antiretroviral treatment.

Simultaneously with the host response, the virus starts a mutation process to escape CD8+ recognition by changing epitopes and to correct the present viral variant. At this moment, a balance between host elimination and replication of new HIV variants is established. However,

CD8+ immune response, as well as humoral response, strongly needs CD4+ T helpers and gradually with CD4+ depletion, the CD8+ control fails to maintain the viremia.

The loss of effective antiviral response leads to a constant stimulation and repeated activation of HIV specific CD8+ T cells. This chronic activation soon exhausts the pool of CD8+ lymphocytes together with CD4+ T cell one.

The elevated activation is characteristic not only for CD8+ and CD4+ T cells, but also for B cells, NK cells, and monocytes. In HIV-seropositive patients, even in early stages of infection, high levels of proinflammatory cytokines (TNF-alpha, IL-6 and IL-1β) and chemokines (MIP-1alpha, MIP-1beta and RANTES) are detected [37].

The HIV life cycle is closely related to the extent of immune system activation. Activation of the immune cells enhances the entry of HIV into the cytoplasm because the auxiliary co-receptors are upregulated under immune stimulation [44]. It also increases the level of provirus transcription together with the normal cellular transcription [45]. The exhausted CD8+ T cells diminish secretion of immune-stimulatory cytokines, slow down proliferation and suspend killing of infected cells [46]. HIV infection stimulates upregulation of CD8+ inhibitory receptors (Programmed Death-1 (PD-1), T cell immunoglobulin, and mucin-domain-containing molecule-3 (Tim-3) [47,48]) that downregulate CD8+ immune response and maintain T cell tolerance.

4.4. Humoral immune response against HIV

The humoral immune response against HIV is mediated by specific anti-HIV antibodies produced from B-lymphocytes several weeks to several months after the initial infection. HIV cannot replicate into B-lymphocytes but influences their activation and apoptosis. Unmatured B-lymphocytes differentiate under the action of Th1 cytokines (IL-4, IL-5, IL-6, IL-10, TGF-beta) into plasma cells producing large amounts of binding and virus-neutralizing antibodies. Antibodies target free viral particles in the HIV-positive blood and a small quantity of them can also eliminate infected cells.

HIV specific antibodies recognize viral envelope (envelope proteins gp120 and gp41) and protect host cells from viral entry, but the virus successfully escapes the antibodies' binding via continual mutations. Memory B cells constantly produce new variants of antibodies and soon become exhausted.

4.5. AIDS

The latent phase can last several years (usually up to ten) and terminates finally with the development of AIDS and death. In the final stage, HIV infection completely exhausts the host immune system and especially the CD4+ T cell pool. AIDS is immunologically diagnosed by a CD4+ count less than 200 per μL or/and clinically by the occurrence of opportunistic HIV-related diseases.

5. Immunology of TB/HIV coinfection

5.1. HIV impact on TB infection

TB is the leading opportunistic infection and major cause of death in HIV-seropositive people. There is some evidence that both HIV-negative and HIV-positive persons have the same chance to be infected with TB [49]. In contrast, other studies have found that already existing HIV infection increased the risk of newly acquired TB [50, 51] and relapse of dormant *M. tuberculosis* [52]. However, there is unanimity that HIV exacerbates TB progress and accelerates the fatal end in coinfected individuals.

Existing data outlines two main hypotheses how HIV influences the course of TB infection: 1. HIV manipulates bactericidal activity of macrophages against *M. tuberculosis*; and 2. HIV kills CD4+ T cells within granulomas and facilitates *M. tuberculosis* survival and dissemination.

HIV impairs macrophages in HIV-positive patients turning them more susceptible to *M. tuberculosis* invasion [53]. First, HIV upregulates some of *M. tuberculosis* receptors on macrophages to favor tubercle bacilli entering into the cell [54]. Second, HIV modulates oxidative stress-dependent bactericidal activity in monocytes by diminishing their capacity to produce ROS [55]. As a result of increased levels of IL-10 (an anti-inflammatory interleukin) and decreased TNF-alpha production, infected macrophages escape apoptosis [53, 56]. Thus, more macrophages are directed towards necrosis, a mechanism that increases the *M. tuberculosis* survival and dissemination in the lungs and other extra pulmonary locations. Furthermore, HIV alters the acidification of phagosomes in *M. tuberculosis*-infected macrophages [57], changing the rate of tubercle bacilli elimination.

HIV manifests its presence by gradual depletion of CD4+ T cells, a main feature of HIV infection and clinical sign for progression towards AIDS. The low CD4+ cell count makes the host more susceptible to tubercle bacilli as the immune system cannot establish an efficient cell-mediated immune response. The risk of reactivation of latent TB, acquirement of new TB infection, and/or of dissemination of TB towards extra pulmonary locations increases with the decrease of CD4+ cell count; patients with CD4+ counts >350 cells/μL have unaltered clinical and radiographic presentation as HIV seronegative patients, while patients with CD4+ counts <350 cells/μL have atypical chest X-ray findings and frequent extra pulmonary TB. HIV-positive patients in South Africa with CD4+ counts <200 cells/μL are more susceptible to *M. tuberculosis* infection than HIV-positive individuals with CD4+ counts >500 cells/μL regardless of antiretroviral therapy applied [58].

The insufficient CD4+ T number fails to control granuloma formation and maintenance, therefore leading to higher incidence of extra pulmonary TB and enlarged risk of reactivation of latent infection in HIV-positive patients. Caseous necrotic granulomas—typical for single TB infection—are rare in TB/HIV coinfected patients. Despite the same number of granulomas and acid-fast stained bacilli in TB infected and TB/HIV coinfected persons [59], granulomas from dual-infected individuals are easy disrupted and infection can readily disseminate into multiple organs to form diffuse lesions [60].

However, HIV influence on TB course may only partially depend on CD4+ depletion, as HIV-positive miners in South Africa had an increased risk (2 to 3 times higher) of developing active TB in the first and second year after HIV seroconversion, when the number of CD4+ T-cell was still high [61]. HIV-positive individuals with preserved CD4+ T cell counts (during an antiretroviral treatment) also have an increased risk of developing TB infection. This suggests that additional immunological changes could happen during HIV infection, making the host more susceptible to TB. Such possible mechanism is the observed uniform distribution of CD8+ T cells within the granuloma, in contrast to the peripheral findings in the single TB infection [62]. HIV also specifically diminishes production of IFN-gamma, IL-2, and IL-12 [63], and suppresses proliferation of TB-specific T cells. Several months after HIV seroconversion, the number of *M. tuberculosis* specific CD4+ memory cells decreases significantly [64].

5.2. TB importance in HIV infection

HIV recognizes immune cells expressing CD4+ glycoprotein on their surface: CD4+ T-cells, macrophages, and dendritic cells. All of these cellular types are involved in TB pathogenesis and immune response. HIV also needs activated immune cells for replication and propagation; such cells are abundantly present during *M. tuberculosis* primary or latent infection. In this way, it can be speculated that TB infection areas (granulomas) create the optimal environment for HIV propagation.

HIV-positive patients who developed TB have an increased viral load during the acute phase of TB disease [65, 66]. Lung tissue samples from patients with TB have increased HIV viral load when compared to HIV-positive patients without lung disease or plasma samples from the same TB patients [67]. This suggests that a TB-infected lung has elevated local HIV replication in vivo. In addition, HIV replication is activated in TB-infected alveolar macrophages [68], lymphocytes, and CD14+ macrophages of the pleural space [69].

Infection with *M. tuberculosis* also enhances the level of inflammatory cytokines and chemokines. Their release stimulates HIV replication and increases viral load. Pleural fluids from patients with active TB provoke HIV replication in vitro via production of TNF-alpha, IL-6, and IFN-gamma [70].

Coinfected individuals have increased incidence and death rate of HIV-related opportunistic infections comparing to HIV-positive but TB-negative patients with the same level of immunosuppression (absolute CD4+ count) [71], indicating that *M. tuberculosis* accelerates the clinical course and outcome of HIV infection.

6. Concluding remarks

TB/HIV coinfection represents a leading threat to public health worldwide. Despite the extreme research effort, many aspects of the exceptionally complicated immunology of concurrent TB and HIV infections still need to be elucidated. Diagnosis of HIV/TB coinfection is challenging as both infections have overlapping clinical manifestations, which often lead to late or misdiagnosis. Furthermore, TB and HIV as well the coinfection mostly affect poor and developing regions where competent health care is hardly accessible.

Changes in both innate and adaptive immune response demand well-organized clinical and laboratory studies to understand possible mechanisms by which HIV and TB disrupt in perfect and fatal cooperation the immune system of the host.

Abbreviatons

AAM – Alternatively activated macrophages

AIDS – Acquired immune deficiency syndrome

CAM – Classically activated macrophages

CCL – CC chemokine ligand

CTL – Cytotoxic T-lymphocytes

DC-SIGN – Dendritic cell-specific intercellular adhesion molecule grabbing nonintegrins

HIV – Human immuno deficiency virus

IFN – Interferon

IL – Interleukin

iNOS – Nitric oxide synthetase

MBTC – *Mycobacterium tuberculosis* complex

MHC – Major histocompatibility complex

MIP – Macrophage inflammatory protein

NK – Natural killer cells

NLR – NOD-like receptors

NO – Nitric oxide

NOD – Nucleotide-binding oligomerization domain

PD-1 – Programmed death-1

RANTES – Regulated on activation, normal T cell expressed and secreted

ROS – Reactive oxygen species

TB – Tuberculosis

TGF – Transforming growth factor

Tim-3 – T cell immunoglobulin and mucin-domain-containing molecule

TLRs – Toll-like receptors

TNF – Tumor necrosis factor

WHO – World Health Organization

Author details

Tatina T. Todorova[1*], Gabriela Tsankova[1], Neli Lodozova[1,2] and Tcvetelina Kostadinova[2]

*Address all correspondence to: tatina.todorova@abv.bg

1 Department of Preclinical and Clinical Sciences, Faculty of Pharmacy, Medical University Varna, Bulgaria

2 TRS "Medical laboratory assistant", Medical College, Medical University Varna, Bulgaria

References

[1] WHO | Global tuberculosis report 2014. World Health Organization; [cited 2015 Jan 15]; Available from: http://www.who.int/tb/publications/global_report/en/.

[2] WHO | HIV/AIDS. World Health Organization; [cited 2015 Jan 15]; Available from: http://www.who.int/mediacentre/factsheets/fs360/en/.

[3] Ahmad S. Pathogenesis, immunology, and diagnosis of latent Mycobacterium tuberculosis infection. Clin Dev Immunol [Internet]. 2011 Jan [cited 2015 Jan 15]; 2011:814943. Available from: http://www.pubmedcentral.nih.gov/articlerender.fcgi?artid=3017943&tool=pmcentrez&rendertype=abstract.

[4] Frieden TR, Sterling T, Pablos-Mendez A, Kilburn JO, Cauthen GM, Dooley SW. The emergence of drug-resistant tuberculosis in New York City. N Engl J Med [Internet]. 1993 Feb 25 [cited 2015 Jan 15];328(8):521–6. Available from: http://www.ncbi.nlm.nih.gov/pubmed/8381207.

[5] Olczak A, Grąbczewska E. Tuberculosis in HIV-infected patients in the HAART era. HIV AIDS Rev [Internet]. 2010 Jan [cited 2015 Jan 15];9(2):41–4. Available from: http://www.sciencedirect.com/science/article/pii/S1730127010600689.

[6] Golub JE, Saraceni V, Cavalcante SC, Pacheco AG, Moulton LH, King BS, et al. The impact of antiretroviral therapy and isoniazid preventive therapy on tuberculosis incidence in HIV-infected patients in Rio de Janeiro, Brazil. AIDS [Internet]. 2007 Jul 11 [cited 2015 Jan 15];21(11):1441–8. Available from: http://www.pubmedcentral.nih.gov/articlerender.fcgi?artid=3063947&tool=pmcentrez&rendertype=abstract.

[7] World Health Organization. Guidelines for intensified tuberculosis case-finding and isoniazid preventive therapy for people living with HIV in resource-constrained settings. World Health [Internet]. 2011;01:142. Available from: http://whqlibdoc.who.int/publications/2011/9789241500708_eng.pdf.

[8] Marais BJ, Rabie H, Cotton MF. TB and HIV in children - advances in prevention and management. Paediatr Respir Rev [Internet]. 2011 Mar [cited 2015 Jan 15];12(1):39–45. Available from: http://www.sciencedirect.com/science/article/pii/S1526054210000709.

[9] Schwander S, Dheda K. Human lung immunity against Mycobacterium tuberculosis: Insights into pathogenesis and protection. Am J Respir Crit Care Med [Internet]. 2011 Mar 15 [cited 2015 Jan 2];183(6):696–707. Available from: http://www.pubmedcentral.nih.gov/articlerender.fcgi?artid=3081283&tool=pmcentrez&rendertype=abstract.

[10] Andersson M, Lutay N, Hallgren O, Westergren-Thorsson G, Svensson M, Godaly G. Mycobacterium bovis bacilli Calmette-Guerin regulates leukocyte recruitment by modulating alveolar inflammatory responses. Innate Immun [Internet]. 2012 Jun 12 [cited 2015 Jan 15];18(3):531–40. Available from: http://ini.sagepub.com/content/early/2012/01/11/1753425911426591.

[11] Jo E-K, Yang C-S, Choi CH, Harding C V. Intracellular signalling cascades regulating innate immune responses to Mycobacteria: Branching out from Toll-like receptors. Cell Microbiol [Internet]. 2007 May [cited 2015 Jan 15];9(5):1087–98. Available from: http://www.ncbi.nlm.nih.gov/pubmed/17359235.

[12] Akira S, Uematsu S, Takeuchi O. Pathogen recognition and innate immunity. Cell [Internet]. 2006 Feb 24 [cited 2014 Jul 9];124(4):783–801. Available from: http://www.ncbi.nlm.nih.gov/pubmed/16497588.

[13] Algood HMS, Chan J, Flynn JL. Chemokines and tuberculosis. Cytokine Growth Factor Rev [Internet]. Elsevier; 2003 Dec 12 [cited 2015 Jan 15];14(6):467–77. Available from: http://www.cgfr.co.uk/article/S1359610103000546/fulltext.

[14] Saunders BM, Cooper AM. Restraining mycobacteria: Role of granulomas in mycobacterial infections. Immunol Cell Biol [Internet]. 2000 Aug [cited 2015 Jan 15];78(4):334–41. Available from: http://www.ncbi.nlm.nih.gov/pubmed/10947857.

[15] Wolf AJ, Linas B, Trevejo-Nunez GJ, Kincaid E, Tamura T, Takatsu K, et al. Mycobacterium tuberculosis Infects Dendritic Cells with High Frequency and Impairs Their Function In Vivo. J Immunol [Internet]. American Association of Immunologists; 2007 Aug 3 [cited 2014 Nov 28];179(4):2509–19. Available from: http://www.jimmunol.org/content/179/4/2509.full.

[16] Giacomini E, Iona E, Ferroni L, Miettinen M, Fattorini L, Orefici G, et al. Infection of Human Macrophages and Dendritic Cells with Mycobacterium tuberculosis Induces a Differential Cytokine Gene Expression That Modulates T Cell Response. J Immunol [Internet]. American Association of Immunologists; 2001 Jun 15 [cited 2015 Jan 15];166(12):7033–41. Available from: http://www.jimmunol.org/content/166/12/7033.full.

[17] Tailleux L, Neyrolles O, Honore-Bouakline S, Perret E, Sanchez F, Abastado J-P, et al. Constrained Intracellular Survival of Mycobacterium tuberculosis in Human Dendritic Cells. J Immunol [Internet]. American Association of Immunologists; 2003 Feb 15 [cited 2015 Jan 15];170(4):1939–48. Available from: http://www.jimmunol.org/content/170/4/1939.full.

[18] Co DO, Hogan LH, Kim S-I, Sandor M. Mycobacterial granulomas: keys to a long-lasting host-pathogen relationship. Clin Immunol [Internet]. 2004 Nov [cited 2015 Jan 15];113(2):130–6. Available from: http://www.ncbi.nlm.nih.gov/pubmed/15451467.

[19] Peyron P, Vaubourgeix J, Poquet Y, Levillain F, Botanch C, Bardou F, et al. Foamy macrophages from tuberculous patients' granulomas constitute a nutrient-rich reservoir for M. tuberculosis persistence. PLoS Pathog [Internet]. 2008 Nov 11 [cited 2014 Dec 27];4(11):e1000204. Available from: http://journals.plos.org/plospathogens/article?id=10.1371/journal.ppat.1000204.

[20] Fulton SA, Reba SM, Martin TD, Boom WH. Neutrophil-Mediated Mycobacteriocidal Immunity in the Lung during Mycobacterium bovis BCG Infection in C57BL/6 Mice. Infect Immun [Internet]. 2002 Sep 1 [cited 2015 Jan 15];70(9):5322–7. Available from: http://iai.asm.org/content/70/9/5322.full.

[21] Lowe DM, Redford PS, Wilkinson RJ, O'Garra A, Martineau AR. Neutrophils in tuberculosis: friend or foe? Trends Immunol [Internet]. 2012 Jan [cited 2015 Jan 9];33(1): 14–25. Available from: http://www.ncbi.nlm.nih.gov/pubmed/22094048.

[22] Sawant K V, McMurray DN. Guinea pig neutrophils infected with Mycobacterium tuberculosis produce cytokines which activate alveolar macrophages in noncontact cultures. Infect Immun [Internet]. 2007 Apr [cited 2015 Jan 15];75(4):1870–7. Available from: http://www.pubmedcentral.nih.gov/articlerender.fcgi?artid=1865707&tool=pmcentrez&rendertype=abstract.

[23] Segovia-Juarez JL, Ganguli S, Kirschner D. Identifying control mechanisms of granuloma formation during M. tuberculosis infection using an agent-based model. J Theor Biol [Internet]. 2004 Dec 7 [cited 2014 Dec 29];231(3):357–76. Available from: http://www.ncbi.nlm.nih.gov/pubmed/15501468.

[24] Schluger NW, Rom WN. The host immune response to tuberculosis. Am J Respir Crit Care Med [Internet]. 1998 Mar [cited 2015 Jan 7];157(3 Pt 1):679–91. Available from: http://www.ncbi.nlm.nih.gov/pubmed/9517576.

[25] Oddo M, Renno T, Attinger A, Bakker T, MacDonald HR, Meylan PR. Fas ligand-induced apoptosis of infected human macrophages reduces the viability of intracellular Mycobacterium tuberculosis. J Immunol [Internet]. 1998 Jun 1 [cited 2015 Jan 15]; 160(11):5448–54. Available from: http://www.ncbi.nlm.nih.gov/pubmed/9605147.

[26] Serbina N V., Lazarevic V, Flynn JL. CD4+ T Cells Are Required for the Development of Cytotoxic CD8+ T Cells During Mycobacterium tuberculosis Infection. J Immunol [Internet]. American Association of Immunologists; 2001 Dec 15 [cited 2015 Jan 7];

167(12):6991–7000. Available from: http://www.jimmunol.org/content/167/12/6991.full.

[27] Cho S, Mehra V, Thoma-Uszynski S, Stenger S, Serbina N, Mazzaccaro RJ, et al. Antimicrobial activity of MHC class I-restricted CD8+ T cells in human tuberculosis. Proc Natl Acad Sci U S A [Internet]. 2000 Oct 24 [cited 2015 Jan 15];97(22):12210–5. Available from: http://www.pubmedcentral.nih.gov/articlerender.fcgi?artid=17320&tool=pmcentrez&rendertype=abstract.

[28] Stenger S, Hanson DA, Teitelbaum R, Dewan P, Niazi KR, Froelich CJ, et al. An antimicrobial activity of cytolytic T cells mediated by granulysin. Science [Internet]. 1998 Oct 2 [cited 2015 Jan 15];282(5386):121–5. Available from: http://www.ncbi.nlm.nih.gov/pubmed/9756476.

[29] Brandes M, Willimann K, Bioley G, Lévy N, Eberl M, Luo M, et al. Cross-presenting human gammadelta T cells induce robust CD8+ alphabeta T cell responses. Proc Natl Acad Sci U S A [Internet]. 2009 Feb 17 [cited 2015 Jan 15];106(7):2307–12. Available from: http://www.pnas.org/content/106/7/2307.full.

[30] Silva Miranda M, Breiman A, Allain S, Deknuydt F, Altare F. The tuberculous granuloma: An unsuccessful host defence mechanism providing a safety shelter for the bacteria? Clin Dev Immunol [Internet]. 2012 Jan [cited 2015 Jan 10];2012:139127. Available from: http://www.pubmedcentral.nih.gov/articlerender.fcgi?artid=3395138&tool=pmcentrez&rendertype=abstract.

[31] Benoit M, Desnues B, Mege J-L. Macrophage polarization in bacterial infections. J Immunol [Internet]. 2008 Sep 15 [cited 2015 Jan 15];181(6):3733–9. Available from: http://www.ncbi.nlm.nih.gov/pubmed/18768823.

[32] Behar SM, Martin CJ, Booty MG, Nishimura T, Zhao X, Gan H-X, et al. Apoptosis is an innate defense function of macrophages against Mycobacterium tuberculosis. Mucosal Immunol [Internet]. 2011 May [cited 2014 Dec 15];4(3):279–87. Available from: http://www.pubmedcentral.nih.gov/articlerender.fcgi?artid=3155700&tool=pmcentrez&rendertype=abstract.

[33] De Vallière S, Abate G, Blazevic A, Heuertz RM, Hoft DF. Enhancement of innate and cell-mediated immunity by antimycobacterial antibodies. Infect Immun [Internet]. 2005 Oct [cited 2015 Jan 15];73(10):6711–20. Available from: http://www.pubmedcentral.nih.gov/articlerender.fcgi?artid=1230956&tool=pmcentrez&rendertype=abstract.

[34] Abebe F, Bjune G. The protective role of antibody responses during Mycobacterium tuberculosis infection. Clin Exp Immunol [Internet]. 2009 Aug [cited 2015 Jan 15];157(2):235–43. Available from: http://www.pubmedcentral.nih.gov/articlerender.fcgi?artid=2730849&tool=pmcentrez&rendertype=abstract.

[35] Maglione PJ, Chan J. How B cells shape the immune response against Mycobacterium tuberculosis. Eur J Immunol [Internet]. 2009 Mar [cited 2014 Dec 30];39(3):676–86.

Available from: http://www.pubmedcentral.nih.gov/articlerender.fcgi?artid=2760469&tool=pmcentrez&rendertype=abstract.

[36] Diedrich CR, Flynn JL. HIV-1/mycobacterium tuberculosis coinfection immunology: How does HIV-1 exacerbate tuberculosis? Infect Immun [Internet]. 2011 Apr [cited 2014 Sep 5];79(4):1407–17. Available from: http://www.pubmedcentral.nih.gov/articlerender.fcgi?artid=3067569&tool=pmcentrez&rendertype=abstract.

[37] Appay V, Sauce D. Immune activation and inflammation in HIV-1 infection: Causes and consequences. J Pathol [Internet]. 2008 Jan [cited 2015 Jan 15];214(2):231–41. Available from: http://www.ncbi.nlm.nih.gov/pubmed/18161758.

[38] Poonia B, Wang X, Veazey RS. Distribution of simian immunodeficiency virus target cells in vaginal tissues of normal rhesus macaques: implications for virus transmission. J Reprod Immunol [Internet]. 2006 Dec [cited 2015 Jan 15];72(1-2):74–84. Available from: http://www.ncbi.nlm.nih.gov/pubmed/16956666.

[39] Hussain LA, Lehner T. Comparative investigation of Langerhans' cells and potential receptors for HIV in oral, genitourinary and rectal epithelia. Immunology [Internet]. 1995 Jul [cited 2015 Jan 15];85(3):475–84. Available from: http://www.pubmedcentral.nih.gov/articlerender.fcgi?artid=1383923&tool=pmcentrez&rendertype=abstract.

[40] Roederer M, Dubs JG, Anderson MT, Raju PA, Herzenberg LA. CD8 naive T cell counts decrease progressively in HIV-infected adults. J Clin Invest [Internet]. 1995 May [cited 2015 Jan 15];95(5):2061–6. Available from: http://www.pubmedcentral.nih.gov/articlerender.fcgi?artid=295794&tool=pmcentrez&rendertype=abstract.

[41] Douek DC, Betts MR, Hill BJ, Little SJ, Lempicki R, Metcalf JA, et al. Evidence for Increased T Cell Turnover and Decreased Thymic Output in HIV Infection. J Immunol [Internet]. American Association of Immunologists; 2001 Dec 1 [cited 2015 Jan 15]; 167(11):6663–8. Available from: http://www.jimmunol.org/content/167/11/6663.full.

[42] Schmitz JE, Kuroda MJ, Santra S, Sasseville VG, Simon MA, Lifton MA, et al. Control of viremia in simian immunodeficiency virus infection by CD8+ lymphocytes. Science [Internet]. 1999 Feb 5 [cited 2015 Jan 15];283(5403):857–60. Available from: http://www.ncbi.nlm.nih.gov/pubmed/9933172.

[43] Hersperger AR, Pereyra F, Nason M, Demers K, Sheth P, Shin LY, et al. Perforin expression directly ex vivo by HIV-specific CD8 T-cells is a correlate of HIV elite control. PLoS Pathog [Internet]. 2010 May 27 [cited 2015 Jan 15];6(5):e1000917. Available from: http://journals.plos.org/plospathogens/article?id=10.1371/journal.ppat.1000917.

[44] Levy JA. Wiley: HIV and the Pathogenesis of AIDS, 3rd Edition - J. A. Levy [Internet]. [cited 2015 Jan 15]. Available from: http://eu.wiley.com/WileyCDA/WileyTitle/productCd-1555813933.html.

[45] Cron RQ, Bartz SR, Clausell A, Bort SJ, Klebanoff SJ, Lewis DB. NFAT1 enhances HIV-1 gene expression in primary human CD4 T cells. Clin Immunol [Internet]. 2000

Mar [cited 2015 Jan 15];94(3):179–91. Available from: http://www.ncbi.nlm.nih.gov/pubmed/10692237.

[46] Wherry EJ, Ahmed R. Memory CD8 T-cell differentiation during viral infection. J Virol [Internet]. 2004 Jun [cited 2015 Jan 15];78(11):5535–45. Available from: http://www.pubmedcentral.nih.gov/articlerender.fcgi?artid=415833&tool=pmcentrez&rendertype=abstract.

[47] Jin H-T, Anderson AC, Tan WG, West EE, Ha S-J, Araki K, et al. Cooperation of Tim-3 and PD-1 in CD8 T-cell exhaustion during chronic viral infection. Proc Natl Acad Sci U S A [Internet]. 2010 Aug 17 [cited 2015 Jan 9];107(33):14733–8. Available from: http://www.pubmedcentral.nih.gov/articlerender.fcgi?artid=2930455&tool=pmcentrez&rendertype=abstract.

[48] Tandon R, Giret MTM, Sengupta D, York VA, Wiznia AA, Rosenberg MG, et al. Age-related expansion of Tim-3 expressing T cells in vertically HIV-1 infected children. PLoS One [Internet]. 2012 Jan [cited 2015 Jan 15];7(9):e45733. Available from: http://www.pubmedcentral.nih.gov/articlerender.fcgi?artid=3454343&tool=pmcentrez&rendertype=abstract.

[49] Whalen CC, Zalwango S, Chiunda A, Malone L, Eisenach K, Joloba M, et al. Secondary attack rate of tuberculosis in urban households in Kampala, Uganda. PLoS One [Internet]. 2011 Jan 14 [cited 2015 Jan 15];6(2):e16137. Available from: http://journals.plos.org/plosone/article?id=10.1371/journal.pone.0016137.

[50] Crampin AC, Mwaungulu JN, Mwaungulu FD, Mwafulirwa DT, Munthali K, Floyd S, et al. Recurrent TB: relapse or reinfection? The effect of HIV in a general population cohort in Malawi. AIDS [Internet]. 2010 Jan 28 [cited 2015 Jan 7];24(3):417–26. Available from: http://www.pubmedcentral.nih.gov/articlerender.fcgi?artid=2917772&tool=pmcentrez&rendertype=abstract.

[51] Sonnenberg P, Murray J, Glynn JR, Shearer S, Kambashi B, Godfrey-Faussett P. HIV-1 and recurrence, relapse, and reinfection of tuberculosis after cure: a cohort study in South African mineworkers. Lancet [Internet]. Elsevier; 2001 Nov 17 [cited 2014 Dec 28];358(9294):1687–93. Available from: http://www.thelancet.com/article/S0140673601067125/fulltext.

[52] Selwyn PA, Hartel D, Lewis VA, Schoenbaum EE, Vermund SH, Klein RS, et al. A prospective study of the risk of tuberculosis among intravenous drug users with human immunodeficiency virus infection. N Engl J Med [Internet]. 1989 Mar 2 [cited 2015 Jan 15];320(9):545–50. Available from: http://www.ncbi.nlm.nih.gov/pubmed/2915665.

[53] Patel NR, Swan K, Li X, Tachado SD, Koziel H. Impaired M. tuberculosis-mediated apoptosis in alveolar macrophages from HIV+ persons: Potential role of IL-10 and BCL-3. J Leukoc Biol [Internet]. 2009 Jul [cited 2015 Jan 15];86(1):53–60. Available

from: http://www.pubmedcentral.nih.gov/articlerender.fcgi?artid=2704623&tool=pmcentrez&rendertype=abstract.

[54] Rosas-Taraco AG, Arce-Mendoza AY, Caballero-Olín G, Salinas-Carmona MC. Mycobacterium tuberculosis upregulates coreceptors CCR5 and CXCR4 while HIV modulates CD14 favoring concurrent infection. AIDS Res Hum Retroviruses [Internet]. 2006 Jan [cited 2015 Jan 15];22(1):45–51. Available from: http://www.ncbi.nlm.nih.gov/pubmed/16438645.

[55] Spear GT, Kessler HA, Rothberg L, Phair J, Landay AL. Decreased oxidative burst activity of monocytes from asymptomatic HIV-infected individuals. Clin Immunol Immunopathol [Internet]. 1990 Feb [cited 2015 Jan 15];54(2):184–91. Available from: http://www.ncbi.nlm.nih.gov/pubmed/1688521.

[56] Patel NR, Zhu J, Tachado SD, Zhang J, Wan Z, Saukkonen J, et al. HIV impairs TNF-alpha mediated macrophage apoptotic response to Mycobacterium tuberculosis. J Immunol [Internet]. 2007 Nov 15 [cited 2014 Dec 23];179(10):6973–80. Available from: http://www.ncbi.nlm.nih.gov/pubmed/17982088.

[57] Mwandumba HC, Russell DG, Nyirenda MH, Anderson J, White SA, Molyneux ME, et al. Mycobacterium tuberculosis resides in nonacidified vacuoles in endocytically competent alveolar macrophages from patients with tuberculosis and HIV infection. J Immunol [Internet]. 2004 Apr 1 [cited 2015 Jan 15];172(7):4592–8. Available from: http://www.ncbi.nlm.nih.gov/pubmed/15034077.

[58] Lawn SD, Myer L, Edwards D, Bekker L-G, Wood R. Short-term and long-term risk of tuberculosis associated with CD4 cell recovery during antiretroviral therapy in South Africa. AIDS [Internet]. 2009 Aug 24 [cited 2015 Jan 15];23(13):1717–25. Available from: http://www.pubmedcentral.nih.gov/articlerender.fcgi?artid=3801095&tool=pmcentrez&rendertype=abstract.

[59] Heyderman RS, Makunike R, Muza T, Odwee M, Kadzirange G, Manyemba J, et al. Pleural tuberculosis in Harare, Zimbabwe: The relationship between human immunodeficiency virus, CD4 lymphocyte count, granuloma formation and disseminated disease. Trop Med Int Health [Internet]. 1998 Jan [cited 2015 Jan 15];3(1):14–20. Available from: http://www.ncbi.nlm.nih.gov/pubmed/9484963.

[60] De Noronha ALL, Báfica A, Nogueira L, Barral A, Barral-Netto M. Lung granulomas from Mycobacterium tuberculosis/HIV-1 co-infected patients display decreased in situ TNF production. Pathol Res Pract [Internet]. 2008 Jan [cited 2015 Jan 15];204(3): 155–61. Available from: http://www.ncbi.nlm.nih.gov/pubmed/18096327.

[61] Sonnenberg P, Glynn JR, Fielding K, Murray J, Godfrey-Faussett P, Shearer S. How soon after infection with HIV does the risk of tuberculosis start to increase? A retrospective cohort study in South African gold miners. J Infect Dis [Internet]. 2005 Jan 15 [cited 2015 Jan 15];191(2):150–8. Available from: http://www.ncbi.nlm.nih.gov/pubmed/15609223.

[62] Shen JY, Barnes PF, Rea TH, Meyer PR. Immunohistology of tuberculous adenitis in symptomatic HIV infection. Clin Exp Immunol [Internet]. 1988 May [cited 2015 Jan 15];72(2):186–9. Available from: http://www.pubmedcentral.nih.gov/articlerender.fcgi?artid=1541541&tool=pmcentrez&rendertype=abstract.

[63] Zhang M, Gong J, Iyer D V, Jones BE, Modlin RL, Barnes PF. T cell cytokine responses in persons with tuberculosis and human immunodeficiency virus infection. J Clin Invest [Internet]. 1994 Dec [cited 2015 Jan 15];94(6):2435–42. Available from: http://www.pubmedcentral.nih.gov/articlerender.fcgi?artid=330075&tool=pmcentrez&rendertype=abstract.

[64] Geldmacher C, Schuetz A, Ngwenyama N, Casazza JP, Sanga E, Saathoff E, et al. Early depletion of Mycobacterium tuberculosis-specific T helper 1 cell responses after HIV-1 infection. J Infect Dis [Internet]. 2008 Dec 1 [cited 2015 Jan 15];198(11):1590–8. Available from: http://www.pubmedcentral.nih.gov/articlerender.fcgi?artid=2650495&tool=pmcentrez&rendertype=abstract.

[65] Toossi Z, Mayanja-Kizza H, Hirsch CS, Edmonds KL, Spahlinger T, Hom DL, et al. Impact of tuberculosis (TB) on HIV-1 activity in dually infected patients. Clin Exp Immunol [Internet]. 2001 Feb [cited 2015 Jan 15];123(2):233–8. Available from: http://doi.wiley.com/10.1046/j.1365-2249.2001.01401.x.

[66] Goletti D, Weissman D, Jackson RW, Graham NM, Vlahov D, Klein RS, et al. Effect of Mycobacterium tuberculosis on HIV replication. Role of immune activation. J Immunol [Internet]. 1996 Aug 1 [cited 2015 Jan 15];157(3):1271–8. Available from: http://www.ncbi.nlm.nih.gov/pubmed/8757635.

[67] Nakata K, Rom WN, Honda Y, Condos R, Kanegasaki S, Cao Y, et al. Mycobacterium tuberculosis enhances human immunodeficiency virus-1 replication in the lung. Am J Respir Crit Care Med [Internet]. 1997 Mar [cited 2015 Jan 15];155(3):996–1003. Available from: http://www.ncbi.nlm.nih.gov/pubmed/9117038.

[68] Hoshino Y, Hoshino S, Gold JA, Raju B, Prabhakar S, Pine R, et al. Mechanisms of polymorphonuclear neutrophil-mediated induction of HIV-1 replication in macrophages during pulmonary tuberculosis. J Infect Dis [Internet]. 2007 May 1 [cited 2015 Jan 15];195(9):1303–10. Available from: http://www.ncbi.nlm.nih.gov/pubmed/17396999.

[69] Lawn SD, Pisell TL, Hirsch CS, Wu M, Butera ST, Toossi Z. Anatomically compartmentalized human immunodeficiency virus replication in HLA-DR+ cells and CD14+ macrophages at the site of pleural tuberculosis coinfection. J Infect Dis [Internet]. 2001 Nov 1 [cited 2015 Jan 15];184(9):1127–33. Available from: http://jid.oxfordjournals.org/content/184/9/1127.long.

[70] Garrait V, Cadranel J, Esvant H, Herry I, Morinet P, Mayaud C, et al. Tuberculosis generates a microenvironment enhancing the productive infection of local lympho-

cytes by HIV. J Immunol [Internet]. 1997 Sep 15 [cited 2015 Jan 15];159(6):2824–30. Available from: http://www.ncbi.nlm.nih.gov/pubmed/9300705.

[71] Whalen C, Horsburgh CR, Hom D, Lahart C, Simberkoff M, Ellner J. Accelerated course of human immunodeficiency virus infection after tuberculosis. Am J Respir Crit Care Med [Internet]. 1995 Jan [cited 2015 Jan 15];151(1):129–35. Available from: http://www.ncbi.nlm.nih.gov/pubmed/7812542.

9

Economic Globalization, HIV and AIDS and Gender Dimensions in the Lesotho Textiles and Garment Industry

Pius Tangwe Tanga, Haruna M. Bello,
Tiisetso J. Makatjane and Tumelo Tsikoane

Abstract

The Kingdom of Lesotho is also experiencing the third highest HIV and AIDS prevalence rate (23.2%) in the world, which poses an internal threat both to the industry and to the workers. The objective of this chapter was to examine workers' economic opportunities, the interplay of HIV and AIDS as well as threats to economic opportunities provided by the industry. This chapter is based on data collected for a study on the economic crisis, globalization and HIV and AIDS nexus in the textiles and garment industry in Lesotho. Data for this chapter were generated from two of the three instruments of the main study using a multistage sampling technique. Data collected were analysed quantitatively using Statistical Package for the Social Sciences (SPSS). The result shows that despite the economic crisis, the textiles and garment industry has enhanced the employment of many *Basotho* (people from Lesotho), especially women. Although workers were economically empowered, HIV and AIDS and the global economic crisis were threats to the industry and workers alike. There is significant rural-urban migration to the industry with almost half of the workers staying away from their traditional family homes.

Keywords: economic globalisation, HIV and AIDS, textiles and garment industry, Lesotho, global economic crisis

1. Introduction

Lesotho is predominantly a mountainous country, with an altitude range of between 1300 and 3500 masl (over 80% of the land is over 1800 m altitude) [1]. The surface area of Lesotho is approximately 30,350 km^2 demarcated into 10 administrative districts. One-quarter of the land is lowlands and the remainder is highlands. Only 9% of the total area is suitable for arable cultivation. Lesotho is described as one of the poorest countries in Sub-Saharan Africa (SSA) with an estimated population of 1.8 million [2]. The majority of the population (77%) resides in the rural and mountainous areas [3, 4]. Lesotho has four seasons with the mountainous areas experiencing heavy snowfall during winters sometimes resulting in loss of livestock and making accessibility to the urban areas almost impossible.

The country has few natural resource endowments but has abundance of labour, water and beautiful landscape whose economic potential remains untapped. There are also concentrations of diamonds. The country enjoys royalties from export of water to the Republic of South Africa (RSA) and remittances resulting from labour migration constituted 28% of the country's GDP in 2010. However, the mine workers have been experiencing increasing retrenchment from the South African mines resulting in an unemployment figure estimated at 45% [5]. This notwithstanding, labour migration, government and textiles and garment industry are the three main forms of employment in the country [3].

The country is faced with a number of challenges but unemployment, HIV and AIDS and retrenchments of Basotho men by the South African mining industry are the main ones. Retrenchments from South African mining industry and the decline in engaging young Basotho men as labour migrants contributed to the high unemployment rate of 45% in 2010 in the country. Employment created by textiles and garment industry is likely to surpass employment created by government in the future hence the need to investigate the impact of economic globalisation on the textiles and garment industry. Furthermore, since the textile and garment industry is a major employer of women (over 70%) in the economy, it is imperative to investigate the nexus between HIV/AIDS and employment in the textile and garment industry in the face of the then on-going economic globalization trend.

Lesotho does not only have the third highest prevalence of HIV and AIDS in the world after Botswana and Swaziland [3, 6–8]; it has also prioritised reduction of HIV as its number one priority among the Millennium Development Goals (MDGs). Available statistics indicate that HIV prevalence sharply increased from around 4% in 1993, to 25% in 1999 and to an estimated 31% in 2002 [9]. According to the 2004 and 2009 Lesotho Demographic Household Survey (DHS) figures, HIV prevalence in Lesotho has remained high at around 23% [10]. It is not surprising that in 2000, HIV was declared a crisis in Lesotho. According to the Ministry of Health and Social Welfare (MoHSW) [11] in the Demographic Health Survey of 2009, it was found that concurrent and multiple sexual partnership is a common feature in Lesotho's society [10]. Six percent of women and 21% of men have had more than two sexual partners in the last 12 months. Within these figures, condom use was only 39% of females and 52% of men having reported using a condom during their last sexual encounter, suggesting unequal sexual power relations disadvantages women in the spread of HIV/AIDS through sexual intercourse [10, 11].

Among a number of attempts to curb the spread of HIV the Lesotho AIDS Programme Coordinating Authority (LAPCA) was established within the office of the Prime Minister in

2001 to coordinate national efforts to address the HIV epidemic. In 2005, the National AIDS Commission (NAC) was established to coordinate implementation of the National HIV and AIDS Strategic Plan, thus superseding LAPCA. An in-depth review of the national response in 2005 resulted in an updated National AIDS Policy and the National Strategic Plan for 2006–2011 as well as the approval of the National Monitoring and Evaluation Plan by the Government of Lesotho (GOL) in December 2006 [12]. Lesotho has also shown consistent political leadership on HIV and AIDS. Since the declaration of HIV and AIDS as an emergency in 2000, the top political leadership has consistently spoken out and supported the HIV and AIDS response at the highest level. At the work place, employers are expected to have HIV policies to address HIV and AIDS issues at the work place including the fight against stigmatization and discrimination.

The Senkatana Centre was opened in 2004 to provide antiretroviral therapy (ART) in the country. In 2005, an HIV paediatric clinical centre—the Baylor-Bristol-Myers Squibb Centre of Excellence—was also opened. Baylor provides state-of-the-art facilities for testing, treating and monitoring patients and training healthcare professionals. At the end of 2007, an estimated 21,710 people were receiving anti-retroviral treatment and the coverage of Prevention of Mother-to-Child Transmission (PMTCT) programmes had increased six-fold from an estimated 5% in 2005 to 31% in 2007 [3]. "Know Your Status" (KYS) campaign was also launched in 2004. In 2007, an estimated 12% of the population had received an HIV test in Lesotho representing a threefold increase from the 2005 figures [7].

Access to the US market under the African Growth and Opportunity Act (AGOA) that made Lesotho the single largest beneficiary from Africa has led to increased employment in the textiles and garment industry [13]. The textiles sector employed about 50,000 workers in 2003/2004, but this significantly declined to 26,475 workers in 2006 [9, 14]. These changes are said to be explained by expiration of preferential trade agreements (PTAs) to which Lesotho has been a beneficiary and the global economic/financial crisis that hit the region in 2007/2008. In 2008, unemployment rate was estimated at 22.7%, of which 21.2% were males against 24.6% females compared to 27.3% in 1999. Economic globalisation could be behind the fluctuations in the employment figures of the textiles and garment industry, hence the interest in how economic globalisation and HIV and AIDS are affecting the textiles and garment industry in Lesotho given that majority of the workers (over 70%) are female with unequal safe and protective sexual power relations. In a study to challenge mainstream theories which present globalization and associated forces as gender neutral, Metcalfe and Rees [15] provide a critical combination of the complexity and interconnections between gender, organization and globalization. The chapter identifies that key stakeholders (transnational corporations, international nongovernmental organizations and government state machineries) need to engage in human rights awareness, equality awareness and raising equality consciousness.

However, the argument pertaining to globalization could be understood in different contexts by different contributors. For example, Townsend, Giorgio, Zembe, Cheyip and Mathews [16] argue that the spread of HIV and AIDS pandemic is closely connected to the process of globalization in the South, and in particular, in Africa where the process happens when human bodies move across borders in search of new economic and educational opportunities or in search of lives free from political conflict and violence. These migrants therefore carry the virus that causes AIDS and often they spread the virus at their destinations. On the other hand, Altman [17] and Tanga [8] state that HIV and AIDS are linked to globalization in a number of ways including the fact that a globalized economy means that vagaries of the market also impact upon spread of infection. The impact of HIV and AIDS is linked to social and economic upheavals which have effectively increased the vulnerability of women, who are more likely to be unable to protect themselves against infection and to carry a greater share of care for those who are sick or infected.

Sapkota [18] conducted a content analysis to identify the degree of mainstreaming of the key elements of globalization in Poverty Reduction Strategy papers in the Asia Pacific region. Trade openness gained the highest priority followed by foreign investment, aid, tourism and lastly migration. Altman [19] and Hirsch [20] highlighted that globalisation has an impact on all aspects of life including sexuality. Sexuality is affected by globalisation in a number of interconnected ways and therefore increases inequalities, acting both as a liberator and an oppressive influence. Pearson [21] argues that people working on gender development in the last third quarter of the twentieth century will lead to the new century realizing the global relevance of gender in development and see that gender analysis is applied in new contexts and to both men and women. According to Sen [22], as quoted by Pearson [21], indications are that the new century will witness an assertion of the global relevance of gender in development institutions and organizations concerned with meeting the challenges of globalisation.

Table 1 shows some socio-economic indicators of Lesotho. With a population of 1.8 million inhabitants, Lesotho has an urbanized population of 25%. Life expectancy has dropped from more than 50 years in the 1990s to 44.9 years in 2008. Furthermore, population poverty line also deteriorated to 56.7%, with a Human Development Index (HDI) ranking of 156 of 182 countries, a GDP per capita of M4795 and an inflation rate of 4.2%. Other important indicators include unemployment figure of 45% as well as high number of orphaned children. The combinations of high levels of poverty and unemployment coupled with high HIV and AIDS prevalence in a population with female majority and an industry that is dependent on female workforce certainly leaves a lot to be desired in terms of the vulnerability that women will go through as a result of global economic crisis.

The objective of this chapter was therefore to review the gender dimensions and interconnectedness of globalization, economic crisis and HIV/AIDS in the textile and garment industry in the Kingdom of Lesotho following the economic financial meltdown of 2008–2009. More specifically, the study aimed to investigate and determine the role of the textile and garment industry as provider of employment opportunities and the nexus between globalization, economic meltdown and HIV/AIDS crisis; determine if HIV/AIDS is an economic threat to the textile and garment industry; and determine if there is a differential in HIV/AIDS vulnerability in the industry based on gender.

Indicator	Value	Year	Source
Population size *(de jure)*	1,862,860	2006	[2]
Population urbanised (%)	23	2006	[2]
Life expectancy at birth	41.2	2006	[14]
Population below poverty line (%)	56.7	2002/3	[23]
Adult (15–49) prevalence of HIV (%)	23.0	2009	[24]
Infant mortality rate (per 1000 live births)	64.6	2007	[25]
Under five mortality rate (per 1000 live births)	98.2	2007	[25]
Maternal mortality rate (per 100,000 live births)	762	2004	[25]
Human Development Index Rank (out of 182 countries)	156	2009	[26]
Population using improved drinking water sources (%)	79	2004	[25]
Population using adequate sanitation facilities (%)	37	2004	[25]
Orphans, children (0–7 years) due to AIDS	130,000	2009	[27]
Orphans, children (0–7 years) due to all causes	200,000	2009	[27]
Crude birth rate per 1000 population	29	2007	[25]
Crude death rate per 1000 population	19.2	2007	[25]
Total fertility rate	3.4	2007	[25]
Skilled attendant at delivery (%)	55.4	1990–2005	[25]
Inflation rate (%)	5.5	2011	[28]
Unemployment rate (%)	45	2010	[5]
GDP growth rate	4.4	2008	[29]
GDP per capita at constant prices (Maloti)	4795	2008	[29]

Table 1. Some socio-economic indicators of Lesotho.

2. Literature review

2.1. Gender dimensions of HIV and AIDS

According to the Ministry of Health and Social Welfare (MoHSW), the bulk of HIV infections in Lesotho have been primarily through heterosexual contact [30] while the National HIV and AIDS Strategic Plan for 2006–2011 reports that the HIV and AIDS epidemic in Lesotho is characterized by high mortality rate estimated at 70 deaths per day, with a resultant increasing number of orphans and vulnerable children [8, 31, 32]. The social, cultural and behavioural factors also contribute to the spread of HIV through concurrent and multiple sexual partnerships [33]. This can better be understood by contextualizing the problem with gender lens. According to Camlin, Kwena, Dworkin, Cohen and Bukusi [34], Sub-Saharan Africa is the only part of the world where HIV prevalence and AIDS deaths are higher for women than for men. They therefore emphasized that gender dimension is crucial to understanding how HIV is spread. The concept facilitates an analysis of how men's and women's roles increase vulnerability to the disease. This is relevant to the Lesotho textiles and garment industry with over 70% of its workforce who are females. Curtis [35] provides a framework for the analysis of the dimension of human diseases within the context of human disease ecology as posited by Meade and Earikson [36]. This context has direct bearing on the gender dimension of HIV and AIDS in Lesotho especially in the textiles and garment industry. They employed the human disease ecology framework to carry out social analysis of HIV and AIDS epidemic in Lesotho highlighting the link between gender inequalities and health. Hlalele and Letsie [37] concluded that there is a general trend in gender inequalities relating to power relations, socialization and cultures as well as legislation in which women remain largely disadvantaged. Nattrass [38] explored the gender dimensions of access to highly active antiretroviral therapy (HAART) in South Africa. Using regression analysis, Natrass found that women are more vulnerable to HIV than men. As a result women access HAART in disproportionately larger numbers compared to men. The findings revealed that fewer men access HAART than women because men in general do not seek treatment for poor health as compared to women. In addition, gender norm makes it difficult for men to admit any health-related weakness and seek medical attention. A number of authors have identified gender inequality as a major driver for the spread of HIV and AIDS [8, 39–42]. Similar views were expressed by Epstein et al. [43] and Mitchell et al. [44] Tanga and Tangwe [9] who claim that gender inequalities fuel HIV and AIDS pandemic and make women more vulnerable to infection. Thus, from the foregoing, understanding the interplay of economic globalization and HIV and AIDS in the textile and garment industry in Lesotho calls for a thorough understanding of the gender dimension in the industry. In the context of Lesotho, socio-cultural differences and power relations between males and females may create gender imbalance in the industry that may predispose women to more vulnerability to the epidemic. Hlalele and Letsie [37] contend that gender inequality and gender-based violence could be promoted by low socio-economic and legal position of women. According to them, this could further be exacerbated by intergenerational sex especially between older males and younger women as a result of their socio-economic vulnerability which appear preponderant in the industry.

Poulsen [45] investigated the gendered impact of HIV and AIDs in South Africa and Swaziland under the auspice of Save the Children. The investigation focused on determining the number and characteristics of children who drop out of school in communities affected by HIV and AIDs as well as primary reasons for drop outs. The result revealed that in most schools teachers acknowledged that HIV and AIDS was a serious issue, particularly in terms of growing numbers of orphans as well as children with sick parents. Parental death was found to be the major cause of disruption of children's home lives. Parental death makes family to be poorer leading children to engage in risky behaviour and more likely to drop out of school. In another study, Bajaj [46] investigated how young women are finding ways to cope with being trapped in a context characterized by severe economic decline and an extensive HIV and AIDS crisis by having "sugar daddies" (rich men). However, the strategies of securing "sugar daddies" result in deadly infection and social isolation of these young women. These studies point to the vulnerability of women and children to the pandemic through unequal power relations. Mindry

[47] thus contends that there is a need to address the HIV crisis in African countries by examining the process in terms of engagement. However, Jewkes [48] recommends that the changes that are needed in school environment should be effective to serve as places for changing sexual practices and gender norms because they are largely the same needed to provide effective education for development. Much more emphasis needs to be given to scaling up delivery interventions to youths in contexts where the curriculum content, skills emphasis, duration, selection of facilitator, use of participatory methods and broader context can be employed.

A baseline study commissioned by the Apparel Lesotho Alliance to Fight AIDS (ALAFA) which assessed the situation of HIV and AIDS among workers in the textile and garment industry in Lesotho revealed a staggering 43.2% rate of prevalence [8, 49]. Further analysis of this study shows that women were significantly more vulnerable than men, with infection levels of 44.2% against 35.6% for men. This finding is important not only due to the significance of the textile and garment industry to the economy of Lesotho but also on account of the demographics of the labour force in the industry where the majority of the workforce are women aged 25–39 years, the age group which has been shown throughout Sub-Saharan Africa to be particularly more vulnerable to HIV infection [4].

2.2. Economic structure, trade and exports

Historic trends of gross domestic product (GDP) growth indicate that Lesotho has performed relatively well over the past two decades, except for 1998 when civil unrest nearly rotted the country [50]. The GDP growth has averaged 3.9% between 1980 and 2006 and stood at 4.4% in 2009. However, challenges still remain. In the past two decades, Lesotho experienced economic transition and has diversified its economy to source growth from other sectors, mainly water development, tourism, manufacturing and mining [51]. Kim et al. [52] identified seven countries in sub-Saharan Africa (Mauritius, Lesotho, South Africa, Madagascar, Kenya, Swaziland and Zimbabwe) as being major exporters of textiles and apparel. They argue that textile and apparel industry is the gate of choice for most countries in the quest to step into industrialization. The US trade policies have been the common factor for the flourishing of the textile and apparel industry in scores of countries of developing countries. It is therefore argued that for the industry to be successful, there should be combined efforts of the local government's industrial and trade policies, the entrepreneurial prowess of the private sector and the flexibility and the work ethic of the labour force. It is on this account that Lesotho took advantage of the African Growth and Opportunity Act (AGOA) to become the largest exporter of garments to the USA from SSA. Exports totalled over $320 million in 2002 [13]. The sector has been an important contributor to economic growth and employment creation. For instance, it contributed about 8% of GDP in the 1980s and reached as high as 16.2% in 2004 [53]. However, despite these positive developments, the removal of textiles quotas and the appreciation of the local currency resulted in decline in the sector's contribution during 2005. The third phase of AGOA in 2007 and the provision of rules of origin of third country have had implications on Lesotho's exports and employment of Basotho by the industry. The expiry of multi-fibre agreement (MFA) implied greater competition in the US market by more efficient countries such as China, also contributed to the problem. As a result, the ratio of textiles and clothing contribution to GDP declined from 9.2% in 2004 to 7.1% in 2005. Exports to the USA have also declined by 13% from 2004 to 2005 although there was a slight improvement from 2005 to 2006 of 2.2% [53]. These fluctuations invariably impacted on the Southern African Customs Union (SACU) revenue and the Lesotho economy, which relies on SACU revenue for most of its income (averaging 55%) [54].

The renegotiation of the SACU agreement and the revenue-sharing formula in the context of Free Trade Agreements (FTA) with the European Union (EU) and United States of America (USA) and the global financial crisis has led to a decline in customs revenues from M4.8 billion in 2009/2010 to about M2.3 billion in 2010/2011. This will mean a reduction in the Government's share in the economy.

3. Research methodology

The study area from which the data for this chapter is derived was comprised of all the textile and garment industry sites located in the districts of Maseru and Leribe. Prior to data collection exercise, the research protocol was submitted to the Lesotho Ministry of Health and Social Welfare Maseru, Ethics Review Committee, which reviewed and gave approval for the data collection. A multistage research design was used for data collection. First, a rapid appraisal questionnaire was administered to 38 factories from which 23 factories served as a sampling frame for the selection of six case study factories. Second, a factory workers' questionnaire, which was a cross-sectional survey instrument, was used to collect data from 640 factory workers among the six selected case-study firms. The number of factory workers interviewed was proportional to the number of workers in a factory. Research assistants were allowed into the factory premises during the lunch break hour, which is between 13.00 and 14.00 H. The original idea of randomly selecting workers for interviews prior to interview proved unworkable since researchers were not allowed access to the factory premises prior to lunch hour. Research assistants were allowed into the factory premises during lunch break to interview the workers. Nonetheless, the lowest response rate for the factories was 90%.

The quantitative data was analysed using descriptive and inferential statistics. Frequency tables were used to summarize pertinent information pertaining to key variables. Logistic regression analysis was employed to determine factors associated with the importance of employment provided by the industry and the likelihood of finding alternative work if retrenched. These analyses were performed using the Statistical Package for Social Sciences (SPSS). All ethical considerations such as confidentiality, informed consent and anonymity of subjects were strictly observed during data collection as well as analysis and dissemination of the findings.

4. Findings and discussion

4.1. Characteristics of firms and socio-demographics of the workers

Out of the 38 firms that received the rapid appraisal questionnaires, 2 firms declined to participate in the study. Of the remaining 36, only 23 completed their questionnaires and returned them while 13 were outstanding giving a response rate of 64%. Attempts to follow up on the remaining questionnaires did not yield positive results. The selection of the study firms was, thus, based on 23 firms that responded to the appraisal questionnaire. Of the 23 firms that responded to the appraisal questionnaire six factories were selected as case study firms guided by three key criteria, namely, factory's exposure to: (1) economic globalization, in this case, focus was on perceived impact on trade and finance; (2) HIV and AIDS response, here the choice was guided by the type of response and the balance was preserved such that all types of responses (comprehensive, none and/or prevention only) were represented; and (3) production process type, whether firms specialise or engage in task shifting processes. **Table 2** presents the characteristics of these factories. From **Table 2**, it can be seen that all the factories were foreign owned with the exception of one. Half of the foreign-owned factories were South African followed by Taiwanese owned factories at 32%. About a tenth of the factories were Chinese owned while one factory was co-owned by Chinese, Taiwanese and other nationalities. Regarding the number of years that the factories have been operating in Lesotho, the result revealed that a fifth of the factories have been operating in Lesotho for 10 or more years while a third (35%) have been in Lesotho for between 5 and 9 years. Forty-four percent of the factories have been working in Lesotho for less than 5 years. There were disparities in the years of operation in Lesotho by factory ownership. Chinese factories have been in Lesotho longest with a mean of 12 years of operation followed by Taiwanese with a mean of 11 years, while the majority of South African factories have been in Lesotho for less than 5 years with a mean of 4 years of operation in Lesotho.

In addition, **Table 2** indicates that employment figures ranged from 260 to over 800 employees. Twenty-six percent of the factories had a workforce of between 500 and 799 followed by those with a workforce of less than 300 and those with a workforce of over 800 workers at 22% each. Workforce disparities were such that Taiwanese factories were employing 45% of the workforce followed by the South African factories with 37%. Chinese factories were employing 11% of the workforce while the other two factories employed 5% or less. Concerning trade patterns, **Table 2** further reveals that United States of America (USA) and the European Union (EU) are the main export destinations (39%) followed by the Southern African Customs Union (SACU) (17.4%) and the rest of the other export destinations constituted less than 10% of the exports. Seventeen percent of the factories were not exporting their products. Thus, the textiles and garment industry is more export oriented, hence more prone to the impact of economic globalization, preferential trade agreements and financial crisis that has hit the industry in recent times. The dominance of the Lesotho textiles industry by foreign firms has additional implications that the global economic crisis may affect the industry very hard due to demand for repatriation of profits abroad which will be affected by the economic crisis.

As regards sources of financial capital, 11 factories were financed from abroad while 8 were partly financed locally and partly from abroad. Only one factory was financed locally. Three factories did not provide information about their sources of financial capital. Of the 18 factories that provided information about the location of their financiers abroad, 44% were located in South Africa, 28% in Asia and 17% in the USA. Eleven percent of the factories had their foreign financiers situated in other countries than South Africa, Asia or the USA. From **Table 2**, 22 of 23 factories (96%) were foreign-owned companies, this coupled with the fact that about

Characteristic		Frequency	Percent
Factory ownership	Chinese	3	13.0
	Taiwanese	7	30.4
	South African	11	47.8
	Basotho	1	4.3
	Chinese + Taiwanese + Other	1	4.3
Years of operation in Lesotho	<5	10	43.5
	5–9	8	34.8
	10 +	5	21.7
	Mean		7.30
Factory employment size	< 300	5	21.7
	300-499	4	17.4
	500-799	6	26.1
	800 and above	5	21.7
	No response	3	13.0
Export destination	Do not export	4	17.4
	SACU	4	17.4
	SADC	2	8.7
	US & EU	9	39.1
	Other destinations	1	4.3
	SADC & US	1	4.3
	US, EU & OTHER	1	4.3
	No response	1	4.3

Table 2. Characteristics of the factories.

19 of the companies have their source of financing from abroad make the operations of the companies more dependent on the success of their operations in the international markets since most have foreign market destinations. Instability in the world economic market will hit these companies very hard unless the companies are well diversified to be able to absorb such a shock.

The distribution of the employees, as evidenced in **Table 3**, reveals that a quarter of the respondents were male compared to three quarters female (75%). Given the role of socialization and culture of the Basotho people that are more patriarchal, power relations and the gender dimensions of the labour force, both the women workforce and the operations of the factories may be at more risks of the HIV and AIDS epidemic unless more precautions and preventative measures are in place. To buttress this point, Hlalele and Letsie [37] posit that "women's minority status, religious and cultural beliefs and adverse economic conditions negatively

Characteristic	Frequency	Percent
Sex		
Male	158	24.7
Female	482	75.3
Experience of working at factories		
<2 years	238	37.2
2–3.99 years	207	32.3
4 years and above	188	29.4
No response	7	1.1
Age		
<20	14	2.2
20–24	118	18.4
25–29	188	29.4
30–34	138	21.6
35+	182	28.4
Educational attainment		
No education	14	2.2
Primary	269	42.0
Junior secondary	247	38.6
Senior secondary or better	110	17.2
Marital status		
Never married	169	26.4
Previous married	114	17.8
Currently married	355	55.5
No response/cohabiting	2	0.3
Total	**640**	**100.0**

Table 3. Some socio-demographic characteristics of the workers.

impact the health status of most Basotho women. This, therefore, makes it difficult for women to negotiate safer or protected sex within their relationships. As a consequence, women face increased chances of contracting sexually transmitted infections (STIs), HIV and AIDS and having undesired pregnancies. Gender-based violence and gender inequality are increasingly cited as important determinants of women's HIV risk." This calls for a stronger HIV and AIDS policy at the workplace and nationally to protect the workforce and women and ensuring sustainability of production. Slightly more than a third (37.2%) of the workforce had worked at the factories for less than 2 years, another third (32.3%) had been with the factories for 2 to less than 4 years and the remaining (29.4%) had worked at the factories for 4 years or more. Less than 5% of the respondents were less than 20 years old, majority (69%) were aged between 20 and 34 years and 28% were aged 35 years and above. Thus, about 70% or more of the workforce are 35 years of age or younger which places them within a more sexually active group with high risk of contracting HIV and AIDS at the workplace given unequal power relations between men and women when it comes to negotiating for protective sexual intercourse. Few (2%) of the workers had no formal education, while those with primary and junior secondary education were 42 and 40%, respectively. Less than 20% had senior secondary education or better. According to marital status, more than half (56%) of the workers were currently married compared to 26% who were never married and 18% previously married. This point bears very well on the socio-cultural dimension of the Basotho people, and at the workplace, as emphasised earlier by Hlalele and Letsie [37] who maintained that with more than 40% of the workforce unmarried, coupled with more patriarchal culture, younger women workforce with more possibility of intergenerational sex preference especially between older men and younger women may be driven by socio-economic conditions as a consequence of unequal power relations. This exposes the workforce to a much greater risk of HIV and AIDS infection detrimental to the workforce, the industry and the nation at large. The low level of educational attainment by the majority of the workforce, which is predominantly women, places the workers and by extension the women employees at more disadvantage in terms of power relations. This can further manifest itself in terms of low economic power and a target for intergenerational sex between older men and younger women with high risk of HIV and AIDS infection with a consequence of reduced productivity either due to sickness themselves or taking care of relatives who may also be infected or affected by the pandemic.

4.2. Economic empowerment

As indicated elsewhere in the chapter, PTAs have made it easier for Lesotho's products to have access to the USA and EU markets. According to results of the rapid appraisal information obtained from the managers and presented in **Table 4**, more than half (52%) of the workforce in the factories are employed by the factories that are exporting solely to the USA and the EU. Considering that some factories are exporting to the USA and or EU and other destinations, the percentage of the workforce employed as a result of the PTAs is over 60%. The success of the economic opportunities created by the PTAs is dependent on sustained market conditions under the economic globalization situation. Any economic instability in the global market can create serious repercussions as experienced during the 2008 global financial crisis which literally led to some of the factories closing down during the data collection phase of this study. Variation in exchange rate of the US$ and the South African Rand also impacts on the operations of the factories in Lesotho which often leads to threats of closure of the factories and loss of jobs. Thus, by implications, because women constitute over 70% of the workforce, they will be more affected and forced into more economic hardship. Besides, the factory job was the first job ever for majority of the women on account of their low level of education which made them not to find jobs in other sectors of the economy.

In assessing how the industry has benefited Basotho economically, the study found that 72% of the workers reported that their present job was their first job ever. Comparative figures were 77% for females and 57% for males and the difference between these percentages was

Export destination	Total employees	Percentage
Do not export	976	7
SACU	1612	11
SADC	536	4
US & EU	7458	52
Other destinations	501	4
SADC & US	1131	8
US & EU & other	1770	12
No response	242	2

Table 4. Distribution of employees by export destination.

statistically significant. Making it evident that the garment and textiles industry is making a positive difference by providing employment to Basotho who otherwise would be without jobs and this is more so among females than males. However, there were no salary differences between male and female employees. To further emphasize the importance of the jobs provided by the industry, of those workers for whom the present job was their first job ever, 81% were dependent on support from either parents or partners for those who were married. Only 5% were supporting themselves from agriculture. To further support the notion that females were benefiting more than their male counterparts, 66% of males compared to 86% of females were dependent on someone before being employed in the garment and textiles industry. In comparing present and previous salaries for those who had worked elsewhere prior to joining the firms, on the average, females were about M300 better off working in the industry while males were M40 worse off. Employment in the factories has enhanced women's economic empowerment and personal autonomy which of course could result into increased HIV vulnerability where there is unprotected sex depending on how the power relations is played out between the sexes following increased economic empowerment.

The logistic regression result in **Table 5** further lends support to the notion that economic opportunities of the garment and textiles industry are benefiting females more than males. The results of the logistic regression analysis indicate that males are less likely to have mentioned that the present job is their first ever implying that they joined the industry having previously worked elsewhere. This indicates that this sector appears to have created more job opportunities for women who previously had no job opportunities than for men. However, the results do confirm that females are the major beneficiaries of economic empowerment provided by the garment and textiles industry. This would not come as a surprise since Basotho men have always benefited from employment provided by the mining industry in South Africa. Recent retrenchments of Basotho men from the mines notwithstanding, mining work is still considered the best option among Basotho men. The logistic regression result also demonstrates that age is negatively associated with getting employment in the textiles and garment industry. One of the reasons why the Basotho males are less schooled than their female counterparts is due to the fact that education was not an important factor for getting

Variable		B	Exp(B)
Location	Maseru	0.265	1.304
	Leribe (RC)		
Sex	Male	−1.134**	0.322
	Female (RC)		
Age		−0.049**	0.952
Years of operation in Lesotho		−0.017	0.983
Type of work	Management	0.208	1.231
	Supervisor	-0.562	0.570
	Unskilled labourer	-0.194	0.824
	Skilled production worker (RC)		
Education	No education	0.350	1.419
	Junior secondary	0.215	1.240
	Senior secondary or better	0.310	1.363
	Primary (RC)		
Marital status	Never married	0.460#	1.584
	Previously married	−0.163	0.850
	Currently married		
Sub-sector	Knitting garments	−0.130	0.878
	Denim/cotton yarn	−0.494#	0.610
	Woven garments (RC)		
Production process	Specialisation and division of labour	0.302	1.352
	Multi-skilling and task shifting (RC)		
Constant		2.706**	
Notes: $^{**}p < 1\%$; $^{*}p < 5\%$ and $^{\#}\ p < 10\%$.			

Table 5. Logistic regression results showing the odds that the current job is the first ever.

a mining job. History would seem to be repeating itself in the textiles and garment industry where education is not an important factor for the industry providing one with the first job ever. It would seem sex and age are the main factors associated with the odds that the present job is the first ever. Marital status and subsector are marginally associated with the odds that the present job is the first ever.

4.3. Threats to economic opportunities

The economic opportunities provided by the industry's jobs are threatened by several factors, both external and internal. For purposes of this chapter, however, only two factors (HIV and

AIDS and economic globalization) were taken into consideration. It is common for firms to cut salaries when ... for self-ill-health workers are absent from work due to self-ill-health. Ninety-one percent of the workers reported that there are salary cuts when they are absent due to ill-health. Over 80% of the workers also reported that absence from work due to reasons other than ill-health attracts salary cuts. Given the high HIV prevalence in Lesotho and among the workers of the industry in particular with more than 40% prevalence rate [49], workers are bound to be away from work because they are either sick themselves or they have to look after sick relatives. On a typical month, the workers are on the average away from work for 6.34 days which is astonishingly high. Salary cuts should be understood in the context where employers have to replace absent workers by temporary staff in order to meet the deadlines of their orders. Absenteeism due to ill-health also impacts on the employers in terms of lost time or having to deal with substitute casual workers whose productivity may be lower than that of regular employees whom they are replacing.

Women are known to be half of the world's migrants and also half of those living with HIV and AIDS [12, 20] and labour migration and other forms of mobility have been associated with increased risk to HIV infection [55, 56]. However, most of the female migrant workers are from the rural mountainous areas of Lesotho. Although most of the respondents were from these areas, there was no indication that there was a breakdown in relationships and the formation of long-term relationships at the factories as has been shown by some studies [55]. This is because most of the women respondents (56%) were married though many stated that they rarely visit home to meet their spouses. Kendall and Pelcastre [55] echoed that internal migration involves the processes of rupture and reformation of social networks. However, there was no evidence pertaining to this in this research. Nonetheless, it can be argued that some migrants apart from the continued economic responsibilities for themselves and their dependents, who have pushed people away from their homes to seek work in the factories, do escape from home community and/or family controls and potential isolation back at home.

It is a widely held view that social vulnerability of poverty contributes to workers, especially women, to the risk of HIV infection [16, 37, 57]. For example, in the context of South Africa, Gilbert and Selikow [58] argue that the HIV epidemic in South Africa and the region at large is increasingly feminized as a growing proportion of new infections occur among women and affect women. It is revealed that in South Africa, a perilous mix of biomedical, political, economic and cultural forces shape the gendered dynamic of the HIV epidemic. The vulnerability can also be attributed to male partners' sexual infidelity having concurrent and multiple sexual partnerships and the lack of condom use which exemplify the link between internal migration and HIV vulnerability and not just international migration which has been the focus of many studies. Therefore, this chapter confirms Webber's [59] assertion that women's biological as well as their social vulnerabilities to the pandemic may be exacerbated within the context of international labour migration and rural-urban migration [4]. The scourge of HIV and AIDS is a complex, multifaceted issue that requires a collaborative effort and hence multidimensional strategies.

The second threat to economic opportunities offered by factory work is global economic crisis. The recent food prices instability on the international market have been at the centre of debates and as Galtier [60] maintains, experts have described the situation in the late 2000s in developing countries as one that is characterized by instability in food prices. One of the causes is globalization which Galtier [60] calls imported instability. Using qualitative design, Uraguchi [61] conducted a study on farming households in Bangladesh and Ethiopia which focused on the vulnerability of women to food insecurity owing to the 2007–2008 food price hikes and their seasonal coping mechanisms. The study confirms that it is gender inequality that makes women more vulnerable to the food price hikes, yet they are resourcefully devising ways to cope with scarcity, access and consumption of food. Women remain highly vulnerable to external shocks and they have fragile intra-household coping mechanisms. In this current study, 91% of the workers who were aware of the global economic crisis reported that the global economic crisis was likely to bring about retrenchment and more economic hardship for them and their families. The economic crisis posed significant threats to the developing countries. Gaerlan et al. [62] argue that global economic crisis has fuelled the continuing job insecurity through "casualisation" in the Philippines, and this has caused women to change their lifestyles by letting go non-essential goods and services. Reductions in employment in the formal economy and escalating food and fuel prices are forcing more and more people into the informal economy as the viable option [63]. In this study, the impact of the global economic crisis has threatened loss of jobs among women employees especially on account of their low level of education with the current job being their first job ever for most of the women. Cohen [63] reports that female traders are insecure and vulnerable since they are earning incomes that are insufficient for supporting a household, reinvesting in their business or saving money. Horn [64] maintains that incomes and employment trend for women in the informal sector are increasing vulnerability and women struggle more to feed their families through cutting back on educational and medical expenses. The women employed in the textile and garment industry in Lesotho were no exception despite the fact that the result of the data analysis revealed women were better off than men from their jobs in the textiles industry. In another study, Mutekwa [65] demonstrated that the discourses of the African renaissances are entangled in the gendered and gendering nature of globalisation discourse since they are framed within it. The study further identified the multifaceted implications and effects of a hegemonic, masculine neoliberal global discourse on the various facets of the African Renaissance concluding that the African Renaissances responses can be either complicit or subversive in addressing key challenges in a globalizing economy with gender sensitivity.

Women and ethnic minority workers have been particularly hard hit, not just by job losses but also by reductions in hours of work, wage rates and non-wage benefits [66]. Similar findings have been documented on the impact of the global crisis on workers in many countries [67–69]. The conundrum even more worrying is that 61% of these workers opined that they are not likely to get a job should they be retrenched due to low level of education and non-availability of jobs. According to the logistic regression results in **Table 6**, age is the only major explanatory variable from the perception of the workers that they would not get a job if retrenched. Education is a marginal explanatory variable except that in factories, the perception of the workers that the likelihood of getting a job if retrenched is low due to low level of education. The poor educational level of participants can be attributed to the difficult economic situation which has truncated their educational opportunities. However, the factories

Variable		B	Exp(B)
Sex	Male	0.288	1.334
	Female		
Age		–0.072**	0.931
Type of work done	Management	–0.668	0.513
	Supervisor	–0.635	0.530
	Unskilled labourer	–0.243	0.784
	Skilled production worker (RC)		
Education	No education	–1.118#	0.327
	Junior secondary	–0.129	0.879
	Senior secondary or better	0.308	1.361
	Primary		
Marital status	Never married	0.349	1.418
	Previously married	0.277	1.319
	Currently married		
Sub-sector	Knitting garment	–0.239	0.788
	Denim fabric/cotton yarn	–0.420	0.657
	Woven garment (RC)		
Years of operation in Lesotho		–0.018	0.982
Number of employees		0.000	1.000
Absence due to ill health	No	–0.234	0.792
	Yes (RC)		
Constant		2.931**	

Notes: $^{**}p < 1\%$; $^{*}p < 5\%$ and $^{\#}\ p < 10\%$.

Table 6. The perceived likelihood of finding alternative work if retrenched.

organize on-the-job training of their semi-skilled employees who easily fit into the production line jobs but due to their low level of education, once retrenched from the factories may not easily get jobs elsewhere.

Furthermore, the findings show that the economic opportunities provided by the industry do not appear to go beyond employment provision. Asked whether they provided employee benefits such as housing, medical aid, funeral cover, pension and life insurance as one way of empowering their workers, employers indicated that they do not provide benefits to their employees with the exception of employees in clerical and management positions. As Pelcastre-Villafuerte et al. [70] aptly put it, the family responsibilities make low-wage factory work the most viable option for women, though these jobs are sometimes without legally mandated medical and social security benefits associated with them. However, the industry does provide minimal benefits stipulated in the labour code.

5. Conclusion and recommendations

The textiles and garment industry attracts a huge number of workers, especially women from the rural mountainous areas of Lesotho who would otherwise be unemployed. This has greatly been as a result of Lesotho enjoying PTAs from the USA and EU. Although the employment of these rural female migrants in this industry provides economic opportunities and economically empowers them, there are challenges posed by both external and internal forces such as the global economic crisis as well as the HIV and AIDS pandemic.

The challenge posed by the global economic crisis has created a sense of job insecurity among workers with 61% of these workers having opined that they are not likely to get a job should they be retrenched due to low level of education. The study found that age was the only major explanatory variable from the perception of the workers that they would not get a job if retrenched. Education is a marginal explanatory variable except that in factories, the perception of the workers that the likelihood of getting a job if retrenched is low due to low level of education. This study also established that it was a common practice for firms in the textile and garment industry in Lesotho to cut salaries whenever workers are absent from work irrespective of whether such absence is due to ill-health. Ninety-one percent of the workers reported that there are salary cuts when they are absent due to ill-health. Over 80% of the workers also reported that absence from work due to reasons other than ill-health attracts salary cuts. Given the high HIV prevalence in Lesotho and among the workers of the industry in particular with more than 40% prevalence rate [49], workers are bound to be away from work because they are either sick themselves or they have to look after sick relatives.

The study also revealed that 75% of the labour force in the industry is made of women as major beneficiaries of employment opportunities although most of them are in their sexually active age (25–39 years old) with unequal gender power relations which make them more vulnerable to the threat posed by the HIV/AIDS pandemic as double-edged sword. This was inferred from the high prevalence rate (43%) of HIV/AIDS infection in the industry with women having prevalence rate of 44% compared to men at 35%. This has major ramifications for sustainability of the industry in both the perspective of the workers and firms without any major policy in place to curb the spread of the HIV/AIDS. Thus, the combined effect of the global economic crisis and the HIV/AIDS pandemic coupled with unequal gender relations in the industry make women more vulnerable than their male counterparts. This outcome is in agreement with a number of authors who identified gender inequality as a major driver for the spread of HIV and AIDS [8, 39–42]. Similar views were expressed by Epstein et al. [43] and Mitchell et al. [44] who claim that gender inequalities fuel HIV and AIDS pandemic and make women more vulnerable to infection. Nonetheless, the opportunities offered by the industry do not go beyond the provision of employment as many workers do not enjoy social insurance and other benefits. Any further retrenchment from this industry would have serious negative impact not only on the economy as a whole but on individual workers and their families since the South African mines have increasingly been retrenching workers, especially foreign-based workers which the Basotho form the majority.

The Department of Labour and Employment has not been able to follow-up with HIV and AIDS responses by the industry neither has it also insisted on various fringe benefits that should accrue to the workers. There is too much reliance by the Government of Lesotho on this industry to provide the necessary jobs at this time of the global economic crisis. The industry is kept afloat because of external capital flow and the end of PTAs can be catastrophic for the government and Basotho and as such dash their hopes for a better economy and decent lives.

The government should invest in diversification of employment opportunities, especially as Lesotho is blessed with abundant natural resources such as mohair and wool, mineral resources and water among many others. Although the Government of Lesotho is already doing much in the area of HIV and AIDS, the Department of Labour and Employment needs to ensure that all factories comply with its stipulations vis-à-vis HIV and AIDS response within the workplace. Also, the department should strive to encourage all the factories to institute fringe benefits not only to a selected few, especially expatriates as is the present case. This gesture needs to be extended to all workers.

Author details

Pius Tangwe Tanga[1]*, Haruna M. Bello[2], Tiisetso J. Makatjane[3] and Tumelo Tsikoane[4]

*Address all correspondence to: ptanga@ufh.ac.za

1 Department of Social Work/Social Development, University of Fort Hare, South Africa

2 Department of Agricultural Economics, University of Namibia, Mandume Ndemufayo Avenue, Winhoek, Namibia

3 Department of Statistics and Demography, National University of Lesotho, Lesotho

4 Department of Development Studies, National University of Lesotho, Lesotho

References

[1] Bello HM, Tsikoane T, Mochebelele M, Tanga PT, Nchake M, Makatjane TJ, Letete J. Economic Globalisation-HIV and AIDS-Nexus in the Textile and Garment Industry in Lesotho (unpublished). Maseru: National University of Lesotho; 2010.

[2] Bureau of Statistics. 2006 Lesotho Population and Housing Census Analytical Report, Volume IIIB Socio Economic Characteristics. Maseru: Bureau of Statistics; 2009.

[3] National AIDS Commission. Report on the National Response to HIV and AIDS (Period: 2006–2010). Maseru: National AIDS Commission; 2010.

[4] Tanga PT, Tangwe MN. The interplay between economic empowerment and HIV and AIDS amongst migrant workers in the textile industry in Lesotho. SAHARA-J: Journal of Social Aspects of HIV/AIDS: An Open Access Journal. 2014; 11 (1): 187–201. DOI:10.1080/17290376.2014.976250.

[5] United Nations Statistics Division. Lesotho Country Responses to HIV/AIDS Prevention. [Internet].2010. Available from: http://www.indexmundi.com/lesotho/hiv-prevention.html [Accessed: 2015/12/10].

[6] UNICEF. Revised country programme document: Lesotho (2008–2012). Maseru: UNICEF; 2007.

[7] UNAIDS. Uniting the World against AIDS. [Internet]. 2009. Available from: http://www.unaids.org/en/CountryResponses/Countries/lesotho.asp. [Accessed: 2012/10/9].

[8] Tanga, PT. The impact of declining extended family support system on the education of orphans in Lesotho. African Journal of AIDS Research. 2013; 12(3):173–183.

[9] Com Mark Trust: Apparel Lesotho Alliance to Fight Aids; 2007. Available from: http//:www.commark.org/pages/Default.asp?SectionID=182. [Accessed 2014/10/23].

[10] Bureau of Statistics. Provisional 2006 Population Figures. Maseru: Bureau of Statistics; 2008.

[11] Ministry of Health and Social Welfare (MOHSW). Lesotho Demographic and Health Survey 2009. Maseru, Lesotho: MOHSW; 2010.

[12] UNAIDS. Report of the global AIDS epidemic. [Internet]. 2008. Available from: http://www.unaids.org/en/KnowledgeCentre/HIVData/GlobalReport/2008/2008_Global_Report.asp. [Accessed 2012/2/12].

[13] Central Bank of Lesotho. Annual Report. Maseru: Central Bank of Lesotho; 2006.

[14] Bureau of Statistics. 2006 Lesotho Population and Housing Census Analytical Report, Volume IIIA Population Dynamics. Maseru: Bureau of Statistics; 2009.

[15] Metcalfe BD, Rees CJ. Gender, globalization and organization: exploring power, relations and intersections. Equality, diversity and Inclusion: International Journal. 2010; 29 (1): 5–22.

[16] Townsend L, Giorgio M, Zembe Y, Cheyip M, Mathews C. HIV Prevalence and Risk Behaviour Among Foreign Migrant Women Residing in Cape Town, South Africa. AIDS Behaviour, Online publication. 2014. DO 10.1007/s10461-014-0784-1.

[17] Altman D. Aids and the globalization of sexuality. Journal of Social Identities. 2008; 14 (2):146–147.

[18] Sapkota JB. Mainstreaming globalization in poverty reduction strategy papers in the Asia-Pacific region. Development in Practice. 2011; 21 (7): 999–1012

[19] Altman D: Sexuality and globalization. Agenda. 2004; 1(62): 22–28.

[20] Hirsch JS. Review: labour migration, externalities and ethics: theorizing the meso-level determinants of HIV vulnerability. Social Science & Medicine. 2014; 100: 38–45.

[21] Pearson R. Moving the goalposts: gender and globalization in the twenty-first century. Gender and Development. 2000; 8(1): 10–19.

[22] Sen G. Globalization in the 21st century: challenges for civil society. University of Amsterdam Development Lecture. Available from the Institute for Development Research Amsterdam (IDRA), University of Amsterdam, Plantage Muidergracht 12, 1018 TV Amsterdam, The Netherlands.

[23] Bureau of Statistics. 2002/03 and 1994/95 Household Budget Survey Analytical Report Volume 1. Maseru: Bureau of Statistics; 2006.

[24] Ministry of Health and Social Welfare [MOHSW], ICF Macro. Lesotho Demographic and Health Survey 2009. Maseru, Lesotho: MOHSW and ICF Macro; 2010.

[25] African Development Bank [ADB]. Kingdom of Lesotho—2008-2012 Country Strategic Paper. Maseru: ADB; 2008.

[26] UNPD. Human Development Report. Geneva: UNDP; 2009.

[27] United Nations Children's Fund [UNICEF]. The State of the World's Children 20118. New York: UNICEF; 2011.

[28] Bureau of Statistics. Consumer Price Index: Statistical Reports No. 19: 2011. Maseru: Bureau of Statistics; 2011.

[29] Bureau of Statistics. National Accounts of Lesotho 1999–2008: Statistical Reports No. 32: 2009. Maseru: Bureau of Statistics; 2009.

[30] Lesotho Review. An Overview of Kingdom of Lesotho's Economy. Maseru, Lesotho: Central Bank of Lesotho; 2008.

[31] National AIDS Commission: National HIV and AIDS Policy. Maseru, Lesotho: National AIDS Commission; 2007.

[32] Government of Lesotho [GOL]. Revised National HIV & AIDS Strategic Plan 2006–2011. Maseru, LS: NAC; 2009.

[33] National AIDS Commission, UNAIDS, Family Health International. Gender and Multiple and Concurrent Sexual Partnerships in Lesotho. Maseru: National AIDS Commission; 2009.

[34] Camlin CS, Kwena ZA, Dworkin SL, Cohen CR, Bukusi EA. She mixes her business: HIV transmission and acquisition risks among female migrants in western Kenya. Social Science & Medicine. 2013, 102: 146–156.

[35] Curtis S. Health and Inequality—Geographical Perspectives. London: Sage; 2004.

[36] Meade MS, Earickson RJ. Medical Geography. 2nd edition. New York/London: The Guilford Press; 2000.

[37] Hlalele D, Letsie PR. Gender Inequality and HIV/AIDS in Lesotho: a human disease ecological perspective. Journal of Human Ecology. 2011; 36(3): 159–165.

[38] Nattrass N. Gender access to antiretroviral treatment in South Africa. Feminist Economics. 2008; 14(4): 19–36.

[39] Poku N. Poverty, debt and Africa's HIV/AIDS crisis. International Affairs. 2002; 78: 531–546.

[40] Natrass N. The Moral Economy of AIDS in South Africa. Cape Town: Cambridge; 2004.

[41] Braun YA, Dreiling MC. From developmentalism to HIV/AIDS crisis: the amplification of women's rights in Lesotho. International Feminist Journal of Politics. 2010; 12(3–4): 464–483.

[42] Hatcher A, de Wet J, Bonell CP, Strange V, Phetla G. Promoting critical consciousness and social mobilisation in HIV/AIDS programmes: lessons and curricular tools from a South African intervention. Health Education Research. 2011; 26(3):542–555.

[43] Epstein D, Morell R, Moletsane R, Unterhalter E. Gender and HIV/AIDS in Africa south of the Sahara: interventions, activism, identities. Transformation: Critical Perspectives on Southern Africa. 2004; 54: 1–16.

[44] Mitchell S, Cockroft A, Lamothe G, Anderson N. Equity in HIV testing: evidence from cross-sectional study in ten Southern African countries. BMC International Health and Human Rights. 2010; 10: 23–33.

[45] Poulsen H. The gendered impact of HIV/AIDS on education in South Africa and Swaziland: save the children's experiences. Gender and Development. 2006; 14 (1): 47–56.

[46] Bajaj M. Sugar daddies and the dangers of sugar: cross-generational relationships, HIV/ AIDS, and secondary schooling in Zambia. In David PB, Alexander WW (eds). Gender, Equality and Education from International and Comparative Perspectives (International Perspectives on Education and Society). West Yorkshire: Emerald Group Publishing Limited; 2009, 10: 123–143.

[47] Mindry D. Engendering care: HIV, humanitarian assistance in Africa and the reproduction of gender stereotypes. Culture, Health & Sexuality. 2010; 12(5): 555–568.

[48] Jewkes R. Where to for sexual health education for adolescents in Sub-Saharan Africa? PLoS Med. 2010; 7(6): e10000288. Doi: 10.1371/journal.pmed.10000288.

[49] ALAFA. Lesotho Apparel Industry Unites to Fight AIDS. Maseru: ALAFA; 2009.

[50] Bennet M. Lesotho's export textile and garment industry. In Jauch H, Traub-Merz (eds). The Future of the Textile and Clothing Industry in Sub-Saharan Africa. Bonn: Friedrich-Ebert-Stiftung; 2006.

[51] Lesotho Review. An Overview of Kingdom of Lesotho's Economy; 2007 edition.

[52] Kim J-O, Traore MK, Warfield C. The textile and apparel industry in developing countries. Textile Progress. 2006; 38 (3): 1–64.

[53] Central Bank of Lesotho. The phasing out of the IMF—Fibre Agreement (MFA): its implications on Lesotho. Economic Review. 2005.

[54] Masenyetse RF, Motelle SI. Government Revenue—expenditure nexus in Lesotho: the decline in SACU revenue. American Journal of Economics. 2012; 2 (1): 8–14.

[55] Kandell T, Pelcastre BE. HIV vulnerability and condom use among migrant workers in Puebla, Mexico. Health Care for Women International. 2010; 31: 515–532.

[56] Jordal M, Wijewardena K, Öhman A, Essen B, Olsson P. Negotiating respectability: migrant women workers' perceptions of relationships and sexuality in free trade zones in Sri Lanka. Health Care for Women International. 2014, 35 (6): 658–676.

[57] Connelly P, Rosen S. Will small and medium enterprises provide HIV and AIDS services to employees? An analysis of market demand. South African Journal of Economics. 2005; 73: 613–626

[58] Gilbert L, Selikow TA. The epidemic in this country has the face of a woman: gender and HIV/AIDS in South Africa. African Journal of Aids Research. 2011; 10 (supplement): 325–334.

[59] Webber G. The impact of migration on HIV prevention for women: constructing a conceptual framework. Health Care for Women International. 2008; 28: 712–731.

[60] Galtier F. Which instruments best tackle food price instability in developing countries? Development in Practice, 2011; 21 (4–5): 526–535.

[61] Uraguchi ZW. Food price hike, food security and gender equality: assessing the roles and vulnerability of women in households of Bangladesh and Ethiopia. Gender and Development. 2010; 18(3): 491–501.

[62] Gaerlan K, Cabrera M, Samla P, Santoalla L. Feminised recession: impact of the global financial crisis on women garment workers in the Philippines. Gender and Development. 2010; 18(2): 229–240.

[63] Cohen J. How the global economic crisis reaches marginalised workers: the case of street traders in Johannesburg, South Africa. Gender and Development. 2010; 18(2): 277–289.

[64] Horn EZ. The effects of global crisis on women in the informal economy: research findings from WIEGO and the Inclusive Cities partners. Gender and Development. 2010; 18(2): 263–276.

[65] Mutekwa A. Gendered globalization discourses: implications for the African Renaissance. International Journal of African Renaissance Studies. 2012; 7(1): 5–21.

[66] Lawson M, King R. If not now, when? [Internet]. 2008. Available from: http:www.oxfam.org.uk/resources/policy/debt_aid/downloads/bn. g20summit%20.pdf [Accessed 2010/2/24].

[67] Arguello R. Securing the fruits of their labours: the effect of the crisis on women in Peru's Ica Valley. Gender and Development. 2010; 18(2): 241–247.

[68] Fernandez B. Cheap and disposable? The impact of the global economic crisis on the migration of Ethiopian women domestic workers to the Gulf. Gender and Development. 2010; 18(2): 249–262.

[69] Espey J, Harper C, Jones N. Crisis, care and childhood: the impact of economic crisis on care work in poor households in the developing world. Gender and Development. 2010; 18(2): 291–307.

[70] Pelcastre-Villafuerte B, Kandell T, Magis C. Las maquiladoras frente al VIH/AIDS, implementacion de programas y percepcion de los empleadores en Puebla. Region y sociedad. 2008; 20 (43): 189–211.

10

The Contextual Environmental Factors Shaping Disclosure of HIV Status across Population Groups in Sub-Saharan Africa

Sphiwe Madiba

Abstract

Disclosure of HIV-positive status is a public health intervention strategy to reduce HIV infections and improve HIV treatment and care. While disclosure occurs for different reasons for different population groups, the focus of studies has been on programmatic concerns such as disclosure to sexual partners to prevent HIV transmission or to prevent mother to child transmission of HIV. However, HIV disclosure occurs within a broad range of social and cultural contexts. Disclosure is facilitated or deterred by relationships at play within the social context beyond just the need for prevention of HIV. This chapter will highlight how the construction of HIV as an incurable, fatal, and contagious disease, stigma and discrimination, cultural and societal norms, secrecy, and the contextual environment influence HIV disclosure across different population groups. The chapter further demonstrated that stigma is the threat that connects the contextual environment and negatively influences disclosure across different population groups. This chapter is based on disclosure studies conducted in South Africa and extensive findings from disclosure research from sub-Saharan Africa. The data comprise qualitative studies on disclosing HIV to perinatally infected children by caregivers, the parental disclosure of own HIV-positive status to HIV-negative children, disclosure to sexual partners, disclosure to parents, and adolescent self-disclosure to romantic partners and friends.

Keywords: disclosure, stigma, secrecy, people living with HIV, cultural context, Southern Africa

1. Introduction

Disclosure has been an area of concern since the beginning of the HIV epidemic and the focus of research for decades. Extensive research has been done to explore the different types of disclosure, the process of disclosure, and patterns of disclosure. HIV disclosure includes an array of behaviors associated with the practice in which HIV-infected persons disclose their HIV serostatus to their partners, family members, or friends; or when a child is informed of her/his own HIV status [1]. Disclosure of HIV-positive serostatus is an integral component of public health prevention and treatment interventions and has been associated with many potential benefits. To sexual partners, disclosure occurs to enable safer sexual choices, to access prevention of mother to child transmission (PMTCT) of HIV programs, to gain emotional and financial support, and to protect the partner from HIV infection. To family members, disclosure occurs to gain various forms of support such as support for treatment adherence, emotional support, and protecting others from HIV. Lastly, to healthcare workers, disclosure occurs to access treatment and care services [2]. Although it is accepted that disclosure is associated with many beneficial outcomes such as increased social support, improved treatment adherence, decreased experienced stigma, greater well-being, and healthier behaviors. HIV disclosure also carries important risks evident by low disclosure rates among different population groups in sub-Saharan Africa (SSA).

The emphasis of most disclosure studies has been on the individual factors affecting low disclosure rates of the different population groups, while disclosure of HIV-positive serostatus is a complex phenomenon in which social, economic, political, cultural, and environmental aspects are interrelated. Disclosure is complicated by the close and complex relationship between disclosure, stigma, and culture which impacts on each other [3]. Furthermore, HIV disclosure is a complex and difficult personal matter that entails communication about a potentially life threatening, stigmatized, and transmissible infection [4]. The attempt to normalize nondisclosure by people affected by and infected with HIV, makes disclosure even more complex, given that the desire to maintain silence about an HIV test persists in many societies. In fact, there seems to be some level of normalcy when people living with HIV (PLHIV) do not talk about their illness when they anticipate and or experience stigma and discrimination [2, 5]. The normalization of silence is also shaped by the general understanding and evidence that disclosure is not always beneficial, positive, or advantageous to the individual. In fact, it is argued that HIV disclosure carries with it higher levels of risk and vulnerability [6], as the individual who discloses can never predict the response or reaction elicited by the disclosure.

The perception of HIV-related stigma shapes people's concerns about what might happen if they disclose. Consequently, people scan their social environment before they decide whether or not they should disclose their HIV status, and disclosure is deterred if individuals live in communities where HIV stigma is present [7, 8]. Steward et al. [9] argue that PLHIV do not need to encounter actual enactments of stigma to fear its social consequences, but being acutely aware of the potential for stigma or having witnessed stigmatization and discrimination against PLHIV raises the fear of stigma and shape their patterns of disclosure. This fear of stigma leads to people affected and infected by HIV adopting coping strategies such as disclosure avoidance or secrecy and silence to protect self from stigma [10].

A general assumption among researchers and policy makers working in the field of HIV prevention was that the availability of antiretroviral treatment (ART) and the beneficial outcomes of ART would increase the rates of disclosure in SSA. However, the low rates of HIV disclosure are an indication that the availability and increased access to ART in SSA are not changing the underlying structural causes of stigma contributing to the reluctance of people to disclose. Extensive research in SSA indicates that HIV-stigma is continuing to deter disclosure [11, 12]. Research indicates that disclosing one's HIV status carries an extraordinary degree of exposure [5], and that by disclosing, the person no longer struggles with concealing a secret, but may now be exposed to stigma [13]. The reluctance of individuals to disclose their HIV status is despite evidence that taking ART assist PLHIV to return to a healthy state by halting or reversing the progression of the diseases thereby hiding the physical and visible stigmatizing attributes of HIV.

Research suggests that the process of normalizing HIV through ART is socially complex, slow, and uneven in many communities in SSA [5, 14, 15]. Since the wide access to ART has not succeeded in increasing the rates of disclosure, there is a need to revisit how disclosure is conceptualized by individuals infected and affected by HIV in their contextual environments under which disclosure is more or less likely to occur.

2. Research on disclosure across populations

While disclosure occurs for different reasons for different population groups, the focus of studies has been on the reasons for disclosure and nondisclosure for the individuals. The chapter will use empirical data to demonstrate that disclosure is not driven by behavior only but by the contextual environment within which disclosure should occur or occurs. The chapter also uses findings from qualitative research conducted from 2009 to 2013 in South Africa to demonstrate how the construction of HIV, stigma and discrimination, secrecy, cultural norms, and the contextual environment influence HIV disclosure across different population groups [16–21].

The chapter will further demonstrate that the contextual environment is comparable across population groups, and that stigma is a constant factor which influences the social context of all population groups and a key factor in the reluctance of people affected and infected with HIV to disclose.

2.1. Study design and population

This chapter reports on the findings of four qualitative studies. The study design employed for three of the studies was qualitative explorative, and the fourth study used grounded theory design. The study participants included caregivers of perinatally infected children aged 6–13 years, HIV-positive parents of negative children aged 7–18 years, HIV-infected postnatal women in PMTCT program, and perinatally infected adolescents aged 12–18 years.

2.2. Study settings

All the studies were conducted in primary health facilities (PHC) and ART clinics of four hospitals in Mpumalanga and Gauteng provinces, South Africa. The four ART clinics were based in three community hospitals and one tertiary hospital and 34 health facilities providing ART services to adults and children living with HIV through the nurse-initiated and managed antiretroviral treatment initiative. The health facilities in Mpumalanga province were located in the rural subdistricts of Nkangala district, whereas the Gauteng province facilities were located in urban Tshwane district.

2.3. Data collection

The studies used focus group discussions (FGDs) and in-depth interviews (IDIs) to collect data with purposely selected participants for all the studies. The investigators (author as a principal investigator and a coinvestigator), Master of Public Health students and research assistants conducted the interviews. All interviews were conducted in local languages.

2.4. Data analysis

Data from three of the studies were analyzed using thematic analysis of the verbatim transcribed interviews. NVivo version 10, qualitative data analysis software, was used for coding. All the analyses were conducted either by the author or under the direct supervision of the author. The grounded theory study was analyzed by the author using constant comparison analysis.

2.5. Ethics

All the studies received ethical clearance from Medunsa Campus Research and Ethics Committee of the University of Limpopo; the author was affiliated with the institution at the time of the conduct of the studies. Permissions to conduct the studies were obtained from relevant provincial, district, and facility authorities of the two provinces. Written informed consent was obtained from all the participants who could legally consent, and assent was obtained from adolescents who were below 18 years of age. Participation for all the participants was voluntary, and privacy and confidentiality were safeguarded.

3. Disclosing a child's HIV status

A grounded theory study was conducted to explore how a sample of caregivers of children receiving ART view and experience HIV disclosure to perinatal infected children. Nine FGDs were conducted with 52 caregivers of children between 6 and 13 years. Data were collected between November 2009 and March 2010. Four main themes emerged from the data: thoughts of death and dying, the influence of media, fear of discrimination, and secrecy illustrate how the contextual environment is influencing disclosure and nondisclosure to infected children.

Caregivers delayed disclosure to children because they believe that their children would live in fear of death and dying. HIV disclosure to children was also influenced by the fear of stigma that the caregivers perceived to be present in their communities, and they feared that the children would be discriminated, mocked, teased, and socially rejected.

The thing is..., whenever you mention HIV, they know that AIDS kills, so..., when you tell her, she will know that she is going to die. That is what we are afraid of..., because the child will live thinking that she is going to die. Isn't it we hear that AIDS kills..., that when you have AIDS, you die? When you tell the child about it she will think she is dying (37-year-old mother of a 6-year-old).

I am afraid it will be known by everyone in my neighborhood and they will start saying "we don't want to play with this one he is HIV positive; he will infect us" (36-year-old mother of an 11-year-old).

Nondisclosed caregivers maintained silence to protect their children from stigma, discrimination, mockery, and social rejection, while disclosed caregivers kept the child's diagnosis secret from families and neighbors. The fear that the child would not keep the secret but would tell other children at school and in the neighborhood that he/she has HIV and subject the family to stigmatization featured strongly as a reason for delaying disclosure to infected children.

When I told him I said this is your secret because I am afraid of stigma, I told him it's only the family that knows because I see the way other people lack knowledge about this thing [HIV]. I am afraid of rejection (32-year-old mother of a 9-year-old).

We didn't tell him to talk or not to talk, but the way I see it, he does not talk, I wouldn't like him to talk (24-year-old brother of an 8-year-old).

4. Disclosing parental status to children

Focus group interviews were conducted to explore the disclosure of parent's own HIV-positive status to HIV-negative children accessing ART from an academic hospital in South Africa. Six FGDs were conducted between November 2010 and January 2011 with 47 HIV-positive parents of children aged between 7 and 18 years. The data present four main themes fear of death and dying, the influence of media, fear of discrimination, and secrecy to highlight the social context influencing disclosure of parental HIV status to children.

Parental disclosure occurs within an environment where children think that AIDS kills and the thoughts of fear of death and dying characterized the discussions of disclosure of parent's HIV status to children. Parents delayed disclosure because they believed that children believe that AIDS kills and would be concerned that their parents may die too.

Children know that people infected with HIV die, you become afraid to tell because the child will say "my mother is going to die" so you become afraid to tell (Mother of 2 children).

I am scared that he will feel miserable and maybe think my mother is dying, my father is dead, my mother is also going to die..., so who are we going to be left with..., what is going to happen? (Widowed mother of 2 children).

Parents perceived the television and media as negatively influencing children's perceptions of HIV-positive people. They were concerned that media portrays HIV as a debilitating, fatal disease. This created fear for parental disclosure of HIV status to children.

My child watches HIV-related drama on TV, many of these dramas show that a person who is HIV positive end up dying. That thing is the one that makes me afraid to tell my child. That is the reason why I am afraid to tell (Father of 3 children).

Fear of stigma and discrimination was one of the main reasons parents delayed HIV status disclosure to children. They had fears that the child may not be able to keep the parent's HIV status secret and were concerned that the family will be subjected to stigma, discrimination, and isolation.

> *The reason for not telling my child is that I have one child who is 7 years old. It is good and not good to tell taking into consideration the child's age and the stigma surrounding this disease (Mother of 1 child).*

> *My reason for not telling is because a child does not have a secret, we have not accepted this disease as a community. Because my child cannot keep a secret, you are going to see people looking down at me (Father of 1child).*

As a result of stigma and discrimination, parents went to considerable lengths to keep their HIV-positive status secret from their children, family members, and community members. Disclosed parents instructed their children to keep the disclosure secret and even when parents did not give their children instructions not to tell other people, they believed that their children understood the nature of the disease and knew that they would not tell people outside the family.

> *Eish..., you know, this child, if you tell him, he is going to tell his friends that my father is going to die; he is having AIDS (Father of 3 children).*

> *At seventeen, she knows that it is a family secret and then if you tell she will never talk (Single mother of 3 children).*

5. Disclosure to sexual partner

The study used FGDs to explore HIV disclosure to sexual partners and significant family members among HIV-positive postnatal women enrolled in a PMTCT program. FGDs were conducted with 25 women aged between 18 and 40 years between November 2010 and January 2011. Three main themes stigma and rejection, protecting the HIV status, and fear of violence highlight the social context influencing disclosure to sexual partners.

The most common reasons for nondisclosure to family members were fear of social rejection and discrimination. Women were fearful of disclosure because they felt that they will be rejected by their family. They further associated disclosure to sexual partners to the risks of discrimination, abandonment, and rejection.

> *My mother has serious problems with HIV-positive people (27yrs single mother).*

> *After I had tested HIV positive, I asked my husband to get tested too, and he was HIV negative. Since that day he never came back home, he has another woman he is staying with now (43yrs married woman).*

> *I told him that I was pregnant and HIV positive, he was happy that I was pregnant, but the issue of me being HIV positive, he did not take it so well. It was the last time I saw him, he left (31yrs single mother).*

Concealing the HIV status was commonly used as a strategy for protecting self from stigma and rejection. However, participating in PMTCT subjected women to scrutiny and questioning and the women devised strategies to continue hiding their HIV status from partners, families, and the community.

> *My grandmother asked me why I was not breastfeeding my baby and I told her that I was having problems with my breasts and I cannot breastfeed (30yrs single mother).*

> *With my tablets, immediately after collecting them from the clinic, I empty them into sachets, and I throw away the ARVs bottles so that if somebody finds me drinking my ART medication, they would not know what I am taking (26yrs single mother).*

The women who did not disclose their HIV-positive status to their sexual partners found disclosure difficult. They were fearful that their partners would react with violence to the disclosure or accuse them of being responsible for the infection.

> *The main thing that is worrying me is how he is going to feel when I tell him. I'm scared to tell him because he is one person that will want to tell everybody about my status in his family that I'm the one who gave it [HIV] to him (24yrs single mother).*

6. Adolescents onward self-disclosure to others

In-depth interviews were conducted with 37 perinatally infected adolescents between December 2012 and July 2013. The study explored how perinatally infected adolescents experienced living with HIV and examined their perceptions and experiences about disclosure and onward self-disclosure to friends, romantic partners, and others. Three themes reaction to knowing HIV diagnosis, fear of stigma and discrimination, and secrecy illustrate the contextual environment within which adolescents receive disclosure and disclose.

Adolescents experienced both positive and negative effects of disclosure. Some described the disclosure event as extremely shocking and hurtful, and some felt like they were dying. They could not figure out how they could have been infected if they did not engage in sexual activities and expressed ambivalent feelings of self-blame.

> *When I discovered about my HIV status, I did not feel good at all. You think about a lot of things. You think that you no longer have a life. You feel that people can see that you are HIV positive (Male participant; 17yrs).*

> *I was very shattered, and I asked myself what I did before God that I should be infected with HIV (Male participant; 17yrs).*

Adolescents were aware of the secret nature of their HIV diagnosis, and they considered their HIV diagnosis a secret. Fear of being gossiped about and stigmatized was an important consideration for keeping their HIV status secret.

> *My status is my secret and will remain my secret until I am older. It is a secret; the only people who need to know are your family (Male participation, 17yrs).*

> *You must only tell your family members who will not tell other people outside because others are gossipers and will tell other people that this child is HIV positive (Female participant, 14yrs).*

Disclosure to friends resulted in stigmatization for some of the adolescents who felt the need to disclose to friends. The subsequent experience of stigma led to secrecy and emotional trauma for the adolescents.

I did not know whom to tell, my mother was always crying, always under stress, and I did not know whom to tell. I told myself that I have to break the silence once and for all, then I told my friends, and they started isolating me (Female participation, 14yrs).

I told my friend, and after I had told him, he told others; whenever I pass them, they bothered me (Male participation; 15yrs).

Adolescents expressed a strong message that their HIV status was truly their secret and expressed anxiety at how difficult disclosure would be. They also feared that their romantic partners and friends would react in a negative way to disclosure.

It will be too painful to me to tell my friends because they will perceive me differently (Female participant; 12yrs).

If I tell him, he will leave me (Female participant; 18yr).

I don't want them judging me, and I am afraid that my best friend will refuse to play with me (Male participation; 14yrs).

7. Environmental contextual factors shaping disclosure

7.1. Construction of HIV

HIV testing and disclosure are influenced by cultural and social contexts and to a greater extent by the understandings of HIV and AIDS which are grounded in broader understandings of the long-term illness, death, and social danger [4, 22]. From the beginning of the HIV epidemic, HIV was conceptualized as highly stigmatizing, incurable, fatal, contagious, a threat to the life of others, physically degenerative and disfiguring, and associated with a painful or anesthetic death [23]. Many decades after the first cases of HIV and AIDS, people continue to perceive HIV and AIDs as meaning death and dying in many societies in SSA. People perceive AIDS as a deadly disease and often make no distinction between HIV and AIDS. Having HIV and AIDS is associated with being sick and approaching death and often people are afraid to test while HIV-positive people see no reasons for disclosure from the anticipation of severe stigma [5, 22, 24–27].

Earlier arguments about the construction of HIV/AIDS as meaning death and dying came from the knowledge that in African settings where ART was not readily available, HIV infection was a death sentence [28]. It was therefore anticipated that with the advent of ART the context of stigmatization due to fear of imminent death might be changing. However, despite the increased access to ART and the positive outcomes of treatment, people continue to perceive HIV as signaling death and dying. Jürgensen et al. argue that the memories of AIDS are embedded in narratives and experiences of the death of people and have been imprinted in people's minds [24].

The fear of death and dying is also evident in the way HIV is constructed by perinatally infected children. HIV is primarily constructed in relation to a language of sickness even when children are on ART and are relatively healthy. Perinatal infected children, who started ART at an early age, have no experience of life pre-HIV [14]. Therefore, their construction of

HIV is influenced by that of the adults whose context of HIV is that of a debilitating illness. Daniel points out that in the case of children, adults ignore to emphasize the positive health that people on ART enjoy. As a consequence, children associate HIV with illness and weakness and horror stories about the physical appearance of other people living with HIV [14, 29]. While this negative view of HIV might have been instilled by the adults who care for them and the society as a whole, Domek argues that for some of the children the association of AIDS with death and dying is real. As some of the children have been exposed to the devastating effects of HIV and had seen their parents or other significant family members die [30].

The first public health prevention campaigns perpetuated negative perceptions and heightened the fear of HIV/AIDS. The original billboards used in HIV/AIDS awareness campaigns depicted HIV/AIDS as debilitating, frightening, and fatal disease, by focusing on negative images of sick, dying, and disfigured persons. The portrayal of HIV as a grossly disfiguring disease resulted in individuals relating an HIV-positive test to a death sentence [31–33]. Research indicates that people continue to have ambiguous feelings about physical contact with HIV-positive people and that HIV stigma is still unintentionally reinforced by campaigns addressing HIV/AIDS [34].

Given the fact that the levels of HIV/AIDS-related knowledge are often inversely correlated with stigma [35], it was anticipated that providing people with factual information about HIV/AIDS would lead to stigma reduction in high HIV prevalence settings [36]. However, stigma lingers on; current research from the Democratic Republic of the Congo shows that the fear of HIV/AIDS prompted people to avoid and stigmatize PLHIV through the use of derogatory labels used to portray PLHIV. Labels commonly used, described PLHIV as walking corpses, dangers to others, or people deserving to die before others get infected. Being labeled made PLHIV suffer in silence and afraid to disclose their status [37].

7.2. Contextual environment

HIV disclosure occurs within a broad range of social and cultural contexts that influence the way individuals infected with HIV and affected by HIV perceive risks, the way they make decisions to take or not to take an HIV test, and the way disclosure takes place [4]. The contextual environment comprises the setting and potential contextual factors under which disclosure is more or less likely to occur. HIV-positive individuals, their families, communities, and their sociocultural and political norms constitute this environment [38]. Bailey and Darak refer to the contextual environment as spaces of disclosure and discrimination and point out that disclosure is influenced by spaces of disclosure which ranges from the clinic or hospital, spouses, family members, relatives, and others [39]. While Hardon et al. identified five social spaces that are considered to shape disclosure practices which include international recommendations, household and family settings, couple relationships, parental relationships, and patient-health worker relationships [40]. According to Bailey and Darak [39], these spaces of disclosure are also spaces of discrimination.

Being able to disclose safely within one space or social environment has been shown to increase disclosure rates and enable people to manage HIV stigma [2, 41]. However, the social contexts influence disclosure in a positive and negative way, and the social relations and family dynamics within the spaces of disclosure play a fundamental role in the decision individuals take to disclose or not disclose. Extensive research shows that stigma is often perpetrated within the family and interpersonal space of marriage. Women, in particular, face unique barriers when disclosing within the marital relationship or to sexual partners in the context of high levels of HIV stigma [36, 42–44]. In many settings in the SSA, the risk of being discriminated and rejected is higher on women because more women get tested for HIV and the burden of disclosing is often on them [45].

The importance of and role of cultural context in the practice of HIV disclosure has been reported upon extensively in research. Cultural values affect decisions on HIV disclosure and different cultural contexts shape the disclosure patterns of individuals, families, and communities [1, 43, 46]. HIV is a socially unacceptable disease and results in the community discriminating against an individual who is perceived to have been infected through their lifestyle and personal behavior [6, 47]. HIV is associated with morally disapproved behavior, and contracting HIV is viewed as the responsibility of the individual, exposing people to blame and judgment [23]. Cultural norms continue to play a significant role in the blame-related stigma and shame associated with HIV/AIDS in many communities in SSA [10, 48]. Community beliefs and societal norms also perpetuate gender inequality, further influencing the social, cultural, and personal spaces for disclosure for women. These shared norms influence a woman's decision regarding HIV disclosure thus shaping HIV and disclosure communication within interpersonal space of marriage and intimate relationships [49].

HIV disclosure to infected children is influenced to a greater extent by the cultural and social contexts in the community [4, 38]. The context of disclosure of HIV status to perinatally infected children is fraught with complexities that relate to the social, familial, and cultural environment of the child in which caregivers are reluctant to discuss the diagnosis with their HIV-infected child [50, 51]. It is argued that parental HIV disclosure to children cannot be expected under circumstances where most PLHIV find it hard to disclose to significant adults such as spouse or partners and family members [52].

7.3. Stigma and HIV

Stigma has been a component of HIV/AIDS since the onset of the pandemic. Stigma compromises AIDS responses and is increasingly regarded as one of the key drivers of the spread of HIV in sub-Saharan Africa. The perception of stigma or the fear of the consequences of stigma prevents people from adopting preventive behavior, getting tested, disclosing their serostatus, accessing treatment and care, and adherence to medication [24, 33, 36, 53]. Alonzo and Reynolds defined stigma as"a powerful discrediting and tainting social label that radically changes the way individuals view themselves and are viewed as persons" [23]. The definition by Parker and Aggleton, describe stigma and stigmatization as being shaped by structures of power and culture and a result of the consequences of collective action by groups rather than that of individual behavior [53]. While HIV stigma is defined as socially shared knowledge about the devalued status of PLHIV [9].

Since HIV is a socially unacceptable disease, it is a highly stigmatized condition compared to many other chronic conditions. HIV stigmatization is not only driven by the physical and visible attributes of an HIV-positive person but by social and cultural processes rooted in communities [27, 47, 54]. HIV stigmatization can include avoidance, exclusion, rejection, isolation, violence, service denial, physical distance, awkward social interaction, and blaming [55]. Nonetheless, the fear of gossip is pronounced as a primary form of HIV stigma throughout SSA [5].

7.4. Stigma and disclosure

HIV stigma affects and is affected by HIV disclosure, while high stigma levels severely hamper disclosure rates and results in silence and secrecy [45], disclosure can lead to stigmatization. Stigmatization is considered a significant barrier to HIV disclosure because HIV disclosure may be deterred if individuals live in communities where HIV stigma is present. The fear of stigma discourages disclosure because PLHIV are more likely to disclose in low-stigma contexts where they expect fewer negative consequences [6, 7, 43, 56].

7.5. Stigma, ART and disclosure

The increasing availability of ART in high prevalence settings did not necessarily reduce stigma and discrimination as anticipated. Extensive research indicates that stigma persists among people on ART and significantly impacts their ability to access treatment and disclose their HIV serostatus [12, 15, 24]. Earlier research on HIV stigma assumed that the increased uptake of ART in many settings in sub-Saharan Africa would reduce some of the stigmatizing characteristics of HIV as disease progression is halted or reversed and PLHIV look healthy. To a lesser extent, ART has made it easier for people to disclose to a closed network particularly within the family setting [5]. However, people still fear, anticipate, and experience stigma from others because ART has not been able to change the underlying causes of stigma, particularly, the moral discourses that judge and blame women and men for contracting HIV [12]. Concerns and fear of being stigmatized are also enduring because HIV stigmatization is not only driven by the physical and visible attributes of an HIV-positive person but also by the underlying structural causes of stigma which ART cannot eliminate [52].

Structural stigma refers to the ways in which societal ideologies and institutions perpetuate or exacerbate a stigmatized status [12]. While structural discrimination relates to accumulated institutional practices that work to the disadvantage of stigmatized groups and can operate in the absence of individual prejudice and discrimination [57]. Research suggests that stigma may be increasing at the individual level for people on ART. It is argued that attending an HIV clinic and adhering to ART medication draw attention to HIV-positive people, making their HIV-positive status visible because of taking ART and regular clinical visits and increase HIV stigma [15, 58].

7.6. Secrecy and silence

Secrecy and silence have characterized the HIV/AIDS epidemic in many societies in sub-Saharan Africa. The perceptions of HIV as a stigmatizing and deadly and contagious disease and the fear of stigma often compels PLWHI people affected by HIV to adopt secrecy and silence as a strategy to manage the HIV stigma [5, 10, 12, 25]. Secrecy is defined as any action taken to attempt to conceal the distinguishing marks that would categorize one in a stigmatized group [59, 60]. In the case of HIV, PLHIV conceal HIV-positive status, clinical signs, ongoing treatment, and visits to the treatment center [61].

Secrecy may be used as a strategic tactic to avoid losing control to others as to how they view one [62]. In these situations, silence is used as a strategy of protecting self and to live as normal a life as possible in social contexts where disclosure would have adverse outcomes [26]. Though the focus of research on the use of silence as a strategy is on individuals, Cohen [63] refers to cultural silence as a strategy that is adopted by the whole community or society. One of the reasons for silence at the cultural level is that the group or the community keeps silent about matters which are based on deep-seated cultural taboos whose open discussion would threaten its self-image. Cultural silence explains the normalization of secrecy and silence around the HIV status among population groups across societies.

Secrecy and silence are also used by caregivers of perinatally infected children to protect the children from discrimination [50, 51, 64]. In SSA, culture is also used to explain silence, particularly in the case of children. Adults use cultural silence as an excuse not to communicate to children by saying that "in our culture, we don't talk to children about death they are too young to understand" [29]. The same argument is used to conceal the HIV diagnosis to perinatally infected children by saying the child is too young to know and understand HIV. As a consequence of the secret nature of HIV and the wide acceptance and adoption of cultural silence, children infected with HIV mimic the behavior of the adults around them. Research has shown that children conceal their HIV diagnosis from friends and people outside of their family network as they have seen their caregivers do and as their caregivers have taught them [29, 41, 65].

However, the use of silence or secrecy as a coping strategy has disadvantages; it can be expensive forcing PLHIV to travel far to access ART. It can also reinforce stigma by not challenging it and fuel gossip and blame. Furthermore, silence can inhibit potential social support, compel PLHIV to conceal medicines, and can lead to death and continued HIV transmission [2, 5, 66, 67]. In the case of children affected by HIV, silence undermines their competence, self-worth, confidence, self-esteem, and increases their anxieties [41].

8. Conclusion

The four case studies highlight that undeniably, disclosure of HIV status across different population groups occurs within the social contexts of thoughts of death and dying, the influence of television, unjust discrimination, and a need for secrecy and silence. Within these contexts, individuals manage the disclosure in such a way as to attempt to keep the situation as normal as possible.

The construction of HIV as signaling a death sentence influence disclosing the child's HIV-positive status, disclosing parental status to HIV-negative children, and disclosing HIV-positive status to family, particularly to elderly parents. The fear of death and dying remains a barrier for caregivers who continue to delay disclosure to perinatally infected children and parental self-disclosure of HIV-positive status to HIV-negative children. The fear of death and dying is intricately linked to the fear-based messaging used on TV campaigns designed to create HIV/AIDS awareness in South Africa. When HIV is perceived as meaning death and dying, disclosure is delayed despite parents and children receiving ART for an extended duration of time and experiencing the positive gains of ART medication.

The construction of HIV as death and dying also influenced the perceptions of perinatally infected adolescents about disclosure significantly. Perinatally infected adolescents experienced receiving disclosure of their HIV diagnosis as painful and traumatic and described their HIV diagnosis as a death sentence.

Fear of death and dying also deterred postnatal women from disclosing their HIV-positive status to their elderly parents. They also described their HIV diagnosis as a death sentence and perceived their parents as too old and frail to deal with the death sentence that their child had just received.

HIV disclosure across the different population groups was surrounded by secrecy and silence. Secrecy was used to a larger extent by caregivers of perinatally infected children and HIV-positive parents to protect children from harmful emotional consequences of disclosure such as fear of death and dying and stigma and discrimination. Postnatal HIV-positive women also used secrecy to protect their HIV status from their family member, partners, and the community as a whole. Caregivers of perinatally infected children, HIV-positive parents, and HIV-positive postnatal women devoted considerable energy to manipulate their social and contextual environments to conceal the HIV status for as long as possible. They commonly substituted HIV for socially accepted diseases and used false names to describe their illness, used various strategies to hide ART medication, or rescheduled the time for taking ART medication.

Perinatally infected children subsequently mimic the behavior of the adult caregivers around them and also conceal their HIV diagnosis. Perinatally infected adolescents argue that their HIV status is their secret and maintained secrecy to be accepted by their peers but also to protect themselves from stigma and isolation. The fear of HIV-related stigma compels HIV infected and affected individuals to adopt coping strategies of secrecy and silence to protect self and or family from stigma and discrimination. Secrecy is viewed as an effective strategy for maintaining a normal life and has been greatly normalized in society.

Stigma and discrimination were a constant barrier for disclosure to sexual partners, family members, perinatally infected children, HIV-negative children, and romantic partners. Since HIV disclosure takes on different meanings for different population groups even within similar contextual environments, the fear of the different manifestation of stigma is experienced differently by population groups. Stigma was more pronounced for disclosing HIV status to infected children and during parental self-disclosure of HIV-positive status to children. The fear of stigma was also a key consideration for nondisclosure to romantic partners and friends by perinatally infected adolescents. Stigma is such a powerful barrier to disclosure such that even when individuals affected and infected with HIV do not experience enactments of stigma, being aware of the potential for stigma in their contextual environments shapes their disclosure pattern.

Given that disclosure of HIV status to perinatally infected children is more complex than that of adults, it is imperative that disclosure of HIV status to others by HIV-positive adults is understood because the social and cultural contexts of the adults providing care to perinatally infected children shapes the disclosure to children. As a result, self-disclosure to romantic partners by perinatally infected adolescents is as complex as that of disclosure among adults because their contextual environment is shaped by that of the adults too. The complexity of disclosure to perinatally infected children is aggravated by the fact that they may experience two aspects of disclosure; first, when they receive disclosure about their HIV-positive status and second when they receive their parental HIV-positive status. Both disclosure occurrences are saddled with sociocultural challenges affecting disclosure to adults within the communities.

A clear understanding of the contextual environment where disclosure occurs should inform interventions to create enabling environments for safe disclosure for the different population groups. It is imperative that the extent and effect of stigma and discrimination should not be underestimated or ignored by healthcare workers and other key stakeholders such as policy makers who have a vital role to play in reducing stigma. The challenge for researchers is to explore how HIV-related stigma could be overcome to enable people to disclose safely within their spaces or contextual environments. The understanding of the contextual environment or the spaces where disclosure and discrimination occurs will greatly influence the development of interventions to address stigma as being influenced by structural factors beyond behavior.

Author details

Sphiwe Madiba

Address all correspondence to: Sphiwe_madiba@embanet.com

School of Public Health, Faculty of Health Sciences, Sefako Makgatho Health Sciences University, Pretoria, South Africa

References

[1] Qiao S, Li X, Stanton B. Disclosure of parental HIV infection to children: a systematic review of global literature. AIDS & Behavior. 2013;17(1):369–89.

[2] Greeff M, Phetlhu R, Makoae LN, Dlamini PS, Holzemer WL, Naidoo JR, et al. Disclosure of HIV status: experiences and perceptions of persons living with HIV/AIDS and nurses involved in their care in Africa. Qualitative Health Research. 2008;18(3):311–24.

[3] Greeff M. Disclosure and stigma: A cultural perspective. In Stigma, discrimination and living with HIV/AIDS, Springer Netherlands; 2013. pp. 71–95.

[4] Lugalla J, Yoder S, Sigalla H, Madihi C. Social context of disclosing HIV test results in Tanzania. Culture, Health & Sexuality. 2012;14(suppl. 1):S53–66.

[5] Bond VA. It is not an easy decision on HIV, especially in Zambia: opting for silence, limited disclosure and implicit understanding to retain a wider identity. AIDS Care. 2010;22(suppl. 1):6–13.

[6] Chaudoir SR, Fisher JD, Simoni JM. Understanding HIV disclosure: a review and application of the disclosure processes model. Social Science & Medicine. 2011;72(10):1618–29.

[7] Wouters E, van Loon F, van Rensburg D, Meulemans H. Community support and disclosure of HIV serostatus to family members by public-sector antiretroviral treatment patients in the Free State Province of South Africa. AIDS Patient Care and STDs. 2009;23(5):357–64.

[8] Derlega VJ, Winstead BA, Greene K, Serovich J, Elwood WN. Reasons for HIV disclosure/nondisclosure in close relationships: testing a model of HIV–disclosure decision making. Journal of Social & Clinical Psychology. 2004;23(6):747–67.

[9] Steward WT, Herek GM, Ramakrishna J, Bharat S, Chandy S, Wrubel J, et al. HIV-related stigma: adapting a theoretical framework for use in India. Social Science & Medicine. 2008;67(8):1225–35.

[10] Roura M, Urassa M, Busza J, Mbata D, Wringe A, Zaba B. Scaling up stigma? The effects of antiretroviral roll-out on stigma and HIV testing. Early evidence from rural Tanzania. Sexually Transmitted Infections. 2009;85(4):308–12.

[11] Mbonye M, Nakamanya S, Birungi J, King R, Seeley J, Jaffar S. Stigma trajectories among people living with HIV (PLHIV) embarking on a life time journey with antiretroviral drugs in Jinja, Uganda. BMC Public Health. 2013;13(1):804.

[12] Russell S, Zalwango F, Namukwaya S, Katongole J, Muhumuza R, Nalugya R, et al. Antiretroviral therapy and changing patterns of HIV stigmatisation in Entebbe, Uganda. Sociology of Health & Illness. 2016;38(1):58–72.

[13] Smith R, Rossetto K, Peterson BL. A meta-analysis of disclosure of one's HIV-positive status, stigma and social support. AIDS Care. 2008;20(10):1266–75.

[14] Bernays S, Seeley J, Rhodes T, Mupambireyi Z. What am I 'living'with? Growing up with HIV in Uganda and Zimbabwe. Sociology of Health & Illness. 2015;37(2):270–83.

[15] Gilbert L, Walker L. My biggest fear was that people would reject me once they knew my status: stigma as experienced by patients in an HIV/AIDS clinic in Johannesburg, South Africa. Health & Social Care in the Community. 2010;18(2):139–46.

[16] Madiba S. Disclosing HIV to infected children in South Africa in the era of HAART: a grounded theory study on the process, reasons and outcomes of disclosure. World Journal of AIDS. 2012; 2(4):319–29.

[17] Madiba S. The impact of fear, secrecy, and stigma on parental disclosure of HIV status to children: a qualitative exploration with HIV positive parents attending an ART clinic in South Africa. Global Journal of Health Science. 2013;5(2):49.

[18] Madiba S, Letsoalo R. HIV disclosure to partners and family among women enrolled in prevention of mother to child transmission of HIV program: implications for infant feeding in poor resourced communities in South Africa. Global Journal of Health Science. 2013;5(4):1.

[19] Madiba S, Matlala C. Disclosure of parental HIV positive status: what, why, when, and how parents tell their children in the era of HAART in South Africa. World Journal of AIDS. 2012;2(03):194.

[20] Madiba S, Mokgatle M. Perceptions and experiences about self-disclosure of HIV Status among adolescents with perinatal acquired HIV in poor-resourced communities in South Africa. AIDS Research and Treatment. 2016;2016:10.

[21] Madiba S, Mokwena K. Caregivers' barriers to disclosing the HIV diagnosis to infected children on antiretroviral therapy in a resource-limited district in South Africa: a grounded theory study. AIDS Research and Treatment. 2012;2012:10.

[22] de Klerk J. The compassion of concealment: silence between older caregivers and dying patients in the AIDS era, northwest Tanzania. Culture, Health & Sexuality. 2012;14(suppl. 1): S27–38.

[23] Alonzo AA, Reynolds NR. Stigma, HIV and AIDS: an exploration and elaboration of a stigma trajectory. Social Science & Medicine. 1995;41(3):303–15.

[24] Jürgensen M, Tuba M, Fylkesnes K, Blystad A. The burden of knowing: balancing benefits and barriers in HIV testing decisions. a qualitative study from Zambia. BMC Health Services Research. 2012;12(1):1.

[25] Mfecane S. Narratives of HIV disclosure and masculinity in a South African village. Culture, Health & Sexuality. 2012;14(suppl. 1):S109–21.

[26] Moyer E. Faidha gani? What's the point: HIV and the logics of (non)-disclosure among young activists in Zanzibar. Culture, Health & Sexuality. 2012;14(suppl. 1):S67–79.

[27] Visser MJ, Makin JD, Vandormael A, Sikkema KJ, Forsyth BW. HIV/AIDS stigma in a South African community. AIDS Care. 2009;21(2):197–206.

[28] Moore A, Kalanzi DN, Amey FK. To disclose or not to disclose? Lower class parents living with HIV/AIDS in Lomé, Togo. International Journal of Sociology & Social Policy. 2008;28(9/10):351–64.

[29] Daniel M. Keeping the secret: how HIV-positive children in Iringa, Tanzania, respond to the perceived need for silence and secrecy. Journal of Child & Adolescent Mental Health. 2015;27(1):11–23.

[30] Domek GJ. Debunking common barriers to pediatric HIV disclosure. Journal of Tropical Pediatrics. 2010;56(6):440–2.

[31] Liamputtong P, Haritavorn N, Kiatying-Angsulee N. HIV and AIDS, stigma and AIDS support groups: perspectives from women living with HIV and AIDS in central Thailand. Social Science & Medicine. 2009;69(6):862–8.

[32] Lyttleton C. Fleeing the fire: transformation and gendered belonging in Thai HIV/AIDS support groups. Medical Anthropology. 2004;23(1):1–40.

[33] Ogden J, Nyblade L. Common at its core: HIV-related stigma across contexts. Washington, DC: International Center for Research on Women (ICRW); 2005.

[34] Gausset Q, Mogensen HO, Yameogo WME, Berthé A, Konaté B. The ambivalence of stigma and the double-edged sword of HIV/AIDS intervention in Burkina Faso. Social Science & Medicine. 2012;74(7):1037–44.

[35] Kalichman SC, Simbayi LC, Jooste S, Toefy Y, Cain D, Cherry C, et al. Development of a brief scale to measure AIDS-related stigma in South Africa. AIDS & Behavior. 2005;9(2):135–43.

[36] Campbell C, Nair Y, Maimane S, Nicholson J. 'Dying twice': a multi-level model of the roots of AIDS stigma in two South African communities. Journal of Health Psychology. 2007;12(3):403–16.

[37] Mupenda B, Duvall S, Maman S, Pettifor A, Holub C, Taylor E, et al. Terms used for people living with HIV in the Democratic Republic of the Congo. Qualitative Health Research. 2014;24(2):209–16.

[38] Eustace RW, Ilagan PR. HIV disclosure among HIV positive individuals: a concept analysis. Journal of Advanced Nursing. 2010;66(9):2094–103.

[39] Bailey A, Darak S. Spaces of disclosure and discrimination: case studies from India. In Stigma, discrimination and living with HIV/AIDS: Springer Netherlands; 2013. pp. 229–45.

[40] Hardon A, Desclaux A, Lugalla J. Disclosure in times of ART: a relational analysis of social practices. SAHARA-J: Journal of Social Aspects of HIV/AIDS. 2013;10(suppl. 1):S1–4.

[41] Daniel M, Malinga Apila H, Bj⊘rgo R, Therese Lie G. Breaching cultural silence: enhancing resilience among Ugandan orphans. African Journal of AIDS Research. 2007;6(2):109–20.

[42] Bott S, Obermeyer CM. The social and gender context of HIV disclosure in sub-Saharan Africa: a review of policies and practices. SAHARA-J: Journal of Social Aspects of HIV/AIDS. 2013;10(suppl. 1):S5–16.

[43] Obermeyer CM, Baijal P, Pegurri E. Facilitating HIV disclosure across diverse settings: a review. American Journal of Public Health. 2011;101(6):1011–23.

[44] Madiba S, Letsoalo B. Disclosure to sexual partner and associated factors among HIV positive adult clinic attendees in Johannesburg, South Africa: perspectives of HIV and AIDS across populations. African Journal for Physical Health Education, Recreation and Dance, Supplement 21. 2015;21:100–11.

[45] Klopper C, Stellenberg E, Van der Merwe A. Stigma and HIV disclosure in the Cape Metropolitan area, South Africa. African Journal of AIDS Research. 2014;13(1):37–43.

[46] Kalichman SC, Simbayi LC. HIV testing attitudes, AIDS stigma, and voluntary HIV counselling and testing in a black township in Cape Town, South Africa. Sexually Transmitted Infections. 2003;79(6):442–7.

[47] Simbayi LC, Kalichman S, Strebel A, Cloete A, Henda N, Mqeketo A. Internalized stigma, discrimination, and depression among men and women living with HIV/AIDS in Cape Town, South Africa. Social Science & Medicine. 2007;64(9):1823–31.

[48] Leclerc-Madlala S. Demonising women in the era of AIDS: On the relationship between cultural constructions of both HIV/AIDS and femininity. Society in Transition. 2001;32(1):38–46.

[49] Ojikutu BO, Pathak S, Srithanaviboonchai K, Limbada M, Friedman R, Li S, et al. Community cultural norms, stigma and disclosure to sexual partners among women living with HIV in Thailand, Brazil and Zambia (HPTN 063). PloS One. 2016;11(5):e0153600.

[50] Lesch A, Swartz L, Kagee A, Moodley K, Kafaar Z, Myer L, et al. Paediatric HIV/AIDS disclosure: towards a developmental and process-oriented approach. AIDS Care. 2007;19(6):811–6.

[51] Mahloko JM, Madiba S. Disclosing HIV diagnosis to children in Odi district, South Africa: reasons for disclosure and non-disclosure. African Journal of Primary Health Care & Family Medicine. 2012;4(1):345.

[52] Tiendrebeogo G, Hejoaka F, Belem EM, Compaoré PLG, Wolmarans L, Soubeiga A, et al. Parental HIV disclosure in Burkina Faso: experiences and challenges in the era of HAART. SAHARA-J: Journal of Social Aspects of HIV/AIDS. 2013;10(suppl. 1): S46–59.

[53] Parker R, Aggleton P. HIV and AIDS-related stigma and discrimination: a conceptual framework and implications for action. Social Science & Medicine. 2003;57(1):13–24.

[54] Herek GM. Hate crimes and stigma-related experiences among sexual minority adults in the United States prevalence estimates from a national probability sample. Journal of Interpersonal Violence. 2009;24(1):54–74.

[55] Lyimo RA, Stutterheim SE, Hospers HJ, de Glee T, van der Ven A, de Bruin M. Stigma, disclosure, coping, and medication adherence among people living with HIV/AIDS in Northern Tanzania. AIDS Patient Care and STDs. 2014;28(2):98–105.

[56] Nyblade LC. Measuring HIV stigma: existing knowledge and gaps. Psychology, Health & Medicine. 2006;11(3):335–45.

[57] Link BG, Phelan JC. Conceptualizing stigma. Annual Review of Sociology. 2001;27:363–85.

[58] Makoae LN, Portillo CJ, Uys LR, Dlamini PS, Greeff M, Chirwa M, et al. The impact of taking or not taking ARVs on HIV stigma as reported by persons living with HIV infection in five African countries. AIDS Care. 2009;21(11):1357–62.

[59] Goffman E. Stigma: Notes on a spoiled identity. Jenkins, JH & Carpenter. 1963.

[60] Herek GM, Capitanio JP, Widaman KF. HIV-related stigma and knowledge in the United States: prevalence and trends, 1991–1999. American Journal of Public Health. 2002;92(3):371–7.

[61] Hardon AP, Akurut D, Comoro C, Ekezie C, Irunde HF, Gerrits T, et al. Hunger, waiting time and transport costs: time to confront challenges to ART adherence in Africa. AIDS Care. 2007;19(5):658–65.

[62] Goffman E. Stigma: Notes on the management of a spoiled identity. New York: Simon & Schuster.

[63] Cohen R. Living and teaching across cultures. International Studies Perspectives. 2001;2(2):151–60.

[64] Oberdorfer P, Puthanakit T, Louthrenoo O, Charnsil C, Sirisanthana V, Sirisanthana T. Disclosure of HIV/AIDS diagnosis to HIV-infected children in Thailand. Journal of Paediatrics & Child Health. 2006;42(5):283–8.

[65] Hejoaka F. Care and secrecy: being a mother of children living with HIV in Burkina Faso. Social Science & Medicine. 2009;69(6):869–76.

[66] George MS, Lambert H. 'I am doing fine only because I have not told anyone': the necessity of concealment in the lives of people living with HIV in India. Culture, Health & Sexuality. 2015;17(8):933–46.

[67] Madiba S, Canti-Sigaqa V. Barriers to participate in support groups for people living with HIV: a qualitative study with men receiving antiretroviral treatment in a HIV clinic in Mthatha, South Africa. Global Journal of Health Science. 2012;4(6):119.

Permissions

All chapters in this book were first published in HIV/AIDSCC, by InTech Open; hereby published with permission under the Creative Commons Attribution License or equivalent. Every chapter published in this book has been scrutinized by our experts. Their significance has been extensively debated. The topics covered herein carry significant findings which will fuel the growth of the discipline. They may even be implemented as practical applications or may be referred to as a beginning point for another development.

The contributors of this book come from diverse backgrounds, making this book a truly international effort. This book will bring forth new frontiers with its revolutionizing research information and detailed analysis of the nascent developments around the world.

We would like to thank all the contributing authors for lending their expertise to make the book truly unique. They have played a crucial role in the development of this book. Without their invaluable contributions this book wouldn't have been possible. They have made vital efforts to compile up to date information on the varied aspects of this subject to make this book a valuable addition to the collection of many professionals and students.

This book was conceptualized with the vision of imparting up-to-date information and advanced data in this field. To ensure the same, a matchless editorial board was set up. Every individual on the board went through rigorous rounds of assessment to prove their worth. After which they invested a large part of their time researching and compiling the most relevant data for our readers.

The editorial board has been involved in producing this book since its inception. They have spent rigorous hours researching and exploring the diverse topics which have resulted in the successful publishing of this book. They have passed on their knowledge of decades through this book. To expedite this challenging task, the publisher supported the team at every step. A small team of assistant editors was also appointed to further simplify the editing procedure and attain best results for the readers.

Apart from the editorial board, the designing team has also invested a significant amount of their time in understanding the subject and creating the most relevant covers. They scrutinized every image to scout for the most suitable representation of the subject and create an appropriate cover for the book.

The publishing team has been an ardent support to the editorial, designing and production team. Their endless efforts to recruit the best for this project, has resulted in the accomplishment of this book. They are a veteran in the field of academics and their pool of knowledge is as vast as their experience in printing. Their expertise and guidance has proved useful at every step. Their uncompromising quality standards have made this book an exceptional effort. Their encouragement from time to time has been an inspiration for everyone.

The publisher and the editorial board hope that this book will prove to be a valuable piece of knowledge for researchers, students, practitioners and scholars across the globe.

List of Contributors

Pius Tangwe Tanga, Princess Khumalo and Priscilla Gutura
University of Fort Hare, Alice, South Africa

Thana Khawcharoenporn
Division of Infectious Diseases, Faculty of Medicine, Thammasat University, Pathumthani, Thailand

Beverly E. Sha
Division of Infectious Diseases, Rush University Medical Center, Chicago, IL, USA

Flavia Matovu Kiweewa
Makerere University School of Public Health, Makerere University College of Health Sciences, Kampala, Uganda University of Witwatersrand, Johannesburg, South Africa

Kenneth K. Mugwanya
Makerere University School of Public Health, Makerere University College of Health Sciences, Kampala, Uganda University of Washington, Seattle, United States

Francis Kiweewa
Makerere University School of Public Health, Makerere University College of Health Sciences, Kampala, Uganda Makerere University-Walter Reed Project, Kampala, Uganda

Jeanne M. Grace
Discipline of Biokinetics, Exercise and Leisure Sciences, College of Health Sciences, University of Kwazulu Natal, Westville, Durban, South Africa

Michael D. Röling, Mateusz Stoszko and Tokameh Mahmoudi
Department of Biochemistry, Erasmus Medical Centre, Rottrerdam, The Netherlands

Ashraf Alqaqa
Tennova Healthcare, Tennessee, USA

Tomoko Omiya, Yoshihiko Yamazaki, Megumi Shimada, Kazuko Ikeda, Seiko Ishiuchi-Ishitani and Katsumi Ohira
Toho University, Tokyo, Japan

Tatina T. Todorova and Gabriela Tsankova
Department of Preclinical and Clinical Sciences, Faculty of Pharmacy, Medical University Varna, Bulgaria

Neli Lodozova
Department of Preclinical and Clinical Sciences, Faculty of Pharmacy, Medical University Varna, Bulgaria TRS "Medical laboratory assistant", Medical College, Medical University Varna, Bulgaria

Tcvetelina Kostadinova
TRS "Medical laboratory assistant", Medical College, Medical University Varna, Bulgaria

Haruna M. Bello
Department of Agricultural Economics, University of Namibia, Mandume Ndemufayo Avenue, Winhoek, Namibia

Tiisetso J. Makatjane
Department of Statistics and Demography, National University of Lesotho, Lesotho

Tumelo Tsikoane
Department of Development Studies, National University of Lesotho, Lesotho

Sphiwe Madiba
School of Public Health, Faculty of Health Sciences, Sefako Makgatho Health Sciences University, Pretoria, South Africa

Index

www.ingramcontent.com/pod-product-compliance
Lightning Source LLC
LaVergne TN
LVHW060555210926
848485LV00005B/1320